KU-544-134

fourth edition

Color Atlas

of

Histology

LESLIE P. GARTNER, Ph.D.
Professor of Anatomy

JAMES L. HIATT, Ph.D.
Associate Professor of Anatomy (Retired)

Department of Biomedical Sciences
Baltimore College of Dental Surgery
Dental School
University of Maryland
Baltimore, Maryland

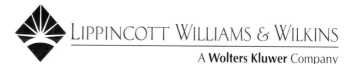

LIPPINCOTT WILLIAMS & WILKINS
A **Wolters Kluwer** Company

Philadelphia • Baltimore • New York • London
Buenos Aires • Hong Kong • Sydney • Tokyo

Acquisitions Editor: Betty Sun
Managing Editor: Crystal Taylor
Marketing Manager: Joseph Schott
Production Editor: Jennifer Glazer
Designer: Risa Clow
Compositor: Maryland Composition
Printer: RR Donnelley–Willard

351 West Camden Street
Baltimore, Maryland 21201-2436 USA

530 Walnut Street
Philadelphia, Pennsylvania 19106-3621 US

First Edition, 1990
Second Edition, 1994
Third Edition, 2000

Translations:
Chinese (Taiwan), Ho-Chi Book Publishing Company, 2002
Chinese (Mainland China), Liaoning Education Press/CITIC, 2004
Greek, Parissianos, 2003
Italian, Masson Italia, 1999
Japanese, Igaku-Shoin, 1997
Portuguese, Editora Guanabara Koogan, 2002
Spanish, Editorial Medica Panamericana, 2002

Library of Congress Cataloging-in-Publication Data

Gartner, Leslie P., 1943–
    Color atlas of histology / Leslie P. Gartner, James L. Hiatt.— 4th ed.
        p ; cm.
    Includes index.
    ISBN 0-7817-5216-7 — ISBN 0-7817-9828-0
    1. Histology—Atlases. I. Hiatt, James L., 1934–   II. Title. [DNLM: 1. Histology—
Atlases. QS 517 G244c 2006]
QM557.G38 2006
611′.018′0222—dc22

                           2005002800

To purchase additional copies of this book, call our customer service department at **(800) 638-3030** or fax orders to **(301) 824-7390**. International customers should call **(301) 714-2324**.

Visit **Lippincott Williams & Wilkins** on the Internet: **http://www.LWW.com**. Lippincott Williams & Wilkins customer service representatives are available from 8:30 am to 6:00 pm, EST.

05 06 07 08 09
1 2 3 4 5 6 7 8 9 10

Dedication

To my wife Roseann,
my daughter Jen,
and my mother Mary
LPG

To my wife Nancy
and my children
Drew, Beth, and Kurt
JLH

Preface

The favorable reception accorded the previous three editions of our *Color Atlas of Histology*, as evidenced by its many reprints and its translations into eight foreign languages, has been most gratifying and has served as an impetus to face the labor of preparing a new edition. We have received numerous suggestions from colleagues and students, many of which were implemented toward the end of improving the atlas and making it more "user friendly."

All of the photomicrographs have been retaken as digital images for the current edition to enhance the quality and clarity of the images presented for the student. Also, we have made several changes in this edition by the addition of new photomicrographs depicting regions of the oral cavity. Moreover, thumbnails of the pertinent four-color illustrations that are present in each chapter are incorporated as illustrative guideposts among the legends to the photomicrographs and have been titled appropriately. These illustrations are designed to trigger the student's memory by providing a three-dimensional representation of the two-dimensional photomicrographs on the facing page. These should prove to be helpful to the student in providing a framework on which the student may base detailed knowledge of histology.

The didactic information appears at the beginning of each chapter, and in this edition we added to the number of relevant clinical considerations to illustrate the importance and the pertinence of Histology to the Medical Sciences. It was our intent to summarize in these few pages that introduce each chapter the essential concepts necessary to the understanding of histology. We also re-titled the section previously entitled "Histological Organization" to its new title "Summary of Histological Organization," to reflect the true intent of that section. We maintained the use of bold-faced type in the text of each chapter, highlighting important words to facilitate a quick recall of the material for the student, and the expanded cross-referenced index to assist the student in locating items of interest.

As in the previous editions, most of the photomicrographs of this atlas are of tissues stained with hematoxylin and eosin. Each figure is supplied with a final magnification, which takes into consideration the photographic enlargement, as well as that achieved by the microscope. Many of the sections were prepared from plastic-embedded specimens, as noted. Most of the exquisite electron micrographs included in this atlas were kindly provided by our colleagues throughout the world as identified in the legends.

As with all of our textbooks, this Atlas has been written with the student in mind, thus the material is complete but not esoteric. We wish to help the student learn and enjoy histology, not be overwhelmed by it. Furthermore, this Atlas is designed not only for use in the laboratory, but also as preparation for both didactic and practical examinations. Although we have attempted to be accurate and complete, we know that errors and omissions may have escaped our attention. Therefore, we welcome criticisms, suggestions, and comments that could help improve this atlas.

INTERACTIVE COLOR ATLAS OF HISTOLOGY CD-ROM

We are pleased to announce that with this edition we have expanded the companion CD-ROM, *Interactive Color Atlas of Histology*. It contains every photomicrograph and electron micrograph and accompanying legends present in the Atlas. The student has the capability to study select chapters or to look up a particular item via a keyword search. Images may be viewed with or without labels and/or legends, enlarged using the "zoom" feature, and compared side-by-side to other images. Also, the updated software now allows students to self-test on all labels using the "hotspot" mode, facilitating learning and preparation for practical examinations. For examination purposes, the CD contains over 300 additional photomicrographs with more than 700 interactive fill-in and true/false questions organized in a fashion to facilitate the student's learning and preparation for practical exams. Additionally, we have included approximately 100 new USMLE Part I format multiple-choice questions, based on photomicrographs created specifically for the questions, that can be accessed in test or study mode. The Student Version of the CD is included with this Atlas. In the Institutional Version, images can be exported for use in PowerPoint presentations. Visit LWW.com or contact your local LWW sales representative for information about purchasing the Institutional Version of the CD.

Acknowledgments

We would like to thank Todd Smith for the rendering of the outstanding full-color plates and thumbnail figures, Jerry Gadd for his paintings of blood cells, and our many colleagues who provided us with electron micrographs. We are especially thankful to Dr. Stephen W. Carmichael of the Mayo Medical School for his suggestions concerning the suprarenal medulla. Additionally, we are grateful to our good friends at Lippincott Williams & Wilkins, including Betty Sun, Executive Acquisitions Editor; Crystal Taylor, Senior Managing Editor; Kathleen Scogna, Senior Developmental Editor; Jennifer Glazer, Production Editor; and Erica Lukenich, Editorial Assistant. We would also like to thank the software developers at Lippincott Williams & Wilkins for their work on the CD-ROM—Craig Jester, Alison Spiegel, and Brad Coleman.

Finally, we wish to thank our families again for encouraging us during the preparation of this work. Their support always makes the labor an achievement.

Contents

1 The Cell   1

2 Epithelium and Glands   25

3 Connective Tissue   45

4 Cartilage and Bone 65

5 Blood and Hemopoiesis 89

6 Muscle 103

7 Nervous Tissue 125

8 Circulatory System 147

9 Lymphoid Tissue 167

10 Endocrine System 193

11 Integument 217

⬦12 Respiratory System 235

⬦13 Digestive System I—Oral Region 255

⬦14 Digestive System II—Alimentary Canal 277

⬦15 Digestive System III—Digestive Glands 303

16 Urinary System   **323**

17 Female Reproductive System   **343**

18 Male Reproductive System   **369**

19 Special Senses   **387**

Index   **409**

The Cell

Cells not only constitute the basic units of the human body but also function in executing all of the activities that the body requires for its survival. Although there are more than 200 different cell types, most cells possess common features, which permit them to perform their varied responsibilities. The living component of the cell is the **protoplasm,** which is subdivided into the **cytoplasm** and the **nucleoplasm** (see Graphic 1-1).

CYTOPLASM

Plasmalemma

Cells possess a membrane, the **plasmalemma,** that provides a selective, structural barrier between the cell and the outside world. The plasmalemma, a phospholipid bilayer with **integral** and **peripheral proteins** and **cholesterol** embedded in it, functions in cell-cell recognition, exocytosis and endocytosis, as a receptor site for signaling molecules, and as an initiator and controller of the secondary messenger system. Materials may enter the cell via **pinocytosis** (nonspecific uptake of molecules in an aqueous solution), **receptor-mediated endocytosis** (specific uptake of substances, such as low density lipoproteins), or **phagocytosis** (uptake of particulate matter). Secretory products may leave the cell via **constitutive** or **regulated secretion. Constitutive secretion,** using non–clathrin-coated vesicles, is the default pathway that does not require an extracellular signal for release and thus the secretory product (e.g., collagen) leaves the cell in a continuous fashion. **Regulated secretion** requires the presence of clathrin-coated storage vesicles whose contents (e.g., pancreatic enzymes) are released only after the initiation of an extracellular signaling process.

Cells possess a number of distinct organelles, many of which are formed from membranes that are similar to but not identical with the biochemical composition of the plasmalemma.

Mitochondria

Mitochondria are composed of two membranes, an outer and an inner with an intervening compartment between them known as the **intermembrane space** (see Graphic 1-2). The inner membrane is folded to form **cristae** and encloses a viscous fluid-filled space known as the **matrix space.** Mitochondria function in the **generation of ATP,** utilizing a chemiosmotic coupling mechanism that employs a specific sequence of enzyme complexes and proton translocator systems (**electron transport chain** and the ATP-synthase containing **elementary particles**) embedded in their cristae. These organelles also assist in the **synthesis** of certain **lipids** and **proteins.** Mitochondria possess the enzymes of the **TCA cycle, circular DNA** molecules, and matrix granules in their matrix space. These organelles increase in number by undergoing **binary fission.**

Ribosomes

Ribososmes are small, bipartite organelles that exist as individual unipartite particles that do not coalesce with each other until protein synthesis begins. These structures are composed of proteins and r-RNA and function as an interactive "workbench" that not only provides a surface upon which protein synthesis occurs but also as a catalyst that facilitates the synthesis of proteins.

Endoplasmic Reticulum

The **endoplasmic reticulum** is composed of tubules, sacs, and flat sheets of membranes that delimit much of the intracellular space (see Graphic 1-2). The **rough endoplasmic reticulum** (RER), whose cytoplasmic surface possesses receptor molecules for ribosomes and signal recognition particles (known as **ribophorins** and **docking protein**, respectively), is continuous with the outer nuclear membrane. The RER functions in the **synthesis and modification of proteins** that are to be **packaged,** as well as in the synthesis of membrane lipids and proteins. **Smooth endoplasmic reticulum** functions in the synthesis of **cholesterols** and **lipids** as well as in the **detoxification** of certain drugs and toxins. Additionally, in skeletal muscle cells this organelle is specialized to sequester and release calcium ions and thus regulate muscle contraction and relaxation.

ERGIC, Golgi Apparatus, and the Trans-Golgi Network

The **Golgi apparatus (complex)** is composed of a specifically oriented cluster of vesicles, tubules, and flattened membrane-bounded cisternae arranged in the following manner: ERGIC, *cis*-Golgi network, *cis*-face, medial face, *trans*-face, and *trans*-Golgi network (see Graphic 1-2). The Golgi complex not only **packages** but also **modifies** macromolecules synthesized on the surface of the rough endoplasmic reticulum. Newly synthesized proteins pass from the rough endoplasmic reticulum to the ERGIC (**E**ndoplasmic **R**eticulum-**G**olgi **I**ntermediate **C**ompartment) by COPII-coated **transfer vesicles** and from there to the *cis*-Golgi Network, probably via COPI-coated vesicles. The proteins continue to travel to the *cis*-, medial-, and to the *trans* faces of the Golgi apparatus by non–clathrin-coated **vesicles** (or, according to some authors, via cisternal maturation). Lysosomal oligosaccharides are phosphorylated in the ERGIC and/or in the *cis* face; mannose groups are removed and other sugar residues are added in the medial face; whereas, the addition of galactose and sialic acid as well as the sulfation of selected residues occur in the *trans* face. **Sorting** and the final **packaging** of the macromolecules are the responsibility of the **trans-Golgi network (TGN).** It should be noted that material can travel through the Golgi complex in an **anterograde fashion,** as just described, as well as in a **retrograde fashion,** which occurs in situations such as when escaped proteins that are residents of the RER or of a particular Golgi-face have to be returned to their compartments of origin.

Endosomes

Endosomes are intermediate compartments within the cell, utilized in the destruction of endocytosed, phagocytosed, or autophagocytosed materials as well as in the formation of lysosomes. Endosomes possess **proton pumps** in their membranes, which pump H^+ into the endosome, thus acidifying the interior of this compartment. Also, these organelles are intermediate stages in the formation of lysosomes. **Early endosomes** are located at the periphery of the cell, contain receptor-ligand complexes, and their acidic contents (pH $\cong$ 6) is responsible for the uncoupling of receptors from ligands. The receptors are usually carried into a system of tubular vesicles, the **recycling endosomes**, from which the receptors are returned to the plasmalemma, whereas the ligands are translocated to **late endosomes**. Within late endosomes the pH is even more acidic (pH $\cong$ 5.5).

Lysosomes

Lysosomes are formed by the utilization of **late endosomes** as an intermediary compartment. Both lysosomal membranes and lysosomal enzymes are packaged in the *trans*-Golgi network and are delivered in separate **clathrin-coated vesicles** to late endosomes, forming **endolysosomes,** which then mature to become **lysosomes**. These membrane-bounded vesicles whose proton pumps are responsible for their very acidic interior (pH $\cong$ 5.0) contain various **hydrolytic enzymes** that function in **intracellular digestion.** They degrade certain macromolecules as well as phagocytosed particulate matter (**phagolysosomes**) and autophagocytosed material (**autophagolysosomes**). Frequently, the indigestible remnants of lysosomal degradation remain in the cell, enclosed in vesicles referred to as **residual bodies.**

Peroxisomes

Peroxisomes are membrane-bounded organelles housing **oxidative enzymes** such as **urate oxidase, D-amino acid oxidase,** and **catalase.** These organelles function in the formation of free radicals (e.g., superoxides) and hydrogen peroxide, which destroy various substances, and in the protection of the cell by degrading hydrogen peroxide by catalase. They also function in **detoxification** of certain toxins and in elongation of some fatty acids during **lipid synthesis.** Most of the proteins intended for inclusions into peroxisomes are synthesized in the cytosol rather than on the RER. All peroxisomes are formed by **fission** from preexisting peroxisomes.

Proteasomes

Proteasomes are small, barrel-shaped organelles that function in the degradation of cytosolic proteins. The practice of cytosolic proteolysis is highly regulated and the candidate protein must be tagged by several ubiquitin molecules before it is permitted to be destroyed by the proteasome system.

Cytoskeleton

The **cytoskeleton** is composed of a filamentous array of proteins that act not only as the structural framework of the cell but also to **transport** material within it from one region of the cell to another and provide it with the capability of **motion** and cell division. Components of the cytoskeleton include **microtubules** (consisting of α- and β-tubulins arranged in 13 protofilaments), **thin** (actin) **filaments** (also known as **microfilaments**), and **intermediate filaments.** Microtubules are also associated with proteins, known as **microtubule-associated proteins** (**MAPs**), which permit organelles, vesicles, and other components of the cytoskeleton to bind to microtubules. Most microtubules originate from **the microtubule-organizing center** (MTOC) of the cell, located in the vicinity of the Golgi apparatus. These elements of the cytoskeleton are pathways for intracellular translocation of organelles and vesicles and, during cell division, chromosomes are moved into their proper locations. Two important MAPs, **kinesin** and **dynein**, are motor proteins that facilitate anterograde and retrograde intracellular vesicular and organelle movement, respectively. The **axoneme** of cilia and flagella, as well as a framework of centrioles, are formed mostly of microtubules.

Inclusions

Cytoplasmic **inclusions,** such as **lipids, glycogen, secretory granules,** and **pigments,** are also consistent constituents of the cytoplasm. Many of these inclusions are transitory in nature, although some pigments, e.g., **lipofuscin,** are permanent residents of certain cells.

NUCLEUS

The **nucleus** is enclosed by the **nuclear envelope,** composed of an **inner** and an **outer nuclear membrane** with an intervening **perinuclear cistern** (see Graphic 1-2). The outer nuclear membrane is studded with **ribosomes** and is continuous, in places, with the rough endoplasmic reticulum. In areas the inner and outer membranes fuse with each other, forming circular profiles, known as **nuclear pores,** that permit communication between the nucleoplasm and the cytoplasm. These perforations of the nuclear envelope are guarded by protein assemblies which, together with the perforations, are known as **nuclear pore complexes,** providing regulated passageways for the transport of materials in and out of the nucleus. The nucleus houses **chromosomes** and is the location of **RNA synthesis.** Both **mRNA** and **tRNA** are transcribed in the nucleus, whereas **rRNA** is transcribed in the **nucleolus.** The nucleolus is also the site of assembly of ribosomal proteins and rRNA into the small and large subunits of **ribosomes.** These ribosomal subunits enter the cytosol individually.

CELL CYCLE

The **cell cycle** is subdivided into four phases, G_1, S, G_2, and M. During the presynthetic phase, G_1, the cell increases its size and organelle content. During the **S phase,** DNA (plus histone and other chromosome-associated protein) synthesis and centriole replication occur. During G_2, ATP is accumulated, centriole replication is completed, and tubulin is accumulated for spindle formation. G_1, S, and G_2 are also referred to as **interphase. M** represents **mitosis,** which is subdivided into prophase, prometaphase, metaphase, anaphase, and telophase. The result is the division of the cell and its genetic material into two identical daughter cells. The sequence of events in the cell cycle is controlled by a number of trigger proteins, known as **cyclins.**

Histophysiology

I. MEMBRANES AND MEMBRANE TRAFFICKING

The fluidity of the plasmalemma is an important factor in the processes of membrane synthesis, endocytosis, exocytosis, as well as in **membrane trafficking** (see Graphic 1-3)—conserving the membrane as it is transferred through the various cellular compartments. The degree of fluidity is influenced directly by temperature and the degree of unsaturation of the fatty acyl tails of the membrane phospholipids and indirectly by the amount of cholesterol present.

Transport across the cell membrane may be **passive** down an ionic or concentration gradient (**simple diffusion** or **facilitated diffusion** via ion channel or carrier proteins; no energy required) or **active** (energy required, usually against a gradient). **Ion channel** proteins may be **ungated** or **gated.** The former are always open, whereas gated ion channels require the presence of a stimulus (alteration in voltage, mechanical stimulus, presence of a ligand, G protein, neurotransmitter substance, etc.) that opens the gate. These **ligands** and **neurotransmitter substances** are types of signaling molecules.

Signaling molecules are either hydrophobic (lipid soluble) or hydrophilic and are used for cell-to-cell communication. Lipid-soluble molecules diffuse through the cell membrane to activate **intracellular messenger systems** by binding to receptor molecules located in either the cytoplasm or the nucleus. Hydrophilic signaling molecules initiate a specific sequence of responses by binding to **receptors** (integral proteins) embedded in the cell membrane.

Receptors permit the endocytosis of a much greater concentration of ligands than would be possible without receptors. This process is referred to as **receptor-mediated endocytosis** and involves the formation of a **clathrin-coated endocytic vesicle,** which, once within the cell, sheds its clathrin coat and fuses with an **early endosome.** The receptors and ligands are uncoupled in this compartment, permitting the receptors to be transported to a system of tubular vesicles, the recycling endosome, from which the receptors are recycled to the cell membrane. The ligands, left in the **early endosome** (pH 6), are ferried to **late endosomes** (pH 5.5), deeper in the cytoplasm. Two groups of clathrin-coated vesicles derived from the *trans*-Golgi network ferry lysosomal enzymes and lyso-

somal membranes (containing additional ATP-energized **proton pumps**) to the late endosome forming an **endolysosome** (or **lysosome**). The newly delivered proton pumps further decrease the pH of the endolysosomal interior (to a pH of 5.0). Hydrolytic enzymes of the lysosome degrade the ligand, releasing the usable substances for use by the cell. The indigestible remnants of the ligand, however, may remain in vesicles, **residual bodies,** within the cytoplasm.

II. PROTEIN SYNTHESIS AND EXOCYTOSIS

Protein synthesis requires the code-bearing mRNA, amino acid-carrying tRNAs, and ribosomes (see Graphic 1-4). Proteins that will not be packaged are synthesized on **ribosomes** in the cytosol, whereas **noncytosolic proteins** (secretory, lysosomal, and membrane proteins) are synthesized on ribosomes on the **rough endoplasmic reticulum (RER).** The complex of mRNA and ribosomes is referred to as a **polysome.**

The **signal hypothesis** states that mRNAs that code for noncytosolic proteins possess a constant initial segment, the **signal codon,** which codes for a **signal protein.** As the mRNA enters the cytoplasm, it becomes associated with the small subunit of a ribosome. The small subunit has a binding site for mRNA, as well as three binding sites (P, A, and E) for tRNAs.

Once the initiation process is completed, the **start codon** (AUG for the amino acid methionine) is recognized, and the **initiator tRNA** (bearing methionine) is attached to the **P site** (peptidyl-tRNA-binding site), the large subunit of the ribosome becomes attached, and protein synthesis may begin. The next codon is recognized by the proper acylated tRNA, which then binds to the **A site** (aminoacyl-tRNA-binding site). Methionine is uncoupled from the initiator tRNA (at the P site) and a **peptide bond** is formed between the two amino acids (forming a **dipeptide**). The initiator tRNA travels to the **E site** (Exit site) on the ribosome eventually to drop off the ribosome, as the tRNA with the attached dipeptide moves from the A site to the recently vacated P site.

The next codon is recognized by the proper acylated tRNA, which then binds to the A site. The dipeptide is uncoupled from the tRNA at the P site, and a peptide bond is formed between the dipeptide and the new amino acid, forming a tripeptide. The empty tRNA again moves to the E site to fall off the ribosome, as the tRNA bearing the tripeptide moves from the A site to the P site. In this fashion, the peptide chain is elongated to form the signal protein.

The cytosol contains proteins known as **signal recognition particles (SRP).** SRP binds to the signal protein and inhibits the continuation of protein synthesis, and the entire polysome proceeds to the RER. A signal recognition particle receptor, known as **docking protein,** located in the membrane of the RER, recognizes and properly positions the polysome. The docking of the polysome, probably assisted by **ribophorin I** and **ribophorin II,** two integral membrane proteins of the RER, results in a pore opening up in the RER membrane, so that the forming protein chain can enter the RER cisterna. The signal recognition particle leaves the polysome, and protein synthesis resumes until the entire protein is formed. During this process the enzyme **signal peptidase,** located in the RER cisterna, cleaves signal protein from the growing polypeptide chain. Once protein synthesis is complete, the two ribosomal subunits fall off the RER and return to the cytosol.

The newly synthesized protein is modified in the RER by glycosylation, as well as by the formation of disulfide bonds, which transforms the linear protein into a globular form. The newly formed protein is transported in COPII-coated **transfer vesicles** to the ERGIC and from there in COPI-coated vesicles to the *cis* Golgi network and from there to the *cis*-face for further processing.

Within the *cis* face, the mannose groups of lysosomal enzymes are phosphorylated. Nonphosphorylated mannose groups are removed, and galactose and sialic acid residues are added (**terminal glycosylation**) in the **medial** compartment of the Golgi apparatus. Final modification occurs in the *trans* compartment, where selected amino acid residues are phosphorylated and sulfated. Modified proteins are then transported from the Golgi apparatus to the trans-Golgi network (TGN) for packaging and sorting.

All transfers between the various faces of the Golgi apparatus including the TGN probably occur via COPI-coated vesicles. (A concurrent theory suggests the possibility of cisternal maturation, that is as the ERGIC matures it is transformed into the various faces of the Golgi and it is replaced by the coalescence of newly-derived transfer vesicles.) Mannose 6-phosphate receptors in the TGN recognize and package enzymes destined for lysosomes. These **lysosomal enzymes** leave the TGN in clathrin-coated vesicles. **Regulated secretory proteins** are separated and are also packaged in clathrin-coated vesicles. **Membrane proteins** and proteins destined for constitutive (unregulated) transport are packaged in non–clathrin-coated vesicles.

Clickal Considerations ▨ ▧ ▨

Certain individuals suffer from **lysosomal storage diseases**, which involve a hereditary deficiency in the ability of their lysosomes to degrade the contents of their endolysosomes. One of the best-characterized examples of these diseases is **Tay-Sachs disease** that occurs mostly in children whose parents are descendants of Northeast European Jews. Since the lysosomes of these children are unable to catabolize GM2 gangliosides, due to hexominidase deficiency, their neurons accumulate massive amounts of this ganglioside in endolysosomes of ever increasing diameters. As the endolysosomes increase in size, they obstruct neuronal function and the child dies by the third year of life.

Zellweger's disease is an inherited autosomal recessive disorder that interferes with normal peroxisomal biogenesis whose characteristics include renal cysts, hepatomegaly, jaundice, hypotonia of the muscular system, and cerebral demyelination resulting in psychomotor retardation.

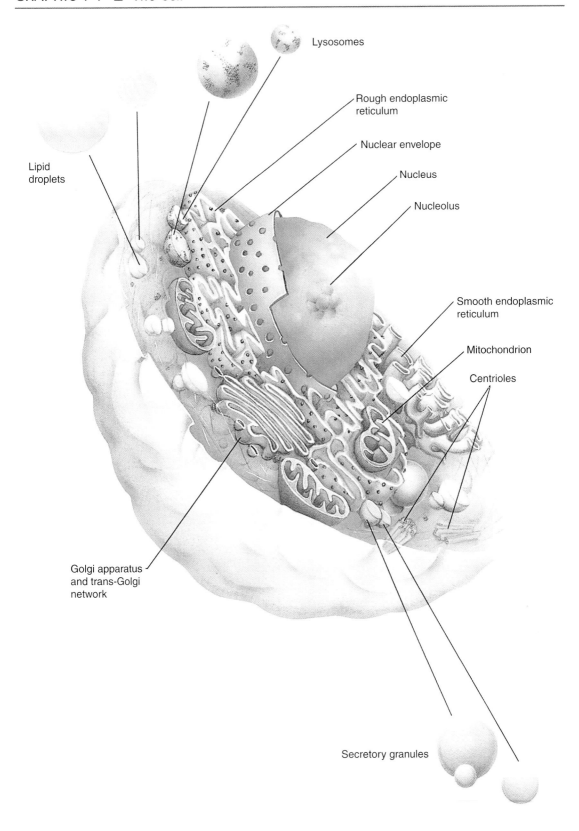

Lysosomes

Rough endoplasmic
reticulum

Nuclear envelope

Nucleus

Nucleolus

Lipid
droplets

Smooth endoplasmic
reticulum

Mitochondrion

Centrioles

Golgi apparatus
and trans-Golgi
network

Secretory granules

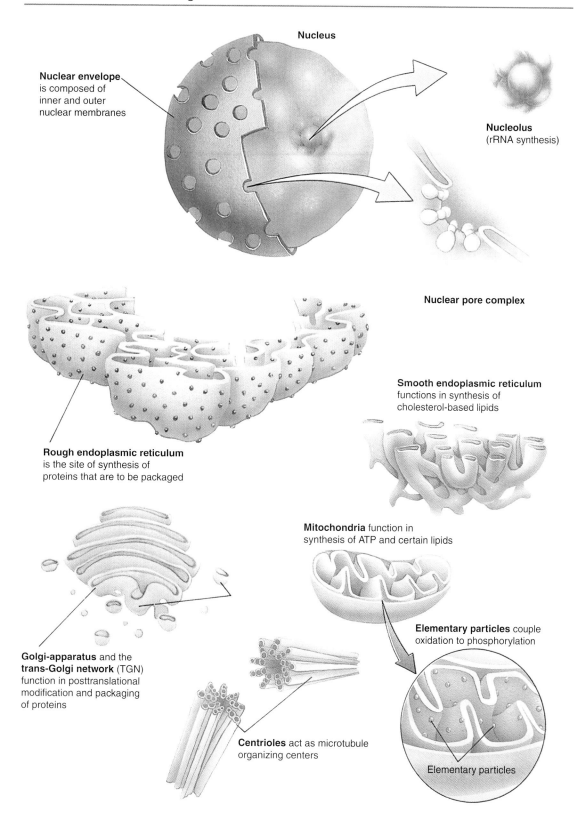

Nucleus

Nuclear envelope is composed of inner and outer nuclear membranes

Nucleolus (rRNA synthesis)

Nuclear pore complex

Rough endoplasmic reticulum is the site of synthesis of proteins that are to be packaged

Smooth endoplasmic reticulum functions in synthesis of cholesterol-based lipids

Mitochondria function in synthesis of ATP and certain lipids

Elementary particles couple oxidation to phosphorylation

Golgi-apparatus and the **trans-Golgi network** (TGN) function in posttranslational modification and packaging of proteins

Centrioles act as microtubule organizing centers

Elementary particles

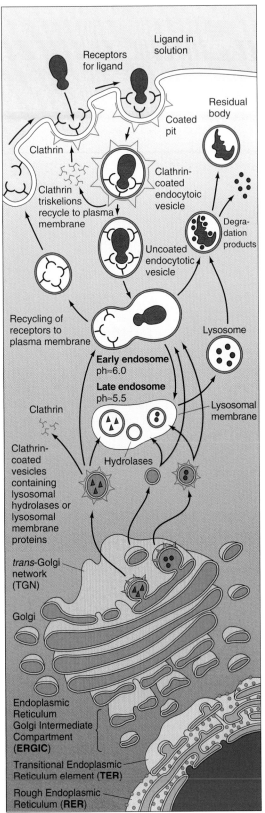

Signaling molecules bind to **receptors** (integral proteins) embedded in the cell membrane and initiate a specific sequence of responses. Receptors permit the endocytosis of a much greater concentration of ligands than would be otherwise possible. This process, **receptor-mediated endocytosis**, involves the formation of **clathrin-coated endocytic vesicles**. Once within the cell, the vesicle sheds its clathrin coat and fuses with an early endosome (pH 6) where the receptor is uncoupled from the ligand. The receptors are carried from the early endosome into a system of tubular vesicles, known as the **recycling endosome**, from which the receptors are returned to the cell membrane.

The ligand is transferred by the use of multivesicular bodies from the early endosome to another system of vesicles late endosomes located deeper in the cytoplasm. **Late endosomes** are more acidic (pH 5.5) and it is here that the ligand begins to be degraded. Late endosomes receive lysosomal hydrolases and lysosomal membranes and in that fashion late endosomes probably are transformed into lysosomes (pH 5.0). Hydrolytic enzymes of the lyosomes degrade the ligand, releasing the usable substances for utilization by the cell, whereas the indigestible remnants of the ligand may remain in vesicles, **residual bodies**, within the cytoplasm.

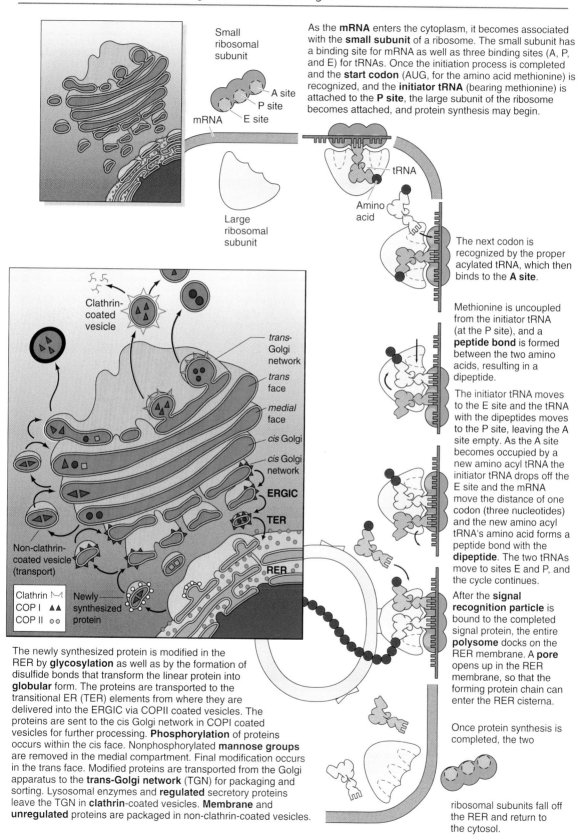

Small ribosomal subunit

A site
P site
E site

mRNA

Large ribosomal subunit

As the **mRNA** enters the cytoplasm, it becomes associated with the **small subunit** of a ribosome. The small subunit has a binding site for mRNA as well as three binding sites (A, P, and E) for tRNAs. Once the initiation process is completed and the **start codon** (AUG, for the amino acid methionine) is recognized, and the **initiator tRNA** (bearing methionine) is attached to the **P site**, the large subunit of the ribosome becomes attached, and protein synthesis may begin.

tRNA

Amino acid

The next codon is recognized by the proper acylated tRNA, which then binds to the **A site**.

Methionine is uncoupled from the initiator tRNA (at the P site), and a **peptide bond** is formed between the two amino acids, resulting in a dipeptide.

The initiator tRNA moves to the E site and the tRNA with the dipeptides moves to the P site, leaving the A site empty. As the A site becomes occupied by a new amino acyl tRNA the initiator tRNA drops off the E site and the mRNA move the distance of one codon (three nucleotides) and the new amino acyl tRNA's amino acid forms a peptide bond with the **dipeptide**. The two tRNAs move to sites E and P, and the cycle continues.

Clathrin-coated vesicle

*trans-*Golgi network

trans face

medial face

cis Golgi

cis Golgi network

ERGIC

TER

Non-clathrin-coated vesicle (transport)

RER

Clathrin
COP I ▲▲
COP II ∘∘

Newly synthesized protein

The newly synthesized protein is modified in the RER by **glycosylation** as well as by the formation of disulfide bonds that transform the linear protein into **globular** form. The proteins are transported to the transitional ER (TER) elements from where they are delivered into the ERGIC via COPII coated vesicles. The proteins are sent to the cis Golgi network in COPI coated vesicles for further processing. **Phosphorylation** of proteins occurs within the cis face. Nonphosphorylated **mannose groups** are removed in the medial compartment. Final modification occurs in the trans face. Modified proteins are transported from the Golgi apparatus to the **trans-Golgi network** (TGN) for packaging and sorting. Lysosomal enzymes and **regulated** secretory proteins leave the TGN in **clathrin**-coated vesicles. **Membrane** and **unregulated** proteins are packaged in non-clathrin-coated vesicles.

After the **signal recognition particle** is bound to the completed signal protein, the entire **polysome** docks on the RER membrane. A **pore** opens up in the RER membrane, so that the forming protein chain can enter the RER cisterna.

Once protein synthesis is completed, the two

ribosomal subunits fall off the RER and return to the cytosol.

PLATE 1-1 ■ *Typical Cell*

FIGURE 1 ■ *Cells. Monkey. Plastic section.* × 1323.

The typical cell is a membrane-bound structure that consists of a **nucleus** (N) and **cytoplasm** (C). Although the cell membrane is too thin to be visualized with the light microscope, the outline of the cell approximates the cell membrane (arrowheads). Observe that the outline of these particular cells more or less approximates a square shape. Viewed in three dimensions, these cells are said to be cuboidal in shape, with a centrally placed nucleus. The **nucleolus** (n) is clearly evident, as are the chromatin granules (arrows) that are dispersed around the periphery, as well as throughout the nucleoplasm.

FIGURE 2 ■ *Cells. Monkey. Plastic section.* × 540.

Cells may possess tall, thin morphologies, like those of a collecting duct of the kidney. Their **nuclei** (N) are located basally, and their lateral cell membranes (arrowheads) are outlined. Since these cells are epithelially derived, they are separated from **connective tissue elements** (CT) by a **basal membrane** (BM).

FIGURE 3 ■ *Cells. Monkey. Plastic section.* × 540.

Cells come in a variety of sizes and shapes. Note that the **epithelium** (E) that lines the **lumen** of the bladder is composed of numerous layers. The surfacemost layer consists of large, dome-shaped cells, some occasionally displaying two **nuclei** (N). The granules evident in the cytoplasm (arrowhead) are glycogen deposits. Cells deeper in the epithelium are elongated and narrow, and their nuclei (arrow) are located in their widest region.

FIGURE 4 ■ *Cells. Monkey. Plastic section.* × 540.

Some cells possess a rather unusual morphology, as exemplified by the **Purkinje cell** (PC) of the cerebellum. Note that the **nucleus** (N) of the cell is housed in its widest portion, known as the soma (perikaryon). The cell possesses several cytoplasmic extensions, **dendrites** (De), and axon. This nerve cell integrates the numerous digits of information that it receives from other nerve cells that synapse on it.

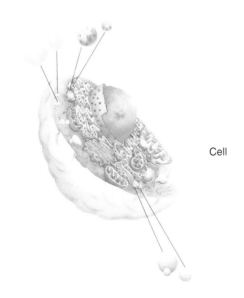

Cell

■ **KEY**

BM	basal membrane	De	dendrite	N	nucleus
C	cytoplasm	E	epithelium	n	nucleolus
CT	connective tissue	L	lumen	PC	Purkinje cell

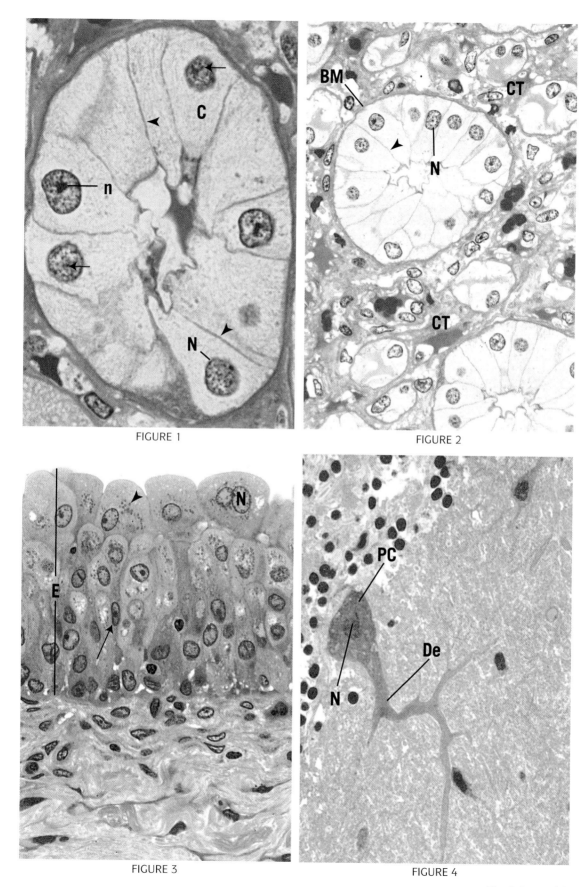

FIGURE 1

FIGURE 2

FIGURE 3

FIGURE 4

PLATE 1-2 ■ *Cell Organelles and Inclusions*

FIGURE 1 ■ *Nucleus and Nissl bodies. Spinal cord. Human. Paraffin section.* × 540.

The motor neurons of the spinal cord are multipolar neurons, since they possess numerous processes arising from an enlarged **soma** (S), which houses the **nucleus** (N) and various organelles. Observe that the nucleus displays a large, densely staining **nucleolus** (n). The cytoplasm also presents a series of densely staining structures known as **Nissl bodies** (NB), which have been demonstrated by electron microscopy to be rough endoplasmic reticulum. The staining intensity is due to the presence of ribonucleic acid of the ribosomes studding the surface of the rough endoplasmic reticulum.

FIGURE 2 ■ *Secretory products. Mast cell. Monkey. Plastic section.* × 540.

The **connective tissue** (CT) subjacent to the epithelial lining of the small intestines is richly endowed with **mast cells** (MC). The granules (arrows) of mast cells are distributed throughout their cytoplasm and are released along the entire periphery of the cell. These small granules contain histamine and heparin, as well as additional substances. Note that the **epithelial cells** (EC) are tall and columnar in morphology, and that **leukocytes** (Le) are migrating, via intercellular spaces, into the **lumen** (L) of the intestines. Arrowheads point to terminal bars, junctions between epithelial cells. The **brush border** (BB) has been demonstrated by electron microscopy to be microvilli.

FIGURE 3 ■ *Zymogen granules. Pancreas. Monkey. Plastic section.* × 540.

The exocrine portion of the pancreas produces enzymes necessary for proper digestion of ingested food materials. These enzymes are stored by the pancreatic cells as **zymogen granules** (ZG) until their release is effected by hormonal activity. Note that the parenchymal cells are arranged in clusters known as **acini** (Ac) with a central lumen into which the secretory product is released. Observe that the zymogen granules are stored in the apical region of the cell, away from the basally located **nucleus** (N). Arrows indicate the lateral cell membranes of adjacent cells of an acinus.

FIGURE 4 ■ *Mucous secretory products. Goblet cells. Large intestines. Monkey. Plastic section.* × 540.

The glands of the large intestine house **goblet cells** (GC), which manufacture a large amount of mucous material that acts as a lubricant for the movement of the compacted residue of digestion. Each goblet cell possesses an expanded apical portion, the **theca** (T), which contains the secretory product of the cell. The base of the cell is compressed and houses the **nucleus** (N), as well as the organelles necessary for the synthesis of the mucus—namely, the rough endoplasmic reticulum and the Golgi apparatus. Arrows indicate the lateral cell membranes of contiguous goblet cells.

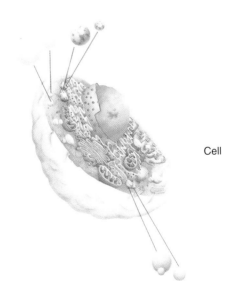

Cell

■ **KEY**

Ac	acinus	L	lumen	NB	Nissl body
BB	brush border	Le	leukocyte	S	soma
CT	connective tissue	MC	mast cell	T	theca
EC	epithelial cell	N	nucleus	ZG	zymogen granule
GC	goblet cell	n	nucleolus		

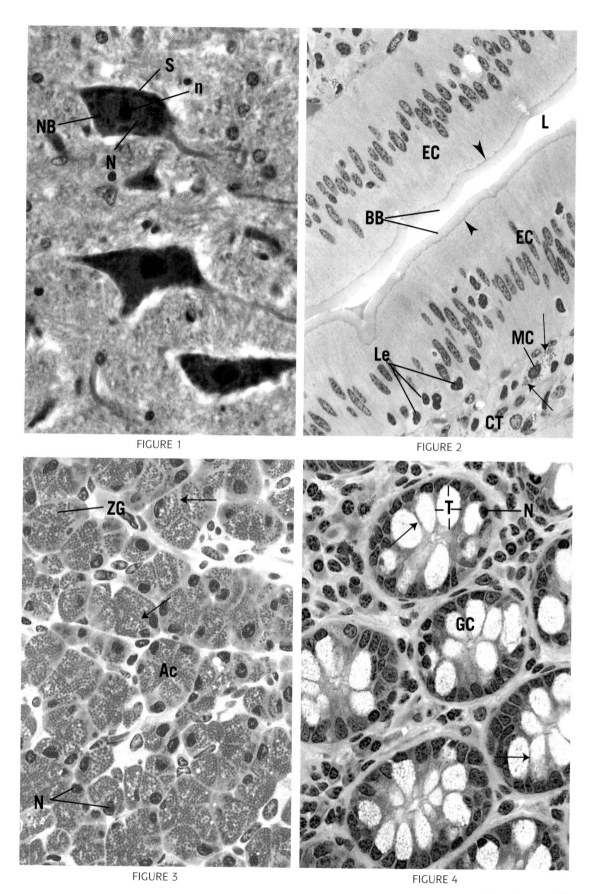

FIGURE 1

FIGURE 2

FIGURE 3

FIGURE 4

PLATE 1-3 ■ *Cell Surface Modifications*

FIGURE 1 ■ *Brush border. Small intestines. Monkey. Plastic section.* × 540.

The cells lining the **lumen** (L) of the small intestine are columnar cells, among which are numerous mucus-producing **goblet cells** (GC). The columnar cells' function is absorbing digested food material along their free, apical surface. In order to increase their free surface area, the cells possess a **brush border** (BB), which has been demonstrated by electron microscopy to be microvilli— short, narrow, finger-like extensions of plasmalemma-covered cytoplasm. Each microvillus bears a glycocalyx cell coat, which also contains digestive enzymes. The core of the microvillus contains longitudinally arranged actin filaments, as well as additional associated proteins.

FIGURE 2 ■ *Cilia. Oviduct. Monkey. Plastic section.* × 540.

The lining of the oviduct is composed of two types of epithelial cells: bleb-bearing **peg cells** (pc), which probably produce nutritional factors necessary for the survival of the gametes, and pale, **ciliated cells** (CC). Cilia (arrows) are long, motile, finger-like extensions of the apical cell membrane and cytoplasm that transport material along the cell surface. The core of the cilium, as shown by electron microscopy, contains the axoneme, composed of microtubules arranged in a specific configuration of nine doublets surrounding a central pair of individual microtubules.

FIGURE 3 ■ *Stereocilia. Epididymis. Monkey. Plastic section.* × 540.

The lining of the epididymis is composed of tall, columnar **principal cells** (Pi) and short **basal cells** (BC). The principal cells bear long stereocilia (arrows) that protrude into the lumen. It was believed that stereocilia were long, nonmotile, cilia-like structures. However, studies with the electron microscope have shown that stereocilia are actually long microvilli that branch as well as clump with each other. The function, if any, of stereocilia within the epididymis is not known. The lumen is occupied by numerous spermatozoa, whose dark heads (asterisks) and pale flagella (arrowhead) are clearly discernible. Flagella are very long, cilia-like structures used by the cell for propulsion.

FIGURE 4 ■ *Intercellular bridges. Skin. Monkey. Plastic section.* × 540.

The epidermis of thick skin is composed of several cell layers, one of which is the stratum spinosum shown in this photomicrograph. The cells of this layer possess short, stubby, finger-like extensions that interdigitate with those of contiguous cells. Before the advent of electron microscopy, these intercellular bridges (arrows) were believed to represent cytoplasmic continuities between neighboring cells; however, it is now known that these processes merely serve as regions of desmosome formation so that the cells may adhere to each other.

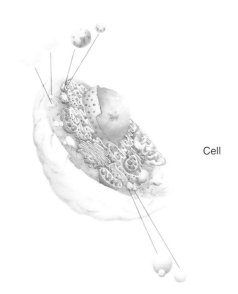

Cell

■ **KEY**

BB	brush border	GC	goblet cell	pc	peg cell
BC	basal cell	L	lumen	Pi	principal cell
CC	ciliated cell				

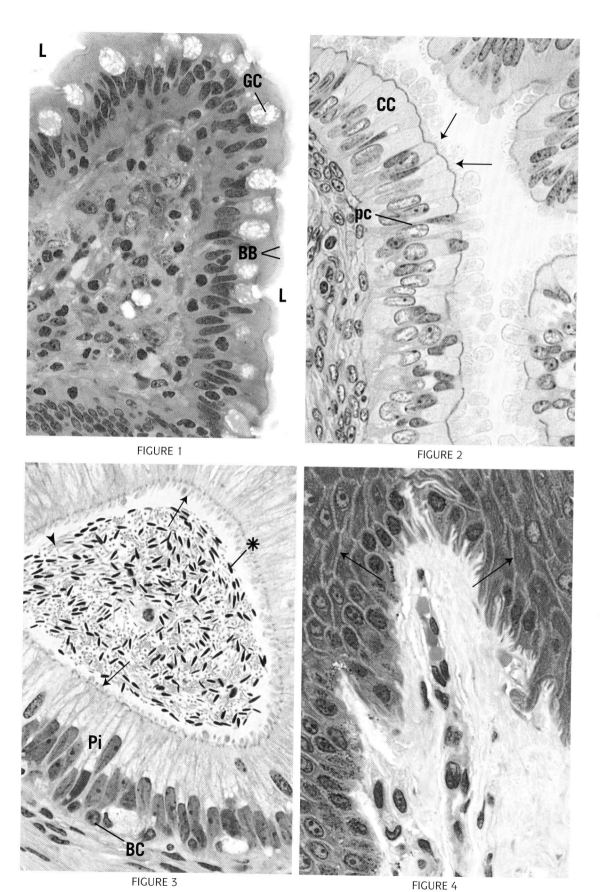

FIGURE 1

FIGURE 2

FIGURE 3

FIGURE 4

PLATE 1-4 ■ *Mitosis, Light and Electron Microscopy*

FIGURE 1 ▦ *Mitosis. Whitefish blastula. Paraffin section.* × 270.

This photomicrograph of whitefish blastula shows different stages of mitosis. The first mitotic stage, **prophase** (P), displays the short, thread-like chromosomes (arrow) in the center of the cell. The nuclear membrane is no longer present. During **metaphase** (M), the chromosomes line up at the equatorial plane of the cell. The chromosomes begin to migrate toward the opposite poles of the cell in early **anaphase** (A) and proceed farther and farther apart as anaphase progresses (arrowheads). Note the dense regions, **centrioles** (c), toward which the chromosomes migrate.

FIGURE 2 ▦ *Mitosis. Whitefish blastula. Paraffin section.* × 540.

During the early telophase stage of mitotic division, the **chromosomes** (Ch) have reached the opposite poles of the cell. The cell membrane constricts to separate the cell into the two new daughter cells, forming a cleavage furrow (arrowheads). The spindle apparatus is visible as parallel, horizontal lines (arrow) that eventually form the mid-body. As telophase progresses, the two new daughter cells will uncoil their chromosomes and the nuclear membrane and nucleoli will become re-established.

FIGURE 3 ▦ *Mitosis. Mouse. Electron microscopy.* × 9423.

Neonatal tissue is characterized by mitotic activity, where numerous cells are in the process of proliferation. Observe that the interphase **nucleus** (N) possesses a typical **nuclear envelope** (NE), perinuclear chromatin (asterisk), nucleolus, and nuclear pores. A cell that is undergoing the mitotic phase of the cell cycle, however, loses its nuclear membrane and nucleolus, while its **chromosomes** (Ch) are quite visible. These chromosomes are no longer lined up at the equatorial plate, but are migrating to opposite poles, indicating that this cell is in the early- to mid-anaphase stage of mitosis. Observe the presence of cytoplasmic organelles, such as mitochondria, rough endoplasmic reticulum, and Golgi apparatus.

■ **KEY**

A	anaphase	M	metaphase	NE	nuclear envelope
c	centriole	N	nucleus	P	prophase
Ch	chromosome				

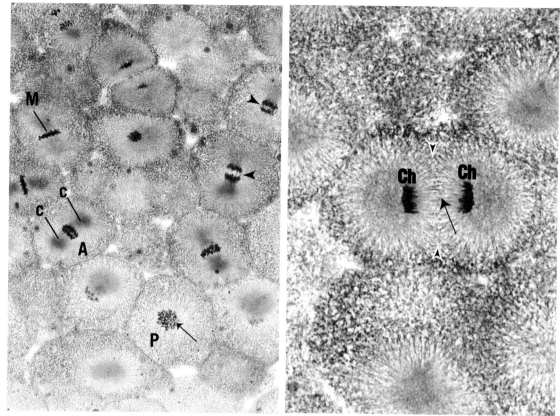

FIGURE 1

FIGURE 2

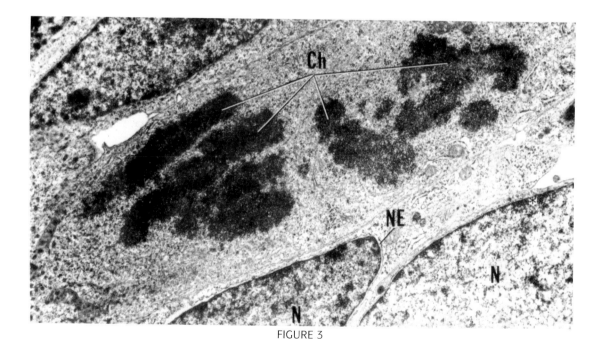

FIGURE 3

PLATE 1-5 ■ *Typical Cell, Electron Microscopy*

FIGURE 1 ■ *Typical cell. Pituitary. Rat. Electron microscopy.* × 8936.

The gonadotrophs of the pituitary gland provide an excellent example of a typical cell, since they house many of the cytoplasmic organelles possessed by most cells. The cytoplasm is limited by a cell membrane (arrowheads) that is clearly evident, especially where it approximates the plasmalemma of the adjacent electron-dense cells. **Mitochondria** (m) are not numerous, but are easily recognizable, especially in longitudinal sections, since their cristae (arrows) are arranged in a characteristic fashion. Since this cell actively manufactures a secretory product that has to be packaged and delivered outside of the cell, it possesses a well-developed **Golgi apparatus** (GA), positioned near the **nucleus** (N). Observe that the Golgi is formed by several stacks of flattened membranes. Additionally, this cell is well-endowed with **rough endoplasmic reticulum** (RER), indicating active protein synthesis.

The cytoplasm also displays secretory products (asterisks), which are transitory inclusions.

The nucleus is bounded by the typical **nuclear envelope** (NE), consisting of a ribosome-studded outer nuclear membrane and an inner nuclear membrane. The peripheral chromatin and chromatin islands are clearly evident, as is the **nucleolus-associated chromatin** (NC). The clear area within the nucleus is the nucleoplasm representing the fluid component of the nucleus. The **nucleolus** (n) presents a sponge-like appearance composed of electron-lucent and electron-dense materials, suspended free in the nucleoplasm. The electron-dense region is composed of the pars granulosa and the pars fibrosa, while the electron-lucent region is probably the nucleoplasm in which the nucleolus is suspended. (From Stokreef JC, Reifel CW, Shin SH: *Cell Tissue Res* 243: 255–261, 1986.)

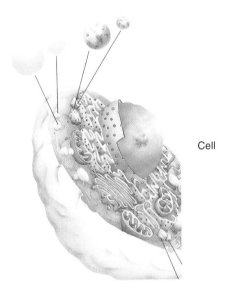

Cell

■ **KEY**

GA	Golgi apparatus	n	nucleolus	NE	nuclear envelope
m	mitochondrion	NC	nucleolus-associated	rER	rough endoplasmic
N	nucleus		chromatin		reticulum

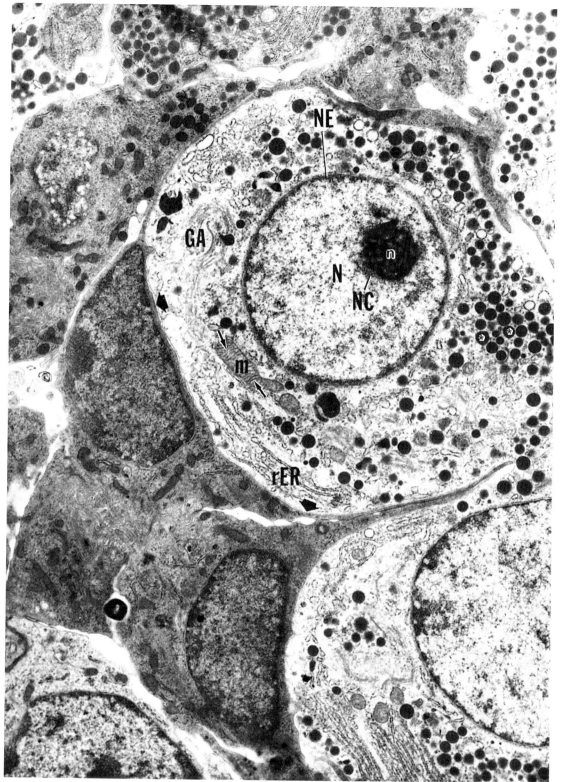

FIGURE 1

PLATE 1-6 ■ *Nucleus and Cytoplasm, Electron Microscopy*

FIGURE 1 ■ *Nucleus and cytoplasm. Liver. Mouse. Electron microscopy.* × 48,176.

The **nucleus** (N) displays its nucleoplasm and **chromatin** (c) to advantage in this electron micrograph. Note that the inner (arrowheads) and outer (double arrows) membranes of the nuclear envelope fuse to form **nuclear** **pores** (NP). The **rough endoplasmic reticulum** (rER) is richly endowed by **ribosomes** (R). Note the presence of numerous **mitochondria** (m), whose double membrane and **cristae** (Cr) are quite evident. Observe the slightly electron-dense **microtubule** (Mi) as it courses through the cytoplasm.

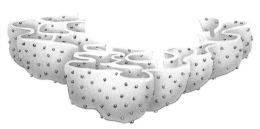

Rough endoplasmic reticulum

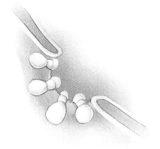

Nuclear pore complex

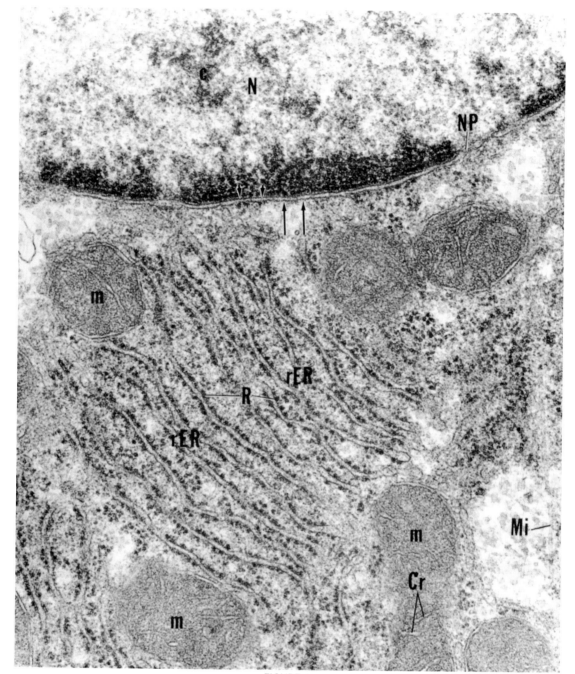

FIGURE 1

PLATE 1-7 ■ *Nucleus and Cytoplasm, Electron Microscopy*

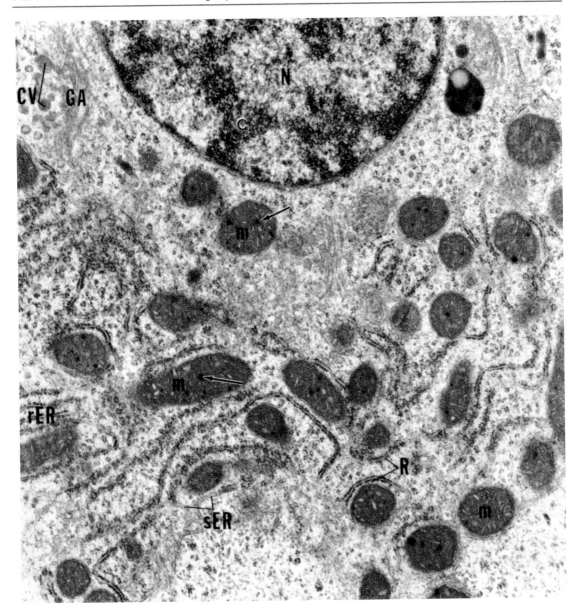

FIGURE 1 ■ *Nucleus and cytoplasm. Liver. Mouse.*
Electron microscopy. × 20,318.

This electron micrograph of a liver cell displays the **nucleus** (N) with its condensed **chromatin** (c), as well as many cytoplasmic organelles. Note that the **mitochondria** (m) possess electron-dense matrix granules (arrows) scattered in the matrix of the intercristal spaces. The perinuclear area presents the **Golgi apparatus** (GA), which is actively packaging material in **condensing vesicles** (CV). The **rough endoplasmic reticulum** (rER) is obvious due to its **ribosomes** (R), whereas the **smooth endoplasmic reticulum** (sER) is less obvious.

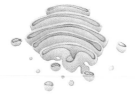

Golgi apparatus

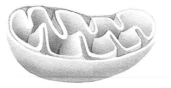

Mitochondrion

PLATE 1-8 ■ *Golgi Apparatus, Electron Microscopy*

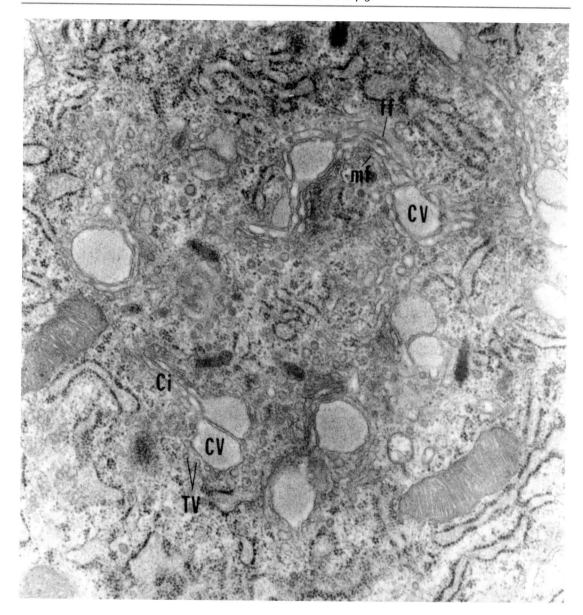

FIGURE 1 ■ *Golgi apparatus. Mouse. Electron microscopy.* × 28,588.

The extensive Golgi apparatus of this secretory cell presents several flattened membrane-bound **cisternae** (Ci), stacked one on top of the other. The convex face (ff) receives **transfer vesicles** (TV) derived from the rough endoplasmic reticulum. The concave, *trans*-**Golgi network** (mf) releases **condensing vesicles** (CV), which house the secretory product. (From Gartner LP, Seibel W, Hiatt JL, Provenza DV: *Acta Anat* 103:16–33, 1979.)

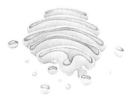

Golgi apparatus

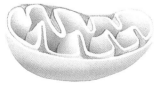

Mitochondrion

PLATE 1-9 ■ *Mitochondria, Electron Microscopy*

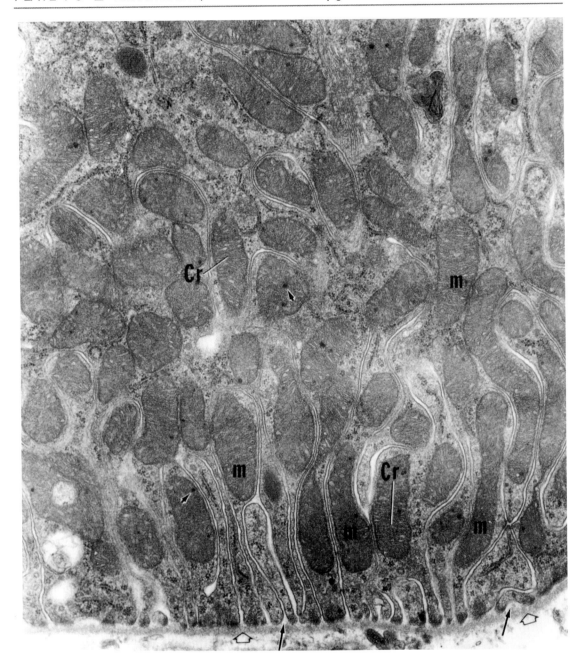

FIGURE 1 ▓ *Mitochondria. Kidney. Mouse.*
Electron microscopy. × 18,529.

The basal aspect of the proximal tubule cell presents numerous interdigitating processes. Many of these processes house longitudinally oriented **mitochondria** (m), whose outer membrane is smooth, while its inner membrane is folded to form **cristae** (Cr). Note that the matrix houses matrix granules (arrowheads). Observe also the basal lamina whose lamina densa (open arrowheads) and lamina lucida (arrows) are clearly evident.

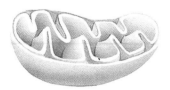

Mitochondrion

Epithelium and Glands

Epithelium is one of the four basic tissues of the body and is derived from all three germ layers. It is composed of very closely packed, contiguous cells, with very little or no intercellular material in the extracellular spaces. Epithelia either form membranes that are represented as sheets covering the body surface and lining its internal surface or occur as secretory elements known as glands. Almost always, epithelia and their derivatives are separated from underlying or surrounding connective tissues by a thin, noncellular layer, the **basal membrane** (**basement membrane**). This is usually composed of an epithelially derived **basal lamina** and the **lamina reticularis**, derived from the connective tissue.

EPITHELIUM

Epithelial Membranes

Epithelial membranes are avascular, deriving their nutrients by diffusion from blood vessels in the underlying connective tissue. These membranes can cover a surface, line a cavity, or line a tube. Surfaces covered may be dry, as the outer body surface, or wet, as the covering of the ovary. All lining epithelia, on the other hand, have a wet surface (e.g., those lining the body cavities, blood vessels, and gastrointestinal tract). Membranes that line serous body cavities are referred to as **mesothelia,** whereas those lining the heart chambers and blood and lymph vessels are known as **endothelia.**

Epithelial membranes are classified according to the shape of the most superficial cell layer, which may be **squamous** (flat), **cuboidal,** or **columnar,** as observed when sectioned perpendicular to the exposed surface of the membrane. Moreover, the number of cell layers composing the epithelium also determines its classification, in that a single layer of cells constitutes a **simple epithelium,** whereas two or more layers of cells are referred to as a **stratified epithelium** (Table 2-1). In a simple epithelium, all of the cells touch the basal lamina and reach the free surface. In **pseudostratified epithelia** (which may or may not possess cilia or stereocilia), however, all of the cells touch the basal lamina, although some cells are much shorter than others and do not reach the free surface. Therefore, this is a simple epithelium that appears to be stratified.

Stratified squamous epithelium may be **keratinized, nonkeratinized,** or even **parakeratinized.** The stratified epithelium found in the urinary tract is known as **transitional epithelium**; its free surface is characterized by large, dome-shaped cells (Table 2-1).

Epithelial cell membranes are frequently specialized. The free surface may form **microvilli (brush border), cilia,** or **stereocilia.** The lateral cell membranes maintain intercellular junctions between contiguous cells. These junctions are the **zonulae occludentes, zonulae adherentes, macula adherentes,** and gap junctions. The basal cell membrane forms **hemidesmosomes,** maintaining the cell's attachment to the basal membrane (see Graphic 2-1).

Epithelial membranes possess numerous functions. These include protection; reduction of friction; absorption; secretion; excretion; synthesis of various proteins, enzymes, mucins, hormones, and a myriad of other substances; and acting in a sensory capacity.

GLANDS

Most glands are formed by epithelial downgrowths into the surrounding connective tissue. Glands that deliver their secretions onto the epithelial surface do so via ducts and are known as **exocrine glands.** Glands that do not maintain a connection to the outside (ductless) and whose secretions enter the vascular system for delivery are known as **endocrine glands.** The secretory cells of a gland are referred to as its **parenchyma** and are separated from surrounding connective tissue and vascular elements

TABLE 2-1 ▦ *Classification of Epithelia*

Type	Surface Cell Shape	Examples (Some)
Simple		
Simple squamous	Flattened	Lining blood and lymphatic vessel walls (endothelium), pleural and abdominal cavities (mesothelium)
Simple cuboidal	Cuboidal	Lining ducts of most glands
Simple columnar	Columnar	Lining much of digestive tract, gall bladder
Pseudostratified	All cells rest on basal lamina with only some reaching the surface. Cells that reach the surface are columnar	Lining of nasal cavity, trachea, bronchi, epididymis
Stratified		
Stratified squamous (nonkeratinized)	Flattened (with nuclei)	Lining mouth, esophagus, vagina
Stratified squamous (keratinized)	Flattened (without nuclei)	Epidermis of the skin
Stratified cuboidal	Cuboidal	Lining ducts of sweat glands
Stratified columnar	Columnar	Conjunctiva of eye, lining some large excretory ducts
Transitional	Large dome-shaped cells when bladder is empty; flattened when bladder is distended	Lining renal calyces, renal pelvis, ureter, urinary bladder, proximal portion of urethra

by a basal membrane. Exocrine glands are classified according to various parameters, e.g., morphology of their functional units, branching of their ducts, types of secretory products they manufacture, and the method whereby their component cells release secretory products. The classification of endocrine glands is much more complex, but morphologically, their secretory units either are composed of **follicles** or are arranged in **cords** and clumps of cells (see Graphic 2-2).

Histophysiology

I. EPITHELIUM

Epithelium is **avascular** and is composed of closely apposed cells with little intercellular space. These cells frequently form epithelial sheets that receive nutrients from the blood vessels of the underlying connective tissue via diffusion through the basal lamina. Epithelium not only **covers** the body but also **lines** body cavities, as well as lumina of vessels and ducts and systems (e.g., digestive tract, urinary tract); consequently, material entering or leaving the body must do so through these epithelial sheets.

Epithelium functions in **protection** from mechanical abrasion, chemical penetration, and bacterial invasion; **absorption** of nutrients as a result of its polarized cells that are capable of performing vectorial functions; **excretion** of waste products; **sensory reception** from the external (or internal) milieu; **forming glands** whose function is the **secreting** enzymes, hormones, lubricants, or other products; and movement of material along the epithelial sheet (such as mucus along the respiratory tract) by the assistance of cilia.

Epithelial cells may present specializations along their various surfaces. These surfaces are **apical** (microvilli, stereocilia, cilia, and flagella), **lateral or basolateral** (junctional complexes, zonula occludens, zonula adherens, macula adherens, gap junctions), and **basal** (hemidesmosomes and basal lamina).

A. Apical Surface Modifications

Microvilli are closely spaced, finger-like extensions of the cell membrane that increase the surface area of cells that function in absorption and secretion. Dense clusters of microvilli are evident in light micrographs, as a striated or brush border.

Stereocilia are located in the epididymis, as well as in a few limited regions of the body. They were named cilia because of their length; however, electron micrography proved them to be elongated microvilli whose functions are, as yet, unknown.

Cilia are elongated, motile, plasmalemma-covered extensions of the cytoplasm that move material along the cell surface. Each cilium arises from a centriole (**basal body**) and possesses an **axoneme** core composed of nine pairs of peripheral (doublets) and two single, centrally placed microtubules (singlets). Microtubules of the doublets possess **dynein** arms with ATPase activity, which functions in energizing ciliary motion.

B. Basolateral Surface Modifications

Junctional complexes, which occupy only a minute region of the basolateral cell surfaces, are visible with light microscopy as **terminal bars,** a structure that encircles the entire cell. Terminal bars are composed of three components: **zonula occludens** (tight or occluding junction), **zonula adherens** (adhering junction), and **macula adheres** (**desmosome**s, also adhering junction). The first two encircle the cell, whereas desmosomes do not. Additionally, another type of junction, the **gap junction**, permits cells to communicate with each other.

C. Basal Surface Modifications

The basal cell membrane of the cell is affixed to the basal lamina by adhering junctions known as the **hemidesmosomes**. Morphologically, this structure resembles half of a desmosome but its biochemical composition and clinical significance demonstrate enough dissimilarity that hemidesmosomes are no longer viewed as being merely a half of a desmosome.

The **basement membrane,** interposed between epithelium and connective tissue, is composed of an epithelially derived component, the **basal lamina,** and a connective tissue-derived region, the **lamina reticularis.** The basal lamina is further subdivided into two regions, the **lamina lucida** and the **lamina densa.** Basal laminae function as structural supports for the epithelium, as molecular filters (e.g., in the renal glomerulus), in regulating the migration of certain cells across epithelial sheaths (e.g., preventing entry to fibroblasts but permitting access to lymphoid cells), in epithelial regeneration (e.g., in wound healing where it forms a surface along which regenerating epithelial cells migrate), and in cell-to-cell interactions (e.g., formation of myoneural junctions).

D. Epithelial Cell Renewal

Epithelial cells usually undergo regular turnover because of their function and location. For example:

cells of the epidermis that are sloughed from the surface, originated approximately 28 days earlier by mitosis from cells of the basal layers. Other cells, such as those lining the small intestine, are replaced every few days. Still others continue to proliferate until adulthood is reached, at which time the mechanism is shut down. However, when large numbers of cells are lost, for example because of injury, certain mechanisms trigger the proliferation of new cells to restore the cell population.

Clinical Considerations ▨ ▨ ▪

Bullous Pemphigoid

Bullous pemphigoid, a rare autoimmune disease, is caused by autoantibodies binding to some of the protein components of hemidesmosomes. Individuals afflicted with this disease exhibit skin blistering of the groin, and axilla about the flexure areas and often in the oral cavity. Fortunately, it can be controlled by steroids and immunosuppressive drugs.

Pemphigus Vulgaris

Pemphigus vulgaris is an autoimmune disease, caused by autoantibodies binding to some of the components of desmosomes. This disease causes blistering and is usually found occurring in middle-aged individuals. It is a relatively dangerous disease since the blistering can easily lead to infections. Frequently this disease also responds to steroid therapy.

Tumor Formation

Under certain pathologic conditions, mechanisms that regulate cell proliferation do not function properly; thus, epithelial proliferation gives rise to tumors that may be benign if they are localized, or malignant if they wander from their original site and metastasize (seed) to another area of the body and continue to proliferate. Malignant tumors that arise from surface epithelium are termed carcinomas, whereas those developing from glandular epithelium are called adenocarcinomas.

Metaplasia

Epithelial cells are derived from certain germ cell layers, possess a definite morphology and location, and perform specific functions; however, under certain pathological conditions, they may undergo metaplasia, transforming into another epithelial cell type. An example of such metaplasia occurs in the lining epithelium of the oral cavity of individuals who smoke or use chewing tobacco.

Summary of Histological Organization

I. EPITHELIUM

A. Types

1. *Simple Squamous*—single layer of uniform flat cells.

2. *Simple Cuboidal*—single layer of uniform cuboidal cells.

3. *Simple Columnar*—single layer of uniform columnar cells.

4. *Pseudostratified Columnar*—single layer of cells of varied shapes and heights.

5. *Stratified Squamous*—several layers of cells whose superficial layers are flattened. These may be nonkeratinized, parakeratinized, or keratinized.

6. *Stratified Cuboidal*—two or more layers of cells whose superficial layers are cuboidal in shape.

7. *Stratified Columnar*—two or more layers of cells whose superficial layers are columnar in shape.

8. *Transitional*—several layers of cells, characterized by large, dome-shaped cells at the free surface, that help maintain the integrity of the epithelium during distention of the various components of the urinary tract.

B. General Characteristics

1. Free Surface Modifications
Cells may possess **microvilli** (brush border, striated border), short finger-like projections that increase the surface area of the cell; **stereocilia** (long anastomosing microvilli), which are only found in the epididymis; and **cilia,** which are long, motile projections of the cell with a 9 + 2 microtubular substructure (**axoneme**).

2. Lateral Surface Modifications
For the purposes of adhesion, the cell membranes form junctional complexes involving the lateral plasmalemma of contiguous cells. These junctions are known as **desmosomes** (maculae adherentes), **zonulae occludentes,** and **zonulae adherentes.** For the purpose of intercellular communication, the lateral cell membranes form **gap junctions (nexus, septate junctions).**

3. Basal Surface Modifications
The basal cell membrane that lies on the basal membrane forms **hemidesmosomes** to assist the cell adhere to the underlying connective tissue.

4. Basal Membrane
The **basal (basement) membrane** of light microscopy is composed of an epithelially derived **basal lamina** (which has two parts, **lamina densa** and **lamina lucida**) and a **lamina reticularis** derived from connective tissue, which may be absent.

II. GLANDS

A. Exocrine Glands

Exocrine glands, which deliver secretions into a system of ducts to be conveyed onto an epithelial surface, may be **unicellular** (goblet cells) or **multicellular.**

Multicellular glands may be classified according to the branching of their **duct system.** If the ducts are not branched, the gland is **simple;** if they are branched, the gland is **compound.** Moreover, the three-dimensional shape of the secretory units may be **tubular, acinar (alveolar),** or a combination of the two, namely **tubuloacinar (alveolar).** Additional criteria include 1) the **type** of secretory product produced: **serous** (parotid, pancreas), **mucous** (palatal glands), and **mixed** (sublingual, submandibular), possessing serous and mucous acini and **serous demilunes;** and 2) the **mode of secretion: merocrine** (only the secretory product is released as in the parotid gland), **apocrine** (the secretory product is accompanied by some of the apical cytoplasm, as perhaps in mammary glands), and **holocrine** (the entire cell becomes the secretory product, as in the sebaceous gland, testes, and ovary). Glands are subdivided by connective tissue septa into lobes and lobules, and the ducts that serve them are interlobar, intralobar, interlobular, and intralobular (striated, intercalated).

Myoepithelial (basket) cells are ectodermally derived myoid cells that share the basement lamina of the glandular parenchyma. These cells possess long processes that surround secretory acini and, by occasional contraction, assist in the delivery of the secretory product into the system of ducts.

B. Endocrine Glands

Endocrine glands are ductless glands that release their secretion into the bloodstream. These glands are described in Chapter 10.

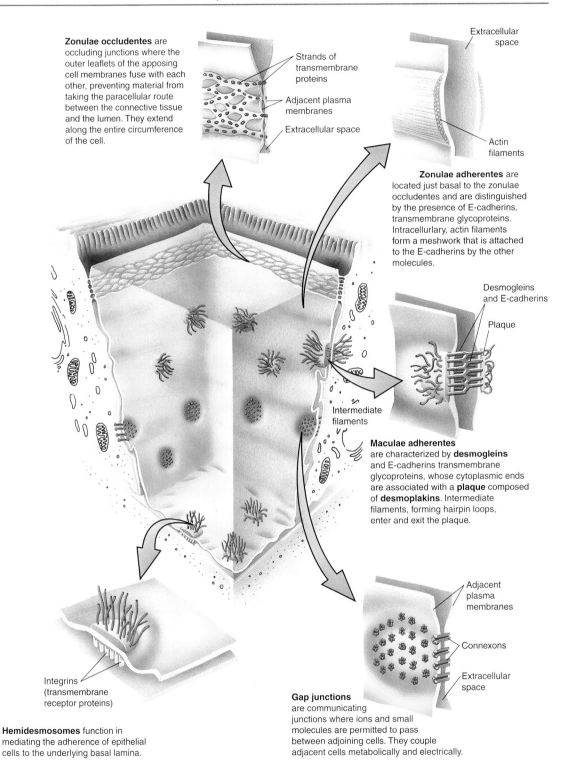

Zonulae occludentes are occluding junctions where the outer leaflets of the apposing cell membranes fuse with each other, preventing material from taking the paracellular route between the connective tissue and the lumen. They extend along the entire circumference of the cell.

Strands of transmembrane proteins

Adjacent plasma membranes

Extracellular space

Extracellular space

Actin filaments

Zonulae adherentes are located just basal to the zonulae occludentes and are distinguished by the presence of E-cadherins, transmembrane glycoproteins. Intracellurlary, actin filaments form a meshwork that is attached to the E-cadherins by the other molecules.

Desmogleins and E-cadherins

Plaque

Intermediate filaments

Maculae adherentes are characterized by **desmogleins** and E-cadherins transmembrane glycoproteins, whose cytoplasmic ends are associated with a **plaque** composed of **desmoplakins**. Intermediate filaments, forming hairpin loops, enter and exit the plaque.

Adjacent plasma membranes

Connexons

Extracellular space

Integrins (transmembrane receptor proteins)

Hemidesmosomes function in mediating the adherence of epithelial cells to the underlying basal lamina.

Gap junctions are communicating junctions where ions and small molecules are permitted to pass between adjoining cells. They couple adjacent cells metabolically and electrically.

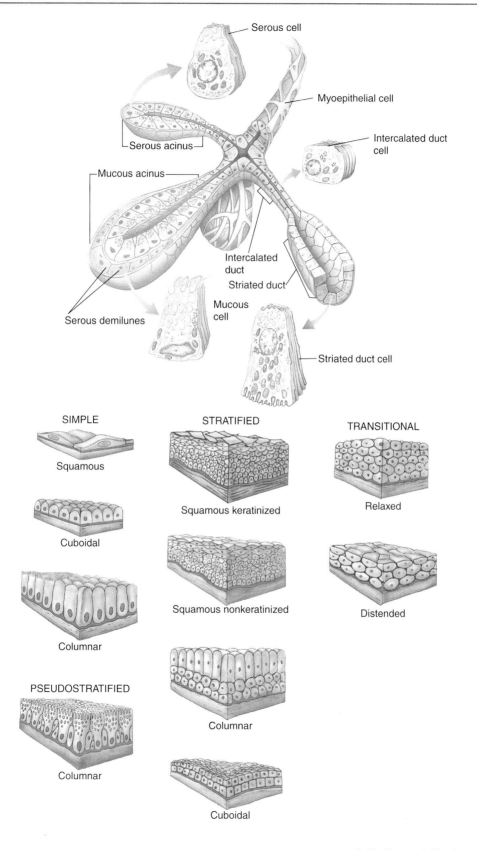

Serous cell

Myoepithelial cell

Serous acinus

Intercalated duct cell

Mucous acinus

Intercalated duct

Striated duct

Serous demilunes

Mucous cell

Striated duct cell

SIMPLE

Squamous

Cuboidal

Columnar

PSEUDOSTRATIFIED

Columnar

STRATIFIED

Squamous keratinized

Squamous nonkeratinized

Columnar

Cuboidal

TRANSITIONAL

Relaxed

Distended

PLATE 2-1 ■ *Simple Epithelia and Pseudostratified Epithelium*

FIGURE 1 ■ *Simple squamous epithelium. Kidney. Monkey. Plastic section.* × 540.

The lining of the **lumen** (L) of this small arteriole is composed of a **simple squamous epithelium** (SE) (known as the endothelium). The cytoplasm of these cells is highly attenuated and can only be approximated in this photomicrograph as a thin line (between the arrowheads). The boundaries of two contiguous epithelial cells cannot be determined with the light microscope. The **nuclei** (N) of the squamous epithelial cells bulge into the lumen, characteristic of this type of epithelium. Note that some of the nuclei appear more flattened than others. This is due to the degree of agonal contraction of the **smooth muscle** (M) cells of the vessel wall.

FIGURE 2 ■ *Simple squamous and simple cuboidal epithelia. x.s. Kidney. Paraffin section.* × 270.

The medulla of the kidney provides ideal representatives of simple squamous and simple cuboidal epithelia. Simple squamous epithelium, as in the previous figure, is easily recognizable due to flattened, but somewhat bulging, **nuclei** (N). Note that the cytoplasm of these cells appears as thin, dark lines (between arrowheads); however, it must be stressed that the dark lines are composed of not only attenuated cells but also the surrounding basal membranes. The **simple cuboidal epithelium** (CE) is very obvious. The lateral cell membranes (arrow) are clearly evident in some areas; even when they cannot be seen, the relationships of the round nuclei permit an imaginary approximation of the extent of each cell. Note that simple cuboidal cells, in section, appear more or less like small squares with centrally positioned nuclei.

FIGURE 3 ■ *Simple columnar epithelium. Monkey. Plastic section.* × 540.

The simple columnar epithelium of the duodenum in this photomicrograph displays a very extensive **brush border** (MV) on the apical aspect of the cells. The **terminal web** (TW), where microvilli are anchored, appears as a dense line between the brush border and the apical cytoplasm. Distinct dots (arrowheads) are evident, which, although they appear to be part of the terminal web, are actually terminal bars, resolved by the electron microscope to be junctional complexes between contiguous cells. Note that the cells are tall and slender, and their **nuclei** (N), more or less oval in shape, are arranged rather uniformly at the same level in each cell. The basal aspects of these cells lie on a basal membrane (arrows), separating the epithelium from the **connective tissue** (CT). The round **nuclei** (rN) noted within the epithelium actually belong to leucocytes migrating into the **lumen** (L) of the duodenum. A few **goblet cells** (GC) are also evident.

FIGURE 4 ■ *Pseudostratified columnar epithelium with cilia. Paraffin section.* × 270.

The first impression conveyed by this epithelium from the nasal cavity is that it is stratified, being composed of at least four layers of cells; however, careful observation of the *inset* (× 540) demonstrates that these are closely packed cells of varying heights and girth, each of which is in contact with the basal membrane. Here, unlike in the previous photomicrograph, the **nuclei** (N) are not uniformly arranged, and they occupy about three-fourths of the epithelial layer. The location and morphology of the nuclei provide an indication of the cell type. The short **basal cells** (BC) display small, round-to-oval nuclei near the basal membrane. The tall, ciliated cells (arrows) possess large, oval nuclei. The **terminal web** (TW) supports tall, slender **cilia** (C), which propel mucus along the epithelial surface. The connective tissue is highly vascularized and presents good examples of simple squamous epithelia (arrowheads) that compose the endothelial lining of **blood** (BV) and **lymph vessels** (LV).

PSEUDOSTRATIFIED

SIMPLE

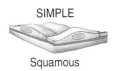
Squamous

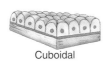
Cuboidal

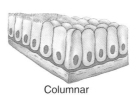
Columnar

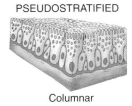
Columnar

■ **KEY**

BC	basal cell	GC	goblet cell	N	nucleus
BV	blood vessel	L	lumen	rN	round nucleus
C	cilia	LV	lymph vessel	SE	simple squamous epithelium
CE	simple cuboidal epithelium	M	smooth muscle		
CT	connective tissue	MV	brush border	TW	terminal web

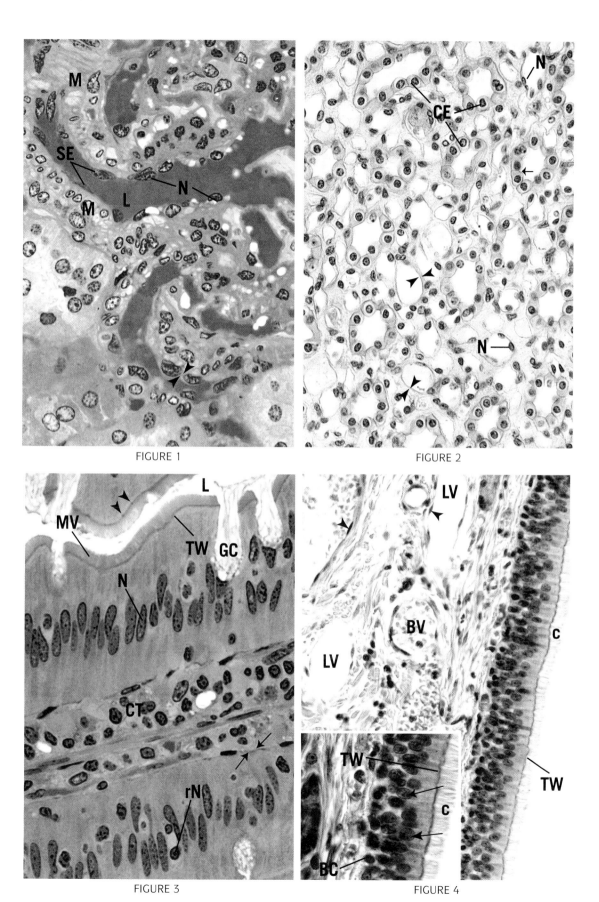

FIGURE 1

FIGURE 2

FIGURE 3

FIGURE 4

Epithelium and Glands ■ 33

PLATE 2-2 ■ *Stratified Epithelia and Transitional Epithelium*

FIGURE 1 ■ *Stratified cuboidal epithelium. Skin. Monkey. Plastic section.* × 540.

Stratified cuboidal epithelium is characterized by two or more layers of cuboid-shaped cells, as illustrated in this photomicrograph of a sweat gland duct. The **lumen** (L) of the duct is surrounded by cells whose cell boundaries are not readily evident, but the layering of the **nuclei** (N) demonstrates that this epithelium is truly stratified. The epithelium of the duct is surrounded by a **basal membrane** (BM). The other thick tubular profiles are tangential sections of the **secretory** (s) portions of the sweat gland, composed of simple cuboidal epithelium. Note the presence of a **capillary** (Cp) containing a single red blood cell, and the bulging nucleus (arrow) of the epithelial cell constituting the endothelial lining. The large empty space in the lower right-hand corner of this photomicrograph represents the lumen of a **lymph vessel** (LV) whose endothelial lining presents a flattened nucleus bulging into the lumen. Note that more cytoplasm is evident near the pole of the nucleus (arrowhead) than elsewhere.

FIGURE 2 ■ *Stratified squamous nonkeratinized epithelium. Plastic section.* × 270.

The lining of the esophagus provides a good example of stratified squamous nonkeratinized epithelium. The lack of vascularity of the epithelium, which is approximately 30–35 cell layers thick, is clearly evident. Nourishment must reach the more superficial cells via diffusion from blood vessels of the **connective tissue** (CT). Note that the deepest cells, which lie on the basal membrane and are known as the **basal layer** (BL), are actually cuboidal in shape. Due to their mitotic activity, they give rise to the cells of the epithelium, which, as they migrate toward the surface, become increasingly flattened. By the time they reach the surface, to be sloughed off into the **esophageal lumen** (EL), they are squamous in morphology. The endothelial lining of a vessel is shown as scattered **nuclei** (N) bulging into the **lumen** (L), providing an obvious contrast between stratified and simple squamous epithelia.

FIGURE 3 ■ *Stratified squamous keratinized epithelium. Skin. Paraffin section.* × 132.

The palm of the hand is covered by a thick stratified squamous keratinized epithelium. The definite difference between this and the preceding photomicrograph is the thick layer of nonliving **keratin** (K), which functions in protecting the deeper living cells and tissues from abrasion, desiccation, and invasion by bacterial flora. Although the various layers of this epithelium will be examined in greater detail in Chapter 11, certain features need to be examined here. Note that the interdigitation between the connective tissue **dermal ridges** (P) and the **epithelial ridges** (R) provides a larger surface area for adhesion and providing nutrients than would be offered by a merely flat interface. The **basal membrane** (BM) is a very definite interval between the epithelium and the connective tissue. The basal layer of this epithelium, composed of cuboidal cells, is known as the stratum germinativum, which possesses a high mitotic activity. Cells originating here press toward the surface, and, while on their way, change their morphology, manufacture proteins, and acquire different names. Note the **duct** (D) of a sweat gland piercing the base of an epidermal ridge as it continues toward the outside (arrows).

FIGURE 4 ■ *Transitional epithelium. Bladder. Monkey. Plastic section.* × 132.

The urinary bladder, as most of the excretory portion of the urinary tract, is lined by a specialized type of stratified epithelium—the transitional epithelium. This particular specimen was taken from an empty, relaxed bladder, as indicated by the large, **round**, dome-**shaped** (rC) **cells,** some of which are occasionally binucleated (arrow), abutting the **lumen** (L). The epithelial cells lying on the **basal membrane** (BM) are quite small, but increase in size as they migrate superficially and begin to acquire a pear shape. When the bladder is distended, the thickness of the epithelium decreases and the cells become flattened, more squamous-like. The connective tissue–epithelium interface is flat with very little interdigitation between them. The **connective tissue** (CT) is very vascular immediately deep to the epithelium, as is evident from the sections of the **arterioles** (A) and **venules** (V) in this field. Observe the simple squamous endothelial linings of these vessels, characterized by their bulging nuclei (arrowheads).

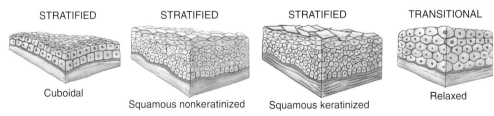

STRATIFIED   STRATIFIED   STRATIFIED   TRANSITIONAL

Cuboidal   Squamous nonkeratinized   Squamous keratinized   Relaxed

■ **KEY**

A	arteriole	EL	esophageal lumen	P	dermal ridge
BL	basal layer	K	keratin	R	epithelial ridge
BM	basal membrane	L	lumen	rC	round-shaped cell
Cp	capillary	LV	lymph vessel	s	secretory portion
CT	connective tissue	N	nucleus	V	venule
D	duct				

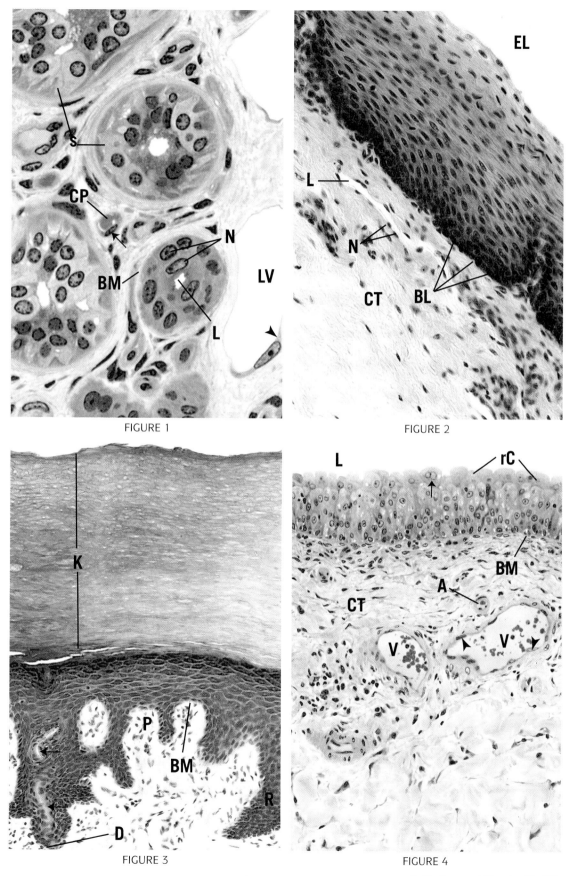

FIGURE 1

FIGURE 2

FIGURE 3

FIGURE 4

FIGURE 1 ■ *Pseudostratified ciliated columnar epithelium. Hamster trachea. Electron microscopy.* × 6480.

The pseudostratified ciliated columnar epithelium of the trachea is composed of several types of cells, some of which are presented here. Since this is an oblique section through the epithelium, it is not readily evident here that all of these cells touch the **basal lamina** (BL). Note that the pale-staining **ciliated cells** (CC) display **rough endoplasmic reticulum** (rER), **mitochondria** (M), **Golgi apparatus** (G), as well as numerous **cilia** (C) interspersed with **microvilli** (MV). Each cilium, some of which are seen in cross-section, displays its plasma membrane and its **axoneme** (A). The cilia are anchored in the terminal web via their **basal bodies** (BB). The mitochondria appear to be concentrated in this area of the cell. The second cell types to be noted are the **mucous cells** (MC), also known as goblet cells. These cells produce a thick, viscous

secretion, which appears as **secretory granules** (SG) within the apical cytoplasm. The protein moiety of the secretion is synthesized on the **rough endoplasmic reticulum** (rER), while most of the carbohydrate groups are added to the protein in the **Golgi apparatus** (G). The mucous cells are nonciliated but do present short, stubby **microvilli** (MV) on their apical surface. When these cells release their secretory product, they change their morphology. They no longer contain secretory granules, and their microvilli become elongated and are known as brush cells. They may be recognized by the filamentous structures within the supranuclear cytoplasm. The lower right-hand corner of this electron micrograph presents a portion of a **capillary** (Ca) containing a **red blood cell** (RBC). Observe that the highly attenuated **endothelial cell** (EC) is outside of but very close to the **basal lamina** (BL) of the tracheal epithelium. (Courtesy of Dr. E. McDowell.)

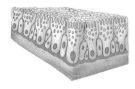

Pseudostratified columnar epithelium

■ **KEY**

A	axoneme	CC	ciliated cell	MV	microvillus
BB	basal body	EC	endothelial cell	RBC	red blood cell
BL	basal lamina	G	Golgi apparatus	rER	rough endoplasmic reticulum
C	cilium	M	mitochondrion		
Ca	capillary	MC	mucous cell	SG	secretory granule

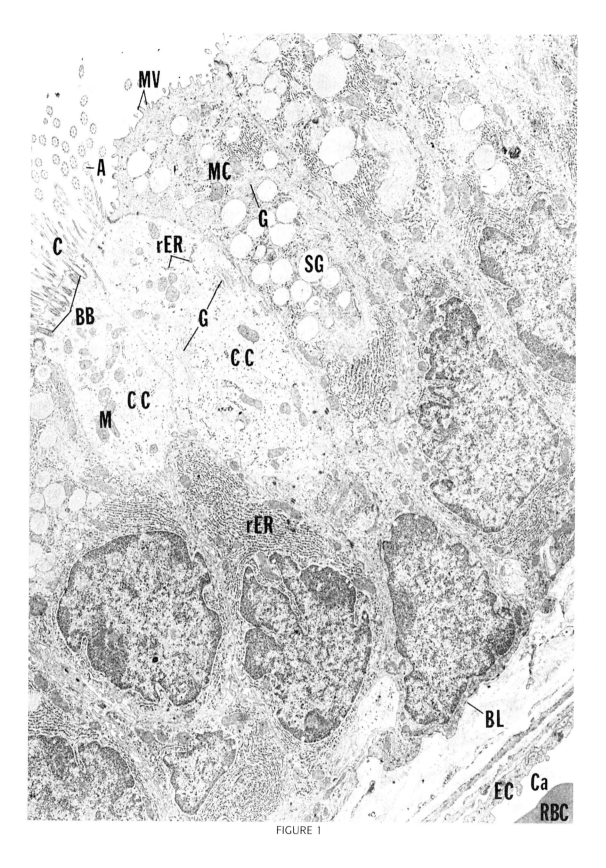

FIGURE 1

PLATE 2-4 ■ *Epithelial Junctions, Electron Microscopy*

FIGURE 1 ■ *Epithelial junction. Human. Electron microscopy.* × 27,815.

This electron micrograph represents a thin section of an intercellular canaliculus between clear cells of a human eccrine sweat gland stained with ferrocyanide-reduced osmium tetroxide. A tight junction (arrows) separates the lumen of the **intercellular canaliculus** (IC) from the basolateral intercellular space. Observe the **nucleus** (N). (From Briggman J, Bank H, Bigelow J, Graves J, Spicer S: *Am J Anat* 162:357–368, 1981.)

FIGURE 2 ■ *Epithelial junction. Zonula occludens. Human. Electron microscopy.* × 83,700.

This is a freeze-fracture replica of an elaborate tight junction along an intercellular canaliculus between two clear cells. Note the smooth transition from a region of wavy, nonintersecting, densely packed junctional elements to an area of complex anastomoses. At the step fracture (arrows), it can be seen that the pattern of ridges on the E face corresponds to that of the grooves on the P face of the plasma membrane of the adjacent clear cell. In certain areas (arrowheads), several of the laterally disposed, densely packed junctional elements are separated from the luminal band. The direction of platinum shadowing is indicated by the circled arrow. (From Briggman J, Bank H, Bigelow J, Graves J, Spicer S: *Am J Anat* 162: 357–368, 1981.)

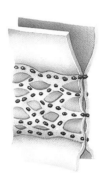

Zonulae occludentes

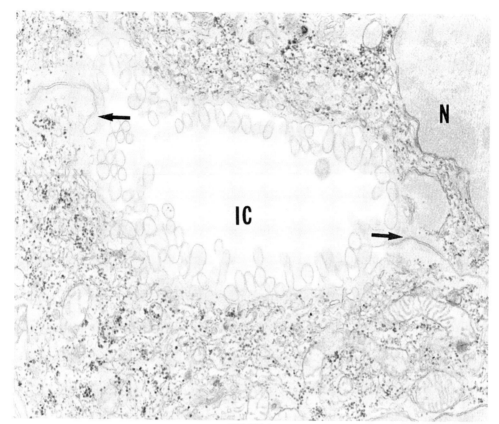

FIGURE 1

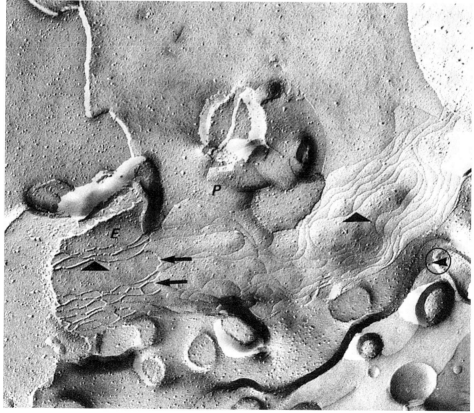

FIGURE 2

PLATE 2-5 ■ *Glands*

FIGURE 1 ■ *Goblet cells. Ileum. Monkey. Plastic section.* × 270.

Goblet cells are unicellular exocrine glands that are found interspersed among simple columnar and pseudostratified columnar epithelia. This photomicrograph of an ileal villus displays numerous **goblet cells** (GC) located among the **simple columnar epithelial cells** (EC). The brush border (arrowhead) of the columnar cells is only scantly present on the goblet cells. The expanded apical region of the goblet cell is known as the **theca** (T) and is filled with **mucin** (m), which, when released into the lumen of the gut, coats and protects the intestinal lining. The lower right-hand corner of the simple columnar epithelium was sectioned somewhat obliquely through the nuclei of the epithelial cells, producing the appearance of a stratified epithelium (asterisk). Looking at the epithelium above the double arrows, however, it is clearly simple columnar. The occasional **round nuclei** (rN) are those of lymphocytes migrating through the epithelium into the **lumen** (L). Figure 2 is a higher magnification of the boxed area.

FIGURE 2 ■ *Goblet cells. Ileum. Monkey. Plastic section.* × 540.

This photomicrograph is a higher magnification of the boxed area of the previous figure, demonstrating the light microscopic morphology of the goblet cell. The **mucin** (m) in the expanded **theca** (T) of the goblet cell has been partly precipitated and dissolved during the dehydration procedure. The **nucleus** (N) of the goblet cell is relatively dense due to the condensed chromatin. Between the nucleus and the theca is the **Golgi zone** (GZ), where the protein product of the cell is modified and packaged into secretory granules for delivery. The **base** (b) of the goblet cell is slender, almost as if it were "squeezed in" between neighboring columnar epithelial cells, but it touches the **basal membrane** (BM). The terminal web and brush border of the goblet cell are greatly reduced, but not completely absent (arrowheads). The **round nuclei** (rN) belong to leucocytes migrating through the epithelium into the **lumen** (L) of the ileum.

FIGURE 3 ■ *Sebaceous gland. Scalp. Paraffin section.* × 132.

Sebaceous glands are usually associated with hair follicles. They discharge their sebum into the follicle, although in certain areas of the body they are present independent of hair follicles. These glands, surrounded by slender connective tissue **capsules** (Ca), are pear-shaped saccules with short ducts. Each saccule is filled with large, amorphous cells with nuclei in various states of degeneration (arrows). The periphery of the saccule is composed of small, cuboidal **basal cells** (BC), which act in a regenerative capacity. As the cells move away from the periphery of the saccule, they enlarge and increase their cytoplasmic **fat** (f) content. Near the duct, the entire cell degenerates and becomes the **secretion** (se). Therefore, sebaceous glands are classified as simple, branched, acinar glands with a holocrine mode of secretion. **Smooth muscles** (M), arrector pili, are associated with sebaceous glands. Observe the **secretory** (s) and **duct** (D) portions of a sweat gland above the sebaceous gland.

FIGURE 4 ■ *Eccrine sweat glands. Skin. Paraffin section.* × 270.

Eccrine sweat glands are the most numerous glands in the body, and they are extensively distributed. The glands are simple, unbranched, coiled tubular, producing a watery solution. The **secretory portion** (s) of the gland is composed of a simple cuboidal type of epithelium with two cell types, a lightly staining cell that makes up most of the secretory portion, and a darker staining cell that usually cannot be distinguished with the light microscope. Surrounding the secretory portion are **myoepithelial cells** (MC) that, with their numerous branching processes, encircle the secretory tubule and assist in expressing the fluid into the ducts. The **ducts** (D) of sweat glands are composed of a stratified cuboidal type of epithelium, whose cells are smaller than those of the secretory unit. In histologic sections, therefore, the ducts are always darker than the secretory units. The large, empty-looking spaces are **adipose** (fat) **cells** (AC). Note the numerous small blood vessels (arrows) in the vicinity of the sweat gland.

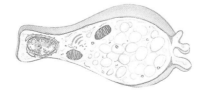

Goblet cell

■ **KEY**

AC	adipose cell	f	fat	MC	myoepithelial cell
b	base	GC	goblet cell	N	nucleus
BC	basal cell	GZ	Golgi zone	rN	round nucleus
BM	basal membrane	L	lumen	s	secretory
Ca	capsule	M	smooth muscle	se	secretion
D	duct	m	mucin	T	theca
EC	simple columnar epithelial cell				

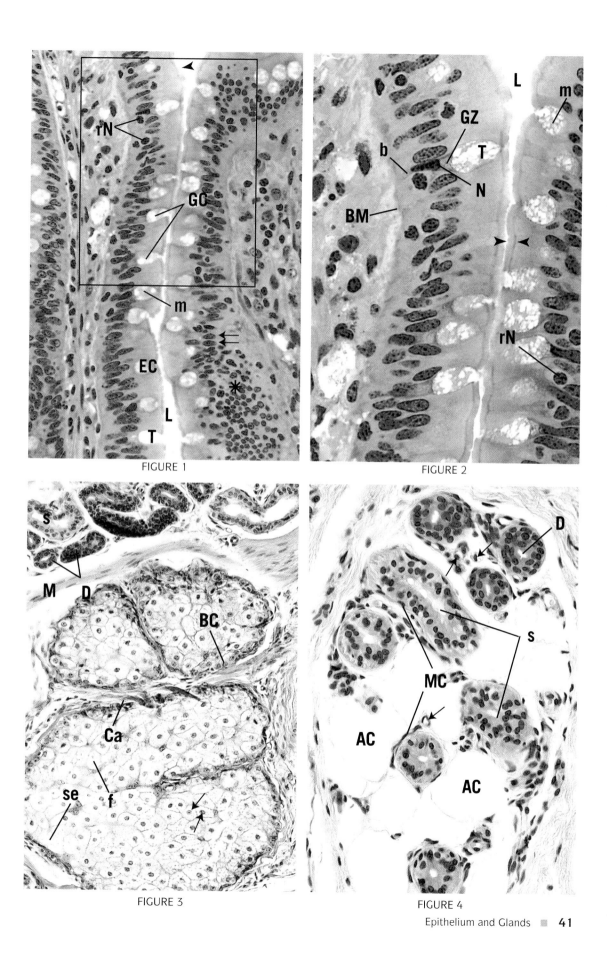

FIGURE 1

FIGURE 2

FIGURE 3

FIGURE 4

PLATE 2-6 ■ *Glands*

FIGURE 1 ■ *Compound tubuloacinar (alveolar) serous gland. Pancreas. Monkey. Plastic section.* × 540.

This is a photomicrograph of the exocrine portion of the pancreas, a compound tubuloacinar (alveolar) serous gland. The duct system of this gland will be studied in Chapter 15 on the Digestive System. Only its secretory cells will be considered at this point. Each acinus, when sectioned well, presents a round appearance with a small central **lumen** (L), with the secretory cells arranged like a pie cut into pieces. The **connective tissue** (CT) investing each acinus is flimsy in the pancreas. The secretory cells are more or less trapezoid-shaped, with a round, basally situated **nucleus** (N). The cytoplasm contains numerous **zymogen granules** (ZG), which are the membrane-bound digestive enzymes packaged by the Golgi apparatus.

FIGURE 2 ■ *Compound tubuloacinar (alveolar) mucous glands. Soft palate. Paraffin section.* × 132.

The compound tubuloacinar glands of the palate are purely mucous and secrete a thick, viscous fluid. The secretory acini of this gland are circular in section and are surrounded by fine **connective tissue** (CT) elements. The **lumina** (L) of the mucous acini are clearly distinguishable, as are the trapezoid-shaped **parenchymal cells** (PC), which manufacture the viscous fluid. The **nuclei** (N) of the trapezoid-shaped cells are dark, dense structures that appear to be flattened against the basal cell membrane. The cytoplasm has an empty, frothy appearance, which stains a light grayish-blue with hematoxylin and eosin.

FIGURE 3 ■ *Compound tubuloacinar (alveolar) mixed gland. Sublingual gland. Monkey. Plastic section.* × 540.

The sublingual gland is a mostly mucous, compound tubuloacinar gland that contains many mucous tubules and acini. These profiles of mucous acini are well represented in this photomicrograph. Note the open **lumen** (L) bordered by several trapezoid-shaped cells whose lateral plasma membranes are clearly evident (double arrows). The **nuclei** (N) of these mucous cells appear to be flattened against the basal plasma membrane and are easily distinguishable from the round nuclei of the cells of serous acini. The cytoplasm appears to possess numerous vacuole-like structures that impart a frothy appearance to the cell. The serous secretions of this gland are derived from the few serous cells that appear to cap the mucous units, known as **serous demilunes** (SD). The secretory products of the serous demilunes gain entrance to the lumen of the secretory unit via small intercellular spaces between neighboring mucous cells.

FIGURE 4 ■ *Compound tubuloacinar (alveolar) mixed gland. Submandibular gland. Monkey. Plastic section.* × 540.

The submandibular gland is a compound tubuloacinar gland that produces a mixed secretion, as does the sublingual gland of the previous figure. However, this gland contains many purely **serous acini** (SA) and very few purely **mucous** ones, namely because the mucous acini are capped by **serous demilunes** (SD). Also this gland possesses an extensive system of **ducts** (D). Note that the cytoplasm of the serous cells appears to be blue when stained with hematoxylin and eosin. Also notice that the lumina of the acini are so small that they are not apparent, while those of mucous units (L) are quite obvious. Observe the difference in the cytoplasms of serous and mucus-secreting cells, as well as the density of the nuclei of individual cells. Finally, note that the lateral cell membranes (arrows) of mucus-producing cells are clearly delineated, while those of the serous cells are very difficult to observe.

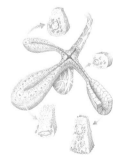

Salivary gland

■ **KEY**

CT	connective tissue	N	nucleus	SD	serous demilunes
D	duct	PC	parenchymal cell	ZG	zymogen granules
L	lumen	SA	serous acini		

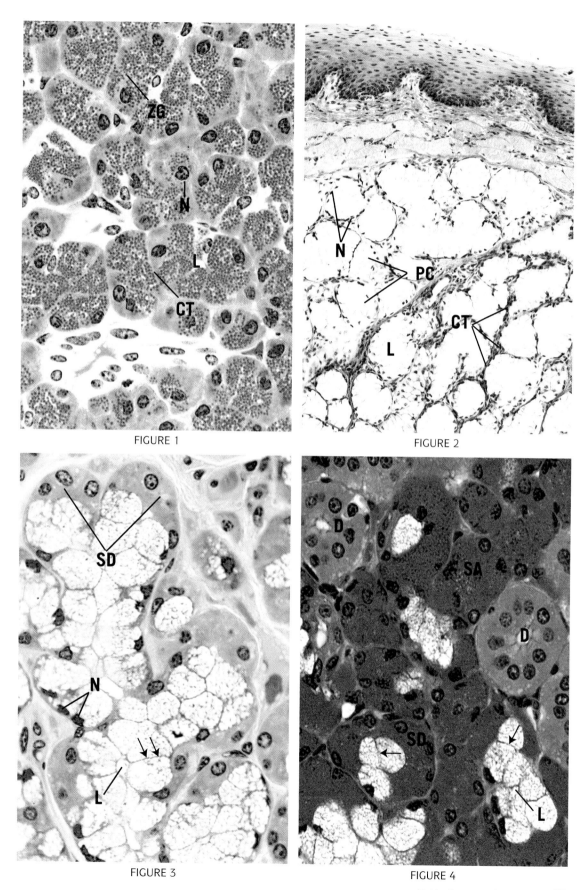

FIGURE 1

FIGURE 2

FIGURE 3

FIGURE 4

Connective Tissue

Connective tissues encompass the major structural constituents of the body. Although seemingly diverse, structurally and functionally they possess many shared qualities; therefore, they are considered in a single category. Most connective tissues are derived from mesoderm, which form the multipotential mesenchyme from which bone, cartilage, tendons, ligaments, capsules, blood and hematopoietic cells, and lymphoid cells develop. Functionally, connective tissues serve in support, defense, transport, storage, and repair, among others. Connective tissues, unlike epithelia, are composed mainly of **intercellular elements** with a limited number of **cells.** They are classified mostly on the basis of their nonliving components rather than on their cellular constituents. Although the precise ordering of the various subtypes differs from author to author, the following categories are generally accepted:

A. Embryonic connective tissues
  1. Mesenchymal
  2. Mucous
B. Adult connective tissues
  1. Connective tissue proper
    a. Loose (areolar)
    b. Reticular
    c. Adipose
    d. Dense irregular
    e. Dense regular
      (1) Collagenous
      (2) Elastic
  2. Specialized connective tissues
    a. Supporting tissues
      (1) Cartilage
      (2) Bone
    b. Blood

EXTRACELLULAR MATRIX

The extracellular matrix of connective tissue proper may be subdivided into **fibers, amorphous ground substance,** and **tissue fluid.**

Three types of fibers are recognized histologically: collagen, reticular, and elastic. **Collagen** fibers usually occur as bundles of nonelastic fibers of varied thickness whose basic subunits, **tropocollagen molecules,** aggregate into specific staggered associations, producing a 67-nm banding once believed to be characteristic of this protein (see Graphic 3-1). Some collagen types, however, such as type IV collagen that is present in basal laminae, do not exhibit this banding characteristic. **Reticular fibers** (once believed to have different composition) are thin, branching, carbohydrate-coated fibers composed of type III collagen that form delicate networks around smooth muscle cells, certain epithelial cells, adipocytes, nerve fibers, and blood vessels. They also constitute the structural framework of certain organs, such as the liver and the spleen. **Elastic fibers** are, as their name implies, highly elastic and may be stretched to about 150% of their resting length without breaking. They are composed of an amorphous protein, **elastin,** surrounded by a **microfibrillar** component. Elastic fibers do not display a periodicity and are found in regions of the body that require considerable flexibility and elasticity.

The **amorphous ground substance** constitutes the gel-like matrix in which the fibers and cells are embedded and through which tissue fluid diffuses. Ground substance is composed of glycosaminoglycans (GAGs), proteoglycans, and glycoproteins. The major GAGs constituents are **hyaluronic acid, chondroitin 4-sulfate, chondroitin 6-sulfate, dermatan sulfate,** and **heparan sulfate. Proteoglycans** are composed of a protein core to which GAGs are covalently bound. **Glycoproteins** have also been localized in connective tissue proper. These substances, especially **fibronectin,** appear to be essential in facilitating the attachment and migration of cells along connective tissue elements, such as collagen fibers.

An additional extracellular region, the **basal lamina (or basement lamina),** is characteristically interposed between epithelia and connective tissues.

Electron microscopy has elucidated this structure, which is composed of a **lamina lucida** and a **lamina densa.** The former is a thin electron-lucent layer directly between the lamina densa and the cell membrane. The major constituents of the basal lamina, **laminin, entactin,** and **type IV collagen,** are epithelially derived, although other components, **fibronectin** and **perlacan,** are probably of connective tissue origin. The basal lamina is frequently associated with a **lamina reticularis,** a reticular fiber network from the underlying connective tissue to which the basal lamina is anchored mostly by fibronectin, type VII collagen, and microfibrils. Together, the basal lamina and lamina reticularis constitute the **basement membrane** of light microscopy.

CELLS

The following are cells of connective tissue proper—or more accurately, loose (areolar) connective tissue (see Graphic 3-2).

Fibroblasts, the predominant cell type, are responsible for the **synthesis** of collagen, elastic and reticular fibers, and much, if not all, of the ground substance. The morphology of these cells appears to be a function of their synthetic activities, and therefore, resting (or inactive fibroblasts) cells were often referred to as fibrocytes, a term that is rapidly disappearing from the literature.

Macrophages (histiocytes) are derived from monocytes in bone marrow. They migrate to the connective tissue and function in ingesting (**phagocytosing**) foreign particulate matter. These cells also participate in enhancing the immunologic activities of lymphocytes.

Plasma cells are the major cell type present during **chronic inflammation.** These cells are derived from a subpopulation of lymphocytes and are responsible for the synthesis and release of humoral antibodies.

Mast cells are usually observed in the vicinity of small blood vessels, although the relationship between them is not understood. These cells house numerous metachromatic granules containing histamine, which is a smooth muscle contractant, and heparin, which is an anticoagulant. Mast cells also release **eosinophilic chemotactic agent** and **leukotriene.** Because of the presence of immunoglobulins on the external surface of the mast cell plasmalemma, these cells, in sensitized individuals, may become degranulated (i.e., release their granules), resulting in **anaphylactic reactions** or even in life-threatening anaphylactic shock.

Pericytes are also associated with minute blood vessels, but much more closely than are mast cells, since they share the basal laminae of the endothelial cells. Pericytes are believed to be **contractile cells** that assist in the regulation of blood flow through the capillaries. Additionally, they may also be **pluripotential cells,** which assume the responsibilities of mesenchymal cells in adult connective tissue. It is now believed that mesenchymal cells are probably not present in the adult.

Fat cells (adipocytes) may form small clusters or aggregates in loose connective tissue. They **store lipids** and form adipose tissue, which protects, insulates, and cushions organs of the body.

Leukocytes (white blood cells) leave the bloodstream and enter the connective tissue spaces. Here they assume various functions, which are discussed in Chapter 5.

CONNECTIVE TISSUE TYPES

Mesenchymal and **mucous connective tissues** are limited to the embryo. The former consists of mesenchymal cells and fine reticular fibers interspersed in a semifluid matrix of ground substance. Mucous connective tissue is more viscous in consistency, contains collagen bundles and numerous fibroblasts, and is found deep to the fetal skin and in the umbilical cord (where it is known as Wharton's jelly), surrounding the umbilical vessels.

Loose (areolar) connective tissue is distributed widely, since it constitutes much of the superficial fascia and invests neurovascular bundles. The cells and intercellular elements described above help form this more or less amorphous, watery tissue.

Reticular connective tissue forms a network of thin reticular fibers that constitute the structural framework of bone marrow and many lymphoid structures, as well as a framework enveloping certain cells.

Adipose tissue is composed of fat cells, reticular fibers, and a rich vascular supply. It acts as a depot for fat, a thermal insulator, and a shock absorber.

Dense irregular connective tissue consists of coarse, almost haphazardly arranged bundles of collagen fibers interlaced with few elastic and reticular fibers. The chief cellular constituents are fibroblasts, macrophages, and occasional mast cells. The dermis of the skin and capsules of some organs are composed of dense irregular connective tissue.

Dense regular connective tissue may be composed either of thick, parallel arrays of collagenous fibers, as in tendons and ligaments, or of parallel bundles of elastic fibers, as in the ligamentum nuchae, the ligamentum flava, and the suspensory ligament of the penis. The cellular constituents of both dense regular collagenous and elastic connective tissues are almost strictly limited to fibroblasts.

Histophysiology

I. EXTRACELLULAR MATRIX

A. Ground Substance

Ground substance is composed of GAGs, proteoglycans, and glycoproteins. **Glycosaminoglycans (GAGs)** are linear polymers of repeating disaccharides, one of which is always a **hexosamine**, while the other is a **hexuronic acid.** All of the GAGs, with the exception of **hyaluronic acid,** are sulfated and, thus, possess a predominantly **negative charge.**

Most GAGs are linked to protein cores, forming huge **proteoglycan** molecules. Many of these proteoglycan molecules are also linked to hyaluronic acid, forming massive molecules of enormous electrochemical **domains** that attract osmotically active cations (e.g., Na^+), forming hydrated molecules that resist compression. The sulfated GAGs include chondroitin sulfate, dermatan sulfate, heparan sulfate, heparin, and keratan sulfate.

Glycoproteins are large polypeptide molecules with attendant carbohydrate side chains. The best characterized are laminin, fibronectin, chondronectin, osteonectin, entactin, and tenascin. Laminin and entactin are derived from epithelial cells, and tenascin is made by glial cells of the embryo, whereas the remainder are manufactured by cells of connective tissue. Many cells possess **integrins,** transmembrane proteins, with receptor sites for one or more of these glycoproteins. Moreover, glycoproteins also bind to collagen, thus facilitating cell adherence to the extracellular matrix.

B. Fibers

1. Collagen

Collagen, the most abundant of the fibers, is inelastic and is composed of a staggered array of the protein **tropocollagen,** composed of three α chains. There are at least twelve different types of collagen, based on the amino acid sequence of their α chains. Interestingly, every third amino acid is **glycine,** and a significant amount of **proline, hydroxyproline, lysine,** and **hydroxylysine** constitute much of the tropocollagen subunit.

The most common collagens are type I (dermis, bone, capsules of organs, fibrocartilage, dentin, cementum), type II (hyaline and elastic cartilages), type III (reticular fibers), type IV (lamina densa of the basal lamina), type V (placenta), and type VII (anchoring fibrils of the basal lamina). With the exception of type IV, all collagen fibers display a **67-nm periodicity** as the result of the specific arrangement of the tropocollagen molecules.

a. Collagen Synthesis

Synthesis of collagen occurs on the rough endoplasmic reticulum, where polysomes possess different mRNAs coding for the three α chains (**preprocollagens**). Within the rough endoplasmic reticulum (RER) cisternae, specific proline and lysine residues are **hydroxylated,** and hydroxylysine residues are **glycosylated.** Each α chain possesses **propeptides (telopeptides)** located at both amino and carboxyl ends. These propeptides are responsible for the precise **alignment** of the α chains, resulting in the formation of the **triple helical procollagen** molecule.

Coatomer-coated transfer vesicles convey the procollagen molecules to the **Golgi apparatus** for modification, mostly the addition of carbohydrate side chains. Subsequent to transfer to the **trans-Golgi network,** the **procollagen** molecule is exocytosed (via non–clathrin-coated vesicles), and the propeptides are cleaved by the enzyme **procollagen peptidase,** resulting in the formation of tropocollagen.

Tropocollagen molecules self-assemble, forming fibrils with 67-nm characteristic banding. Type IV collagen is composed of procollagen rather than tropocollagen subunits, hence the absence of periodicity and fibril formation in this type of collagen.

b. Reticular Fibers

Reticular fibers (type III collagen) are thinner than type I collagen and possess a higher content of carbohydrate moieties than do the remaining collagen types. As a result, when stained with silver stain, the silver preferentially deposits on these fibers giving them a brown to black appearance in the light microscope.

2. Elastic Fibers

Elastic fibers may be stretched up to 150% of their resting length before breaking. They are composed of **microfibrils** (whose chief constituent is fibrillin) and the protein **elastin,** where the latter has **desmosine** and **isodesmosine,** that are responsible for this fiber's elasticity. Individual elastin molecules are cross-linked via their lysine residues, forming sizable networks of molecules.

C. Extracellular Fluid

Extracellular fluid (tissue fluid) is the fluid component of blood, similar to plasma, that percolates throughout the ground substance, carrying nutrients, oxygen, and other blood-borne materials to and carbon dioxide and waste products from cells. Extracellular fluid leaves the vascular supply at the arterial end of the capillaries and returns into the circulatory system at the venous end of capillaries, the venules, and the excess fluid enters lymphatic capillaries.

II. ADIPOSE TISSUE

There are two types of adipose tissue, white (unilocular) and brown (multilocular).

A. Unilocular Adipose Tissue

Cells of **unilocular adipose tissue** store triglycerides in a single, large fat droplet that occupies most of the cell. Fat cells of adipose tissue make the enzyme **lipoprotein lipase,** which is transported to the luminal surface of the capillary endothelial cell membrane, where it hydrolyzes chylomicrons and very low density lipoproteins. The fatty acids and monoglycerides are transported to the adipocytes, diffuse into their cytoplasm, and are reesterified into triglycerides. **Hormone-sensitive lipase,** activated by cAMP, hydrolyzes the stored lipids into fatty acids and glycerol, which are released from the cell as the need arises, to enter the capillaries for distribution to the remainder of the body.

B. Multilocular Adipose Tissue

Multilocular adipose cells are rare in the adult human. They are present in the neonate, as well as in animals that hibernate. These cells possess numerous droplets of lipid in their cytoplasm and a rich supply of mitochondria. These mitochondria are capable of uncoupling oxidation from phosphorylation, and instead of producing ATP, they release heat, thus arousing the animal from hibernation.

Clinical Considerations ▪ ▪ ▪

Keloid Formation
Surgical wounds are repaired by the body first with weak type III collagen that is later replaced by type I collagen, which is much stronger. Some individuals, especially blacks, form an overabundance of collagen in the healing process, thus developing elevated scars called keloids.

Scurvy
Scurvy, a condition characterized by bleeding gums and loose teeth among other symptoms, results from a vitamin C deficiency. Vitamin C is necessary for hydroxylation of proline for proper tropocollagen formation giving rise to fibrils necessary for maintaining teeth in their bony sockets.

Marfan's Syndrome
Patients with Marfan's syndrome, a genetic defect in chromosome 15 that codes for fibrillin, possess undeveloped elastic fibers in their body and are predisposed to rupture of the aorta.

Edema
The release of histamine and leukotrienes from mast cells during an inflammatory response elicits increased capillary permeability, resulting in an excess accumulation of tissue fluid and, thus, gross swelling (edema).

Obesity
There are two types of obesity—hypertrophic obesity, which occurs when adipose cells increase in size from storing fat (adult onset), and hyperplastic obesity, which is characterized by an increase in the number of adipose cells resulting from overfeeding a new-born for a few weeks after birth. This type of obesity is usually life long.

Systemic Lupus Erythematosus
Systemic lupus erythematosus is an autoimmune connective tissue disease that results in the inflammation in the connective tissue elements of certain organs as well as of tendons and joints. The symptoms depend on the type and number of antibodies present and can be anywhere from mild to severe and, due to the variety of symptoms, lupus may resemble other conditions such as growing pains, arthritis, epilepsy, and even psychologic diseases. The characteristic symptoms include facial and skin rash, sores in the oral cavity, joint pains and inflammation, kidney malfunction, neurologic conditions, anemia, thrombocytopenia, fluid on the lungs. For mild cases the usual choice of treatment is nonsteroidal anti-inflammatory drugs, whereas in severe cases initially steroids and immunosuppressants are administered.

Summary of Histological Organization

I. EMBRYONIC CONNECTIVE TISSUE

A. Mesenchymal Connective Tissue

1. Cells
Stellate to spindle-shaped **mesenchymal cells** have processes that touch one another. Pale scanty cytoplasm with large clear nuclei. Indistinct cell membrane.

2. Intercellular Materials
Delicate, empty-looking matrix, containing fine **reticular fibers.** Small blood vessels are evident.

B. Mucous Connective Tissue

1. Cells
Fibroblasts, with their numerous flattened processes and oval nuclei, constitute the major cellular component. In section, these cells frequently appear spindle-shaped, and resemble or are identical with mesenchymal cells when viewed with a light microscope.

2. Intercellular Materials
When compared with mesenchymal connective tissue, the intercellular space is filled with coarse **collagen bundles,** irregularly arranged, in a matrix of precipitated jelly-like material.

II. CONNECTIVE TISSUE PROPER

A. Loose (Areolar) Connective Tissue

1. Cells
The most common cell types are **fibroblasts,** whose spindle-shaped morphology closely resembles the next most numerous cells, the **macrophages.** The oval nuclei of macrophages are smaller, darker, and denser than those of fibroblasts. **Mast cells,** located in the vicinity of blood vessels, may be recognized by their size, the numerous small granules in their cytoplasm, and their large, round, centrally located nuclei. Occasional **fat cells** resembling round, empty spaces bordered by a thin rim of cytoplasm may also be present. When sectioned through its peripherally squeezed, flattened nucleus, a fat cell has a ring-like appearance.

Additionally, in certain regions such as the subepithelial connective tissue (lamina propria) of the intestines, plasma cells and leukocytes are commonly found. **Plasma cells** are small, round cells with round, acentric nuclei, whose chromatin network presents a clockface (cartwheel) appearance. These cells also display a clear, paranuclear Golgi zone. **Lymphocytes, neutrophils,** and occasional **eosinophils** also contribute to the cellularity of loose connective tissue.

2. Intercellular Materials
Slender bundles of long, ribbon-like bands of **collagen fibers** are intertwined by numerous thin, straight, long, branching **elastic fibers** embedded in a watery matrix of **ground substance,** most of which is extracted by dehydration procedures during preparation. **Reticular fibers,** also present, are usually not visible in sections stained with hematoxylin and eosin.

B. Reticular Connective Tissue

1. Cells
Reticular cells are found only in reticular connective tissue. They are stellate in shape and envelop the reticular fibers, which they also manufacture. They possess large, oval, pale nuclei, and their cytoplasm is not easily visible with the light microscope. The other cells in the interstitial spaces are **lymphocytes, macrophages,** and other **lymphoid cells.**

2. Intercellular Materials
Reticular fibers constitute the major portion of the intercellular matrix. With the use of a silver stain, they are evident as dark, thin, branching fibers.

C. Adipose Tissue

1. Cells
Unlike other connective tissues, adipose tissue is composed of adipose cells so closely packed together that the normal spherical morphology of these cells becomes distorted. Groups of fat cells are subdivided into lobules by thin sheaths of loose connective tissue septa housing **mast cells, endothelial cells** of blood vessels, and other components of **neurovascular elements.**

2. Intercellular Materials
Each fat cell is invested by **reticular fibers,** which, in turn, are anchored to the **collagen fibers** of the connective tissue septa.

D. Dense Irregular Connective Tissue

1. Cells

Fibroblasts, macrophages, and cells associated with neurovascular bundles constitute the chief cellular elements.

2. Intercellular Materials

Haphazardly oriented thick, wavy bundles of collagen fibers, as well as occasional elastic and reticular fibers are found in dense irregular connective tissue.

E. Dense Regular Collagenous Connective Tissue

1. Cells

Parallel rows of flattened fibroblasts are essentially the only cells found here. Even these are few in number.

2. Intercellular Materials

Parallel fibers of densely packed collagen are regularly arranged in dense regular collagenous connective tissue.

F. Dense Regular Elastic Connective Tissue

1. Cells

Parallel rows of flattened fibroblasts are usually difficult to distinguish in preparations that use stains specific for elastic fibers.

2. Intercellular Materials

Parallel bundles of thick elastic fibers, surrounded by slender elements of loose connective tissue, comprise the intercellular components of dense regular elastic connective tissue.

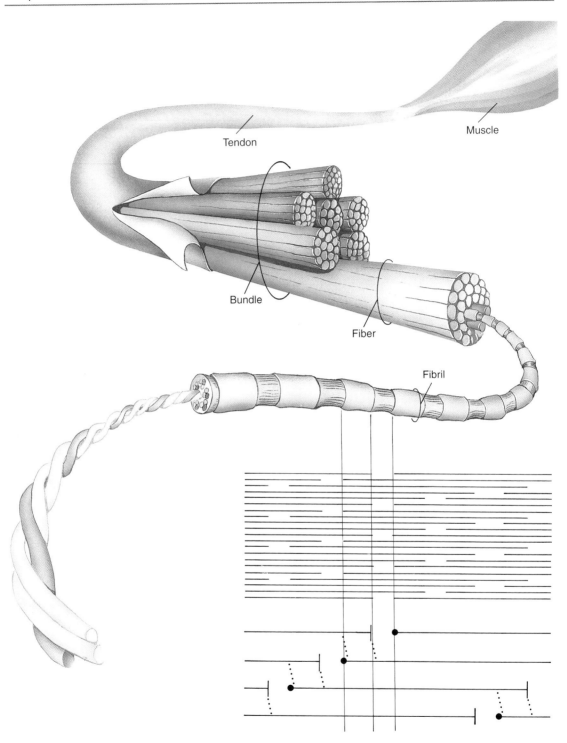

Each collagen fiber bundle is composed of smaller fibrils, which in turn consist of aggregates of **tropocollagen molecules**. Tropocollagen molecules self-assemble in the extracellular environment in such a fashion that there is a gap between the tail of the one and the head of the succeeding molecule of a single row. As fibrils are formed, tails of tropocollagen molecules overlap the heads of tropocollagen molecules in adjacent rows. Additionally, the **gaps** and **overlaps** are arranged so that they are in register with those of neighboring (but not adjacent) rows of tropocollagen molecules. When stained with a heavy metal, such as osmium, the stain preferentially precipitates in the gap regions, resulting in the repeating **light** and **dark** banding of collagen.

GRAPHIC 3-2 ■ *Connective Tissue Cells*

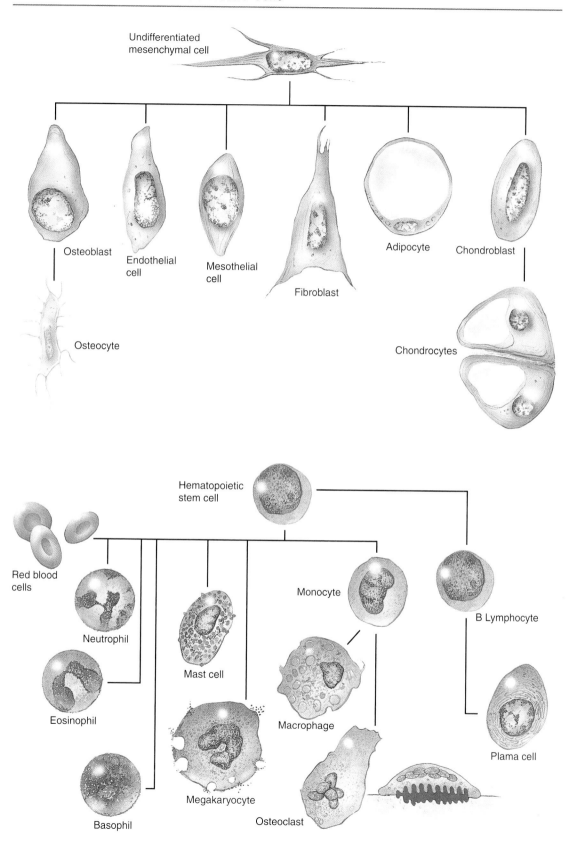

Undifferentiated mesenchymal cell

Osteoblast

Endothelial cell

Mesothelial cell

Fibroblast

Adipocyte

Chondroblast

Osteocyte

Chondrocytes

Hematopoietic stem cell

Red blood cells

Neutrophil

Mast cell

Monocyte

B Lymphocyte

Eosinophil

Macrophage

Basophil

Megakaryocyte

Osteoclast

Plama cell

PLATE 3-1 ■ *Embryonic and Connective Tissue Proper I*

FIGURE 1 ■ *Loose (areolar) connective tissue. Paraffin section.* × 132.

This photomicrograph depicts a whole mount of mesentery, through its entire thickness. The two large **mast cells** (MC) are easily identified, since they are the largest cells in the field and possess a granular cytoplasm. Although their cytoplasms are not visible, it is still possible to recognize two other cell types due to their nuclear morphology. **Fibroblasts** (F) possess oval nuclei that are paler and larger than the nuclei of **macrophages** (M). The semifluid **ground substance** (GS) through which tissue fluid percolates is invisible, since it was extracted during the preparation of the tissues. However, two types of fibers, the thicker, wavy, ribbon-like, interlacing **collagen fibers** (CF) and the thin, straight, branching **elastic fibers** (EF) are well demonstrated.

FIGURE 2 ■ *Mesenchymal connective tissue. Fetal pig. Paraffin section.* × 540.

Mesenchymal connective tissue of the fetus is very immature and cellular. The **mesenchymal cells** (MeC) are stellate-shaped to fusiform cells, whose **cytoplasm** (c) can be distinguished from the surrounding matrix. The **nuclei** (N) are pale and centrally located. The ground substance is semifluid in consistency and contains slender reticular fibers. The vascularity of this tissue is evidenced by the presence of **blood vessels** (BV).

FIGURE 3 ■ *Mucous connective tissue. Umbilical cord. Human. Paraffin section.* × 132.

This example of mucous connective tissue (Wharton's jelly) was derived from the umbilical cord of a fetus. Observe the obvious differences between the two embryonic tissues. The matrix of mesenchymal connective tissue (Fig. 2) contains no collagenous fibers, while this connective tissue displays a loose network of haphazardly arranged **collagen fibers** (CF). The cells are no longer mesenchymal cells; instead, they are **fibroblasts** (F), although morphologically they resemble each other. The empty-looking spaces (arrows) are areas where the ground substance was extracted during specimen preparation.

Inset. **Fibroblast. Umbilical cord. Human. Paraffin section.** × 270.

Note the centrally placed **nucleus** (N) and the fusiform shape of the **cytoplasm** (c) of this fibroblast.

FIGURE 4 ■ *Reticular connective tissue. Silver stain. Paraffin section.* × 270.

Silver stain, used in the preparation of this specimen, was deposited on the carbohydrate coating of the **reticular fibers** (RF). Note that these fibers are thin, long, branching structures that ramify throughout the field. Note that in this photomicrograph of a lymph node, the reticular fibers in the lower right-hand corner are oriented in a circular fashion. These form the structural framework of a cortical **lymphatic nodule** (LN). The small round cells are probably **lymphoid cells** (LC), while the larger cells, closely associated with the reticular fibers, may be **reticular cells** (RC), although definite identification is not possible with this stain. It should be noted that reticular connective tissue is characteristically associated with lymphatic tissue.

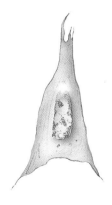

Fibroblast

■ **KEY**

BV	blood vessel	GS	ground substance	MeC	mesenchymal cell
C	cytoplasm	LC	lymphoid cell	N	nucleus
CF	collagen fiber	LN	lymphatic nodule	RC	reticular cell
EF	elastic fiber	M	macrophage	RF	reticular fiber
F	fibroblast	MC	mast cell		

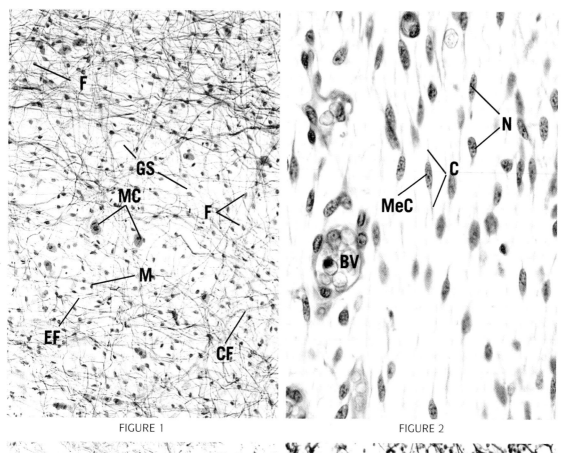

FIGURE 1

FIGURE 2

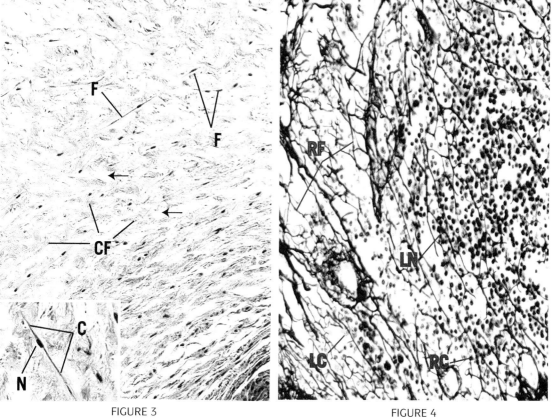

FIGURE 3

FIGURE 4

PLATE 3-2 ■ *Connective Tissue Proper II*

FIGURE 1 ■ *Adipose tissue. Hypodermis. Monkey. Plastic section.* × 132.

This photomicrograph of adipose tissue is from monkey hypodermis. The **adipocytes** (A), or fat cells, appear empty due to tissue processing that dissolves fatty material. The **cytoplasm** (c) of these cells appears as a peripheral rim, and the **nucleus** (N) is also pressed to the side by the single, large **fat droplet** (FD) within the cytoplasm. Fat is subdivided into lobules by **septa** (S) of connective tissue conducting **vascular elements** (BV) to the adipocytes. Fibroblast nuclei (arrows) are clearly evident in the connective tissue septa. Note the presence of the secretory portions of a **sweat gland** (SG) in the upper aspect of this photomicrograph.

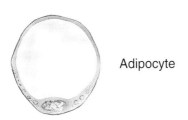

Adipocyte

FIGURE 2 ■ *Dense irregular collagenous connective tissue. Palmar skin. Monkey. Plastic section.* × 132.

The dermis of the skin provides a good representation of dense irregular collagenous connective tissue. The thick, coarse, intertwined bundles of **collagen fibers** (CF) are arranged in a haphazard fashion. Although this tissue has numerous **blood vessels** (BV) and **nerve fibers** (NF) branching through it, it is not a very vascular tissue. Dense irregular connective tissue is only sparsely supplied with cells, mostly fibroblasts and macrophages, whose **nuclei** (N) appear as dark dots scattered throughout the field. At this magnification, it is not possible to identify the cell types with any degree of accuracy. The large epithelial structure in the upper center of the field is the **duct** (d) of a sweat gland. At higher magnification (Inset, × 540), the coarse bundles of collagen fibers are composed of a conglomeration of **collagen fibrils** (Cf) intertwined around each other. The three cells, whose **nuclei** (N) are clearly evident, cannot be identified with any degree of certainty, even though the **cytoplasm** (c) of the two on the left-hand side is visible. It is possible that they are macrophages, but without employing special staining techniques, the possibility of their being fibroblasts cannot be ruled out.

FIGURE 3 ■ *Dense regular collagenous connective tissue. l.s. Tendon. Monkey. Plastic section.* × 270.

Tendons and ligaments present the most vivid examples of dense regular collagenous connective tissue. This connective tissue type is composed of regularly oriented parallel **bundles of collagen fibers** (CF), where individual bundles are demarcated by parallel rows of **fibroblasts** (F). Nuclei of these cells are clearly evident as thin, dark lines, while their **cytoplasm** (c) is only somewhat discernible. With hematoxylin and eosin, the collagen bundles stain a more or less light shade of pink with parallel rows of dark blue nuclei of fibroblasts interspersed among them.

FIGURE 4 ■ *Dense regular collagenous connective tissue. x.s. Tendon. Paraffin section.* × 270.

Transverse sections of tendon present a very typical appearance. Tendon is organized into fascicles that are separated from each other by the **peritendineum** (P) surrounding each fascicle. **Blood vessels** (BV) may be observed in the peritendineum. Collagen bundles within the fascicles are regularly arranged; however, shrinkage due to preparation causes an artifactual layering (arrows), although in some preparations swelling of the tissue results in a homogenous appearance. The nuclei of **fibroblasts** (F) appear to be strewn about in a haphazard manner.

■ **KEY**

A	adipocyte	d	duct	P	peritendineum
BV	blood vessel	F	fibroblast	S	septum
C	cytoplasm	FD	fat droplet	SG	sweat gland
Cf	collagen fibril	N	nucleus		
CF	bundle of collagen fibers	NF	nerve fiber		

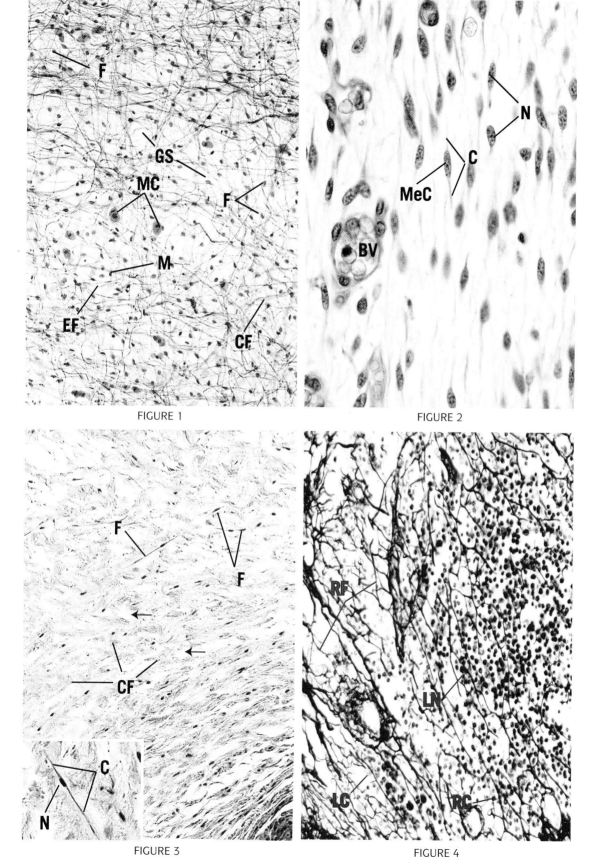

FIGURE 1

FIGURE 2

FIGURE 3

FIGURE 4

PLATE 3-2 ■ *Connective Tissue Proper II*

FIGURE 1 ▓ *Adipose tissue. Hypodermis. Monkey. Plastic section.* × 132.

This photomicrograph of adipose tissue is from monkey hypodermis. The **adipocytes** (A), or fat cells, appear empty due to tissue processing that dissolves fatty material. The **cytoplasm** (c) of these cells appears as a peripheral rim, and the **nucleus** (N) is also pressed to the side by the single, large **fat droplet** (FD) within the cytoplasm. Fat is subdivided into lobules by **septa** (S) of connective tissue conducting **vascular elements** (BV) to the adipocytes. Fibroblast nuclei (arrows) are clearly evident in the connective tissue septa. Note the presence of the secretory portions of a **sweat gland** (SG) in the upper aspect of this photomicrograph.

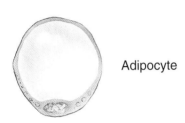

Adipocyte

FIGURE 2 ▓ *Dense irregular collagenous connective tissue. Palmar skin. Monkey. Plastic section.* × 132.

The dermis of the skin provides a good representation of dense irregular collagenous connective tissue. The thick, coarse, intertwined bundles of **collagen fibers** (CF) are arranged in a haphazard fashion. Although this tissue has numerous **blood vessels** (BV) and **nerve fibers** (NF) branching through it, it is not a very vascular tissue. Dense irregular connective tissue is only sparsely supplied with cells, mostly fibroblasts and macrophages, whose **nuclei** (N) appear as dark dots scattered throughout the field. At this magnification, it is not possible to identify the cell types with any degree of accuracy. The large epithelial structure in the upper center of the field is the **duct** (d) of a sweat gland. At higher magnification (Inset, × 540), the coarse bundles of collagen fibers are composed of a conglomeration of **collagen fibrils** (Cf) intertwined around each other. The three cells, whose **nuclei** (N) are clearly evident, cannot be identified with any degree of certainty, even though the **cytoplasm** (c) of the two on the left-hand side is visible. It is possible that they are macrophages, but without employing special staining techniques, the possibility of their being fibroblasts cannot be ruled out.

FIGURE 3 ▓ *Dense regular collagenous connective tissue. l.s. Tendon. Monkey. Plastic section.* × 270.

Tendons and ligaments present the most vivid examples of dense regular collagenous connective tissue. This connective tissue type is composed of regularly oriented parallel **bundles of collagen fibers** (CF), where individual bundles are demarcated by parallel rows of **fibroblasts** (F). Nuclei of these cells are clearly evident as thin, dark lines, while their **cytoplasm** (c) is only somewhat discernible. With hematoxylin and eosin, the collagen bundles stain a more or less light shade of pink with parallel rows of dark blue nuclei of fibroblasts interspersed among them.

FIGURE 4 ▓ *Dense regular collagenous connective tissue. x.s. Tendon. Paraffin section.* × 270.

Transverse sections of tendon present a very typical appearance. Tendon is organized into fascicles that are separated from each other by the **peritendineum** (P) surrounding each fascicle. **Blood vessels** (BV) may be observed in the peritendineum. Collagen bundles within the fascicles are regularly arranged; however, shrinkage due to preparation causes an artifactual layering (arrows), although in some preparations swelling of the tissue results in a homogenous appearance. The nuclei of **fibroblasts** (F) appear to be strewn about in a haphazard manner.

■ **KEY**

A	adipocyte	d	duct	P	peritendineum
BV	blood vessel	F	fibroblast	S	septum
C	cytoplasm	FD	fat droplet	SG	sweat gland
Cf	collagen fibril	N	nucleus		
CF	bundle of collagen fibers	NF	nerve fiber		

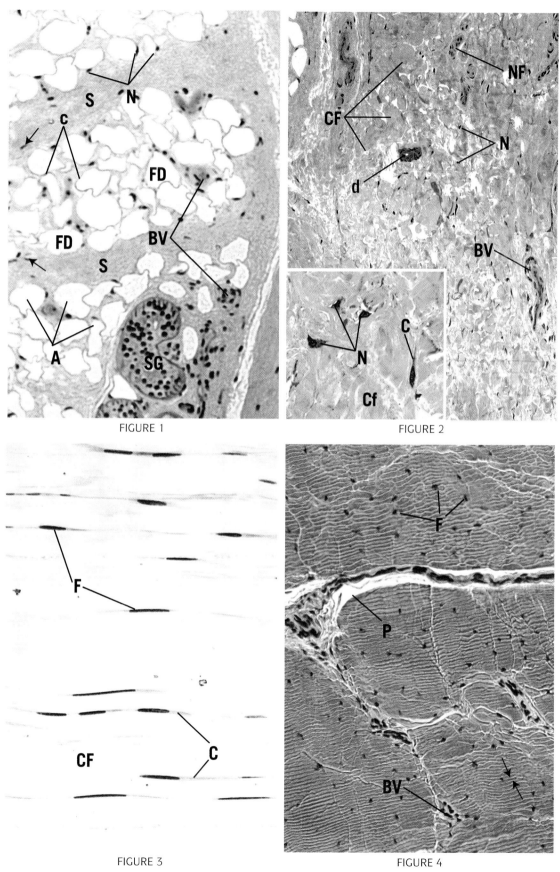

FIGURE 1

FIGURE 2

FIGURE 3

FIGURE 4

Connective Tissue ■ 57

PLATE 3-3 ■ *Connective Tissue Proper III*

FIGURE 1 ■ *Dense regular elastic connective tissue. l.s. Paraffin section.* × 132.

This longitudinal section of dense regular elastic tissue demonstrates that the **elastic fibers** (EF) are arranged in parallel arrays. However, the fibers are short and are curled at their ends (arrows). The white spaces among the fibers represent the loose connective tissue elements that remain unstained. The cellular elements are composed of parallel rows of flattened fibroblasts. These cells are also unstained and cannot be distinguished in this preparation.

FIGURE 2 ■ *Dense regular elastic connective tissue. x.s. Paraffin section.* × 132.

A transverse section of dense regular elastic connective tissue displays a very characteristic appearance. In some areas the fibers present precise cross-sectional profiles as dark dots of various diameters (arrows). Other areas present oblique sections of these fibers, represented by short linear profiles (arrowhead). As in the previous figure, the white spaces represent the unstained loose connective tissue elements. The large clear area (middle left) is also composed of loose connective tissue surrounding **blood vessels** (BV).

FIGURE 3 ■ *Elastic laminae (membranes). Aorta. Paraffin section.* × 132.

The wall of the aorta is composed of thick, concentrically arranged **elastic membranes** (EM). Since these sheet-like membranes wrap around within the wall of the aorta, in transverse sections they present discontinuous, concentric circles, which in this photomicrograph are represented by more or less parallel, wavy dark lines (arrows). The connective tissue material between membranes is composed of ground substance, **collagen fibers** (CF) and reticular fibers. Also present are fibroblasts and smooth muscle cells, whose nuclei may be discerned.

FIGURE 4 ■ *Mast cells, plasma cells, macrophages.*

Mast cells (MC) are conspicuous components of connective tissue proper, **Figure 4a** (Tendon. Monkey. Plastic section. × 540.), although they are only infrequently encountered. Note the round to oval nucleus, and numerous small granules in the cytoplasm. Observe also, among the bundles of **collagen fibers** (CF), the nuclei of several fibroblasts. **Mast cells** (MC) are very common components of the subepithelial connective tissue (lamina propria) of the digestive tract, **Figure 4b** (Jejunum. Monkey. Plastic section. × 540). Note the **basal membrane** (BM) separating the connective tissue from the **simple columnar epithelium** (E), whose nuclei are oval in shape. The denser, more amorphous nuclei (arrows) belong to lymphoid cells, migrating from the connective tissue into the intestinal lumen. The lamina propria also houses numerous **plasma cells** (PC), as evidenced in **Figure 4c** (Jejunum. Monkey. Plastic section. × 540). Plasma cells are characterized by clockface ("cart-wheel") nuclei, as well as by a clear paranuclear Golgi zone (arrowhead). **Figure 4d** (Macrophage. Liver, injected. Paraffin section. × 270.) is a photomicrograph of liver that was injected with India ink. This material is preferentially phagocytosed by macrophages of the liver, known as **Kupffer cells** (KC). These cells appear as dense, black structures in the liver sinusoids, vascular channels represented by clear areas (arrow). An individual Kupffer cell (Inset. Paraffin section. × 540.) displays the **nucleus** (N), as well as the granules of India ink (arrowhead) in its cytoplasm.

Mast cell

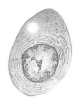

Plasma cell

■ **KEY**

BM	basal membrane	EF	elastic fiber	KC	Kupffer cell
BV	blood vessel	EM	elastic membrane	N	nucleus
CF	collagen fiber	MC	mast cell	PC	plasma cell

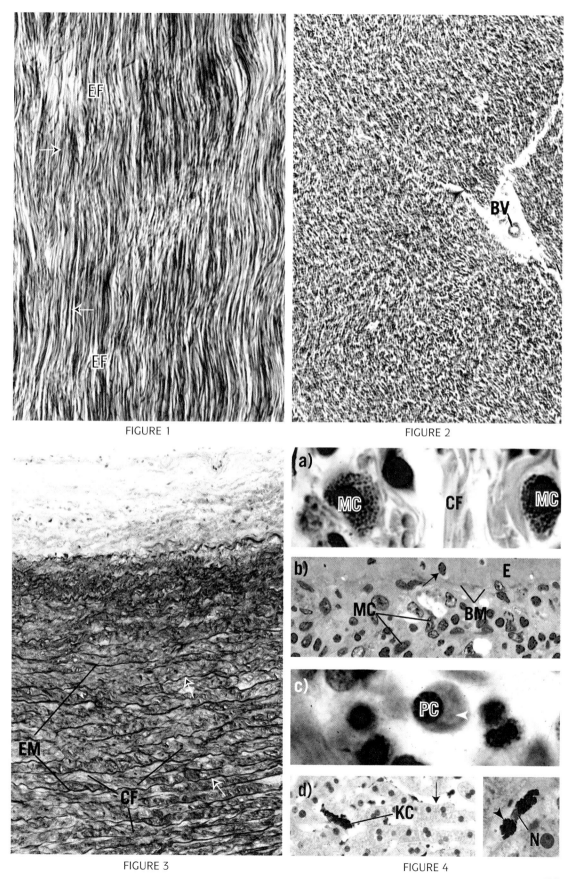

FIGURE 1

FIGURE 2

FIGURE 3

a)

b)

c)

d)

FIGURE 4

PLATE 3-4 ■ *Fibroblasts and Collagen, Electron Microscopy*

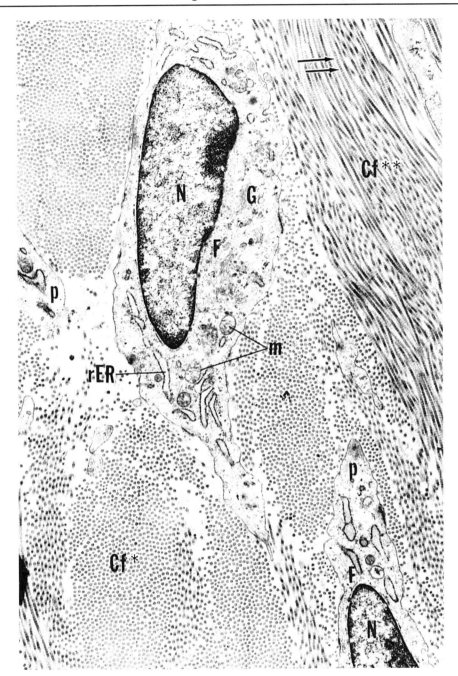

FIGURE 1 ▦ *Fibroblast. Baboon. Electron microscopy.* × 11,070.

This electron micrograph of **fibroblasts** (F) demonstrates that they are long, fusiform cells whose **processes** (p) extend into the surrounding area, between bundles of collagen fibrils. These cells manufacture collagen, reticular, and elastic fibers, and the ground substance of connective tissue. Therefore, they are rich in organelles, such as **Golgi apparatus** (G), **rough endoplasmic reticulum** (rER), and **mitochondria** (m); however, in the quiescent stage, as in tendons, where they no longer actively synthesize the intercellular elements of connective tissue, the organelle population of fibroblasts is reduced in number, and the plump, euchromatic **nucleus** (N) becomes flattened and heterochromatic. Note that the bundles of **collagen fibrils** (Cf) are sectioned both transversely (asterisk) and longitudinally (double asterisks). Individual fibrils display alternating transverse dark and light banding (arrows) along their length. The specific banding results from the ordered arrangement of the tropocollagen molecules constituting the collagen fibrils. (From Simpson D, Avery B: *J Periodontol* 45:500–510, 1974.)

PLATE 3-5 ■ *Mast Cell, Electron Microscopy*

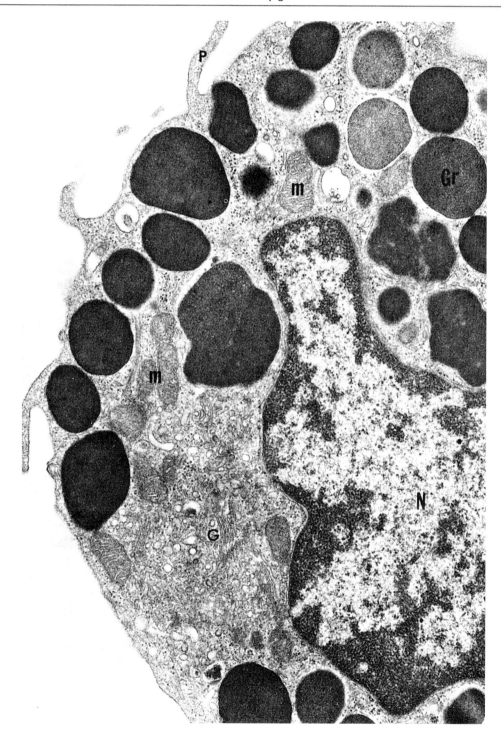

FIGURE 1 ■ *Mast cell. Rat. Electron microscopy.*
× 14,400.

This electron micrograph of a rat peritoneal mast cell displays characteristics of this cell. Note that the **nucleus** (N) is not lobulated, and the cell contains organelles, such as **mitochondria** (m) and **Golgi apparatus** (G). Numerous **processes** (p) extend from the cell. Observe that the most characteristic component of this cell is that it is filled with numerous membrane-bound **granules** (Gr) of more or less uniform density. These granules contain heparin, histamine, and serotonin (although human mast cells do not contain serotonin). Additionally, mast cells release a number of unstored substances that act in allergic reactions. (From Lagunoff D: *J Invest Dermatol* 58:296–311, 1972.)

PLATE 3-6 ■ *Mast Cell Degranulation, Electron Microscopy*

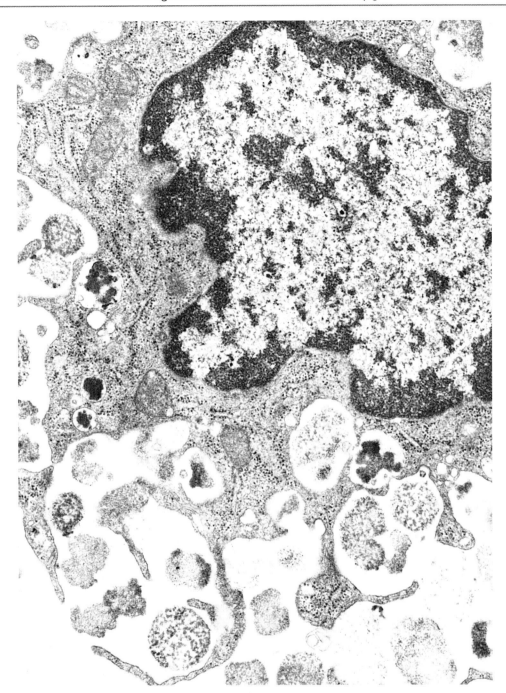

FIGURE 1 ■ *Mast cell degranulation. Rat. Electron microscopy.* × 20,250.

Mast cells possess receptor molecules on their plasma membrane, which are specific for the constant region of IgE antibody molecules. These molecules attach to the mast cell surface and, as the cell comes in contact with those specific antigens to which it was sensitized, the antigen binds with the active regions of the IgE antibody. Such antibody-antigen binding on the mast cell surface causes degranulation, i.e., the release of granules, as well as the release of the unstored substances that act in allergic reactions. Degranulation occurs very quickly, but requires both ATP and calcium. Granules at the periphery of the cell are released by fusion with the cell membrane, while granules deeper in the cytoplasm fuse with each other, forming convoluted intracellular canaliculi that connect to the extracellular space. Such a canaliculus may be noted in the bottom left-hand corner of this electron micrograph. (From Lagunoff D: *J Invest Dermatol* 58: 296–311, 1972.)

PLATE 3-7 ■ *Developing Fat Cell, Electron Microscopy*

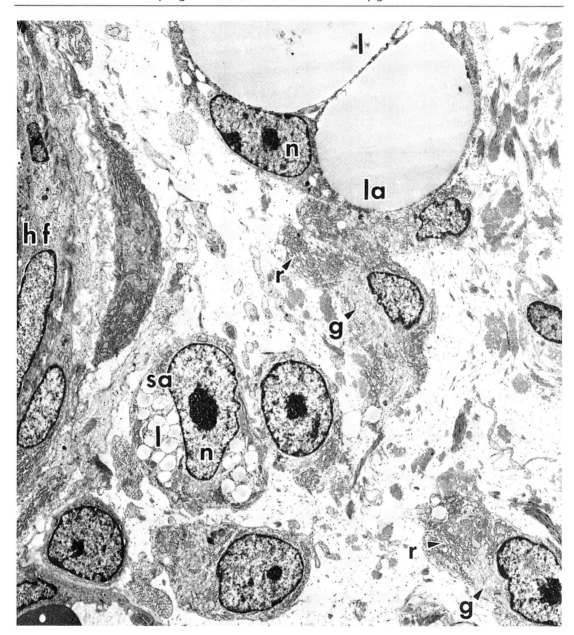

FIGURE 1 ▨ *Developing fat cell. Rat. Electron microscopy.* × 3060.

This electron micrograph from the developing rat hypodermis displays a region of the developing **hair follicle** (hf). The peripheral aspect of the hair follicle presents a **small adipocyte** (sa) whose **nucleus** (n) and nucleolus are clearly visible. Although white adipose cells are unilocular, in that the cytoplasm of the cell contains a single, large droplet of lipid, during development lipid begins to accumulate as small **droplets** (l) in the cytoplasm of the small adipocyte. As the fat cell matures to become a **large adipocyte** (la), its **nucleus** (n) is displaced peripherally, and the lipid **droplets** (l) fuse to form several large droplets, which will eventually coalesce to form a single, central fat deposit. The nucleus displays some alterations during the transformation from small to large adipocytes, in that the nucleolus becomes smaller and less prominent. Immature adipocytes are distinguishable, since they possess as well-developed **Golgi apparatus** (g) that is actively functioning in the biosynthesis of lipids. Moreover, the **rough endoplasmic reticulum** (r) presents dilated cisternae, indicative of protein synthetic activity. Note the capillary, whose lumen displays a red blood cell in the lower left-hand corner of this photomicrograph. (From Hausman G, Campion D, Richardson R, Martin R: *Am J Anat* 161:85–100, 1981.)

4

(chapter marker with squares)

Cartilage and Bone

Cartilage and bone form the supporting tissues of the body. In these specialized connective tissues, as in other connective tissues, the intercellular elements dominate their microscopic appearance.

CARTILAGE

Cartilage forms the supporting framework of certain organs, the articulating surfaces of bones, and the greater part of the fetal skeleton, although most of that will be replaced by bone (see Graphic 4-2).

There are three types of cartilage in the body, namely, hyaline cartilage, elastic cartilage, and fibrocartilage. **Hyaline cartilage** is found at the articulating surfaces of most bones; the C rings of the trachea; and the laryngeal, costal, and nasal cartilages, among others. **Elastic cartilage,** as its name implies, possesses a great deal of elasticity, which is due to the elastic fibers embedded in its matrix. This cartilage is found in areas like the epiglottis, external ear and ear canal, and some of the smaller laryngeal cartilages. **Fibrocartilage** is found in only a few places, namely, in some symphyses, the eustachian tube, intervertebral (and some articular) disks, and certain areas where tendons insert into bone (Table 4-1).

Cartilage is a nonvascular, strong, and somewhat pliable structure composed of a firm matrix of **proteoglycans** whose main **glycosaminoglycans** are chondroitin-4-sulfate and chondroitin-6-sulfate. The fibrous and cellular components of cartilage are embedded in this matrix. The fibers are either solely collagenous or a combination of elastic and collagenous, depending on the cartilage type. The cellular components are the **chondrocytes,** which are housed in small spaces known as **lacunae,** interspersed within the matrix, as well as **chondroblasts** and **chondrogenic cells,** both of which are in the **perichondrium.**

Most cartilage is surrounded by a connective tissue membrane, the perichondrium, which has an outer fibrous layer and an inner chondrogenic layer.

The **fibrous layer,** although poor in cells, is composed mostly of fibroblasts and collagen fibers. The inner cellular or **chondrogenic layer** is composed of chondroblasts and chondrogenic cells. The latter give rise to chondroblasts, cells that are responsible for secreting the **cartilage matrix.** It is from this layer that the cartilage may grow **appositionally.**

As the chondroblasts secrete matrix and fibers around themselves, they become incarcerated in their own secretions and are then termed chondrocytes. The space that they occupy within the matrix is known as a lacuna. These **chondrocytes,** at least in young cartilage, possess the capacity to undergo cell division, thus contributing to the growth of the cartilage from within (**interstitial growth**). When this occurs, each lacuna may house several chondrocytes and is referred to as a cell nest (**isogenous group**).

Hyaline cartilage is surrounded by a well-defined **perichondrium.** The type II collagen fibers of this cartilage are mostly very fine and are, therefore, fairly well masked by the surrounding **glycosaminoglycans,** giving the matrix a smooth, glassy appearance.

Elastic cartilage possesses a perichondrium. The matrix, in addition to the type II collagen fibers, contains a wealth of coarse elastic fibers that impart to it a characteristic appearance.

Fibrocartilage differs from elastic and hyaline cartilage in that it has no perichondrium. Additionally, the chondrocytes are smaller and are usually oriented in parallel longitudinal rows. The matrix of this cartilage contains a large number of thick type I collagen fiber bundles between the rows of chondrocytes (Table 4-1).

BONE

Bone has many functions, including support, protection, mineral storage, and hemopoiesis. At the specialized cartilage-covered ends, it permits articulation or movement. Bone, a vascular connective tissue consisting of cells and calcified intercellular

TABLE 4-1 ■ Cartilage—Types, Characteristics, Locations

Type	Characteristics	Perichondrium	Locations (Major Samples)
Hyaline	Chondrocytes arranged in groups within a basophilic matrix containing Type II collagen	Usually present except at articular surfaces	Articular ends of long bones, ventral rib cartilage, templates for endochondral bone formation
Elastic	Chondrocytes compacted in matrix containing Type II collagen and elastic fibers	Present	Pinna of ear, auditory canal, laryngeal cartilages
Fibrocartilage	Chondrocytes arranged in rows in an acidophilic matrix containing Type I collagen bundles in rows	Absent	Intervertebral discs, pubic symphysis

materials, may be dense (compact) or sponge-like (cancellous). Cancellous bone, like that found inside the epiphysis or head of long bones, is always surrounded by compact bone. **Cancellous bone** has large, open spaces surrounded by thin, anastomosing plates of bone. The large spaces are **marrow spaces,** and the plates of bones are **trabeculae** composed of several layers or **lamellae.** Compact bone is much more dense than cancellous bone. Its spaces are much reduced in size, and its lamellar organization is much more precise and thicker. The calcified matrix is composed of 50% minerals (mostly **calcium hydroxyapatite**), 50% organic matter (**collagen and protein-associated glycosaminoglycans**), and bound water.

Bone is always covered and lined by soft connective tissues. The marrow cavity is lined by an **endosteum** composed of **osteoprogenitor cells** (previously known as osteogenic cells), **osteoblasts,** and occasional **osteoclasts.** The periosteum covering the bone surface is composed of an outer fibrous layer consisting mainly of collagen fibers and populated by fibroblasts. The inner osteogenic layer consists of some collagen fibers and mostly osteogenic cells and their progeny, the osteoblasts. The periosteum is affixed to bone via **Sharpey's fibers,** collagenous bundles trapped in the calcified bone matrix during ossification.

Bone matrix is produced by osteoblasts, cells derived from their less differentiated precursors, the **osteoprogenitor cells.** As osteoblasts elaborate bone matrix, they become trapped, and as the matrix calcifies, the trapped osteoblasts become known as **osteocytes.** Osteocytes, occupying lenticular-shaped spaces known as **lacunae,** possess long processes that are housed in tiny canals or tunnels known as **canaliculi.** Since bone, unlike cartilage, is a vascular hard tissue whose blood vessels penetrate and perforate it, canaliculi eventually open into channels known as **haversian canals** housing

the blood vessels. Each haversian canal with its surrounding lamellae of bone containing canaliculi radiating to it from the osteocytes trapped in the lacunae is known as an **osteon** or **haversian canal system.**

The canaliculi of the osteon extend to the haversian canal in order to exchange cellular waste material for nutrients and oxygen. Haversian canals, which more or less parallel the longitudinal axis of long bones, are connected to each other by **Volkmann's canals.**

The bony lamellae of compact bone are organized into four lamellar systems: **external** and **internal circumferential lamellae, interstitial lamellae,** and the **osteons** (see Graphic 4-1).

Osteogenesis

Histogenesis of bone occurs via either **intramembranous** or **endochondral ossification.** The former arises in a richly vascularized mesenchymal membrane where **mesenchymal cells** differentiate into osteoblasts (possibly via osteprogenitor cells), which begin to elaborate bone matrix, thus forming trabeculae of bone. As more and more trabeculae form in the same vicinity, they will become interconnected. As they fuse with each other, they form **cancellous bone,** which will be remodeled to give rise to **compact bone.** The surfaces of these trabeculae are populated with osteoblasts. Frequently, an additional cell type, the **osteoclast,** may be evident. These large, multinuclear cells derived from **monocytes** are found in shallow depressions on the trabecular surface (**Howship's lacunae**) and function to resorb bone. It is through the integrated interactions of these cells and osteoblasts that bone is remodeled. The region of the mesenchymal membrane that does not participate in the ossification process will remain the soft tissue component of bone (i.e., periosteum, endosteum).

Newly formed bone is called **primary** or **woven bone,** since the arrangement of collagen fibers lacks the precise orientation present in older bone. The integrated interaction between osteoblasts and osteoclasts will act to replace the woven bone with **secondary** or **mature bone.**

Endochondral ossification, responsible for the formation of long and short bones, relies on the presence of a hyaline cartilage model that is used as a template on and within which bone is made (see Graphic 4-2). However, cartilage does not become bone. Instead, a **bony subperiosteal collar** is formed (via intramembranous ossification) around the midriff of the cartilaginous template. This collar increases in width and length. The chondrocytes in the center of the template hypertrophy and resorb some of their matrix, thus enlarging their lacunae so much that some lacunae become confluent. The **hypertrophied chondrocytes,** subsequent to assisting in calcification of the cartilage, degenerate and die. The newly formed spaces are invaded by the **periosteal bud** (composed of blood vessels, mesenchymal cells, and osteoprogenitor cells). Osteoprogenitor cells differentiate into osteoblasts, and these cells elaborate a bony matrix lining on the calcified cartilage. As the subperiosteal bone collar increases in thickness and length, osteoclasts resorb the calcified cartilage-calcified bone complex, leaving an enlarged space, the future marrow cavity (which will be populated by marrow cells). The entire process of ossification will spread away from this primary ossification center, and eventually most of the cartilage template will be replaced by bone, forming the **diaphysis** of a long bone. The formation of the **bony epiphysis** (secondary ossification center) occurs in a modified fashion so that a cartilaginous covering may be maintained at the articular surface. The growth in length of a long bone is due to the presence of epiphyseal plates of cartilage located between the epiphysis and the diaphysis.

Histophysiology

I. CARTILAGE

A. Cartilage Matrix

Hyaline cartilage is an avascular connective tissue whose pliable matrix provides a conduit for nutrients and waste products to and from its perichondrium and its chondrocytes. The matrix consists of **type II collagen** embedded in an amorphous ground substance composed of the glycosaminoglycan, **hyaluronic acid,** to which proteoglycans are bound. The glycosaminoglycan components of the proteoglycans are mainly **chondroitin-4-sulfate** and **chondroitin-6-sulfate.** The acidic nature of the proteoglycans, combined with the enormous size of the proteoglycan—hyaluronic acid complex, results in these molecules possessing huge **domains** and tremendous capacity for binding cations and water. Additionally, the matrix contains **glycoproteins** that help the cells maintain contact with the intercellular matrix.

Elastic cartilage is similar to hyaline cartilage, but it also possesses **elastic fibers. Fibrocartilage** possesses no perichondrium, only a limited amount of acidophilic matrix, and an abundance of **type I collagen** arranged in parallel rows.

B. Chondrocytes

The **chondrocytes** of hyaline and elastic cartilage resemble each other, in that they may be arranged individually in their **lacunae** or in **cell nests** (in young cartilage). Peripherally located chondrocytes are lenticular in shape, whereas those located centrally are round. The cells completely fill their lacunae. They possess an abundance of glycogen, frequent large lipid droplets, and a well-developed protein synthetic machinery (rough endoplasmic reticulum, Golgi apparatus, trans-Golgi network), as well as mitochondria, since these cells continuously turn over the cartilage matrix.

II. BONE

A. Bone Matrix

Bone is a **calcified,** vascular connective tissue. Its cells are located in the surrounding periosteum, in the endosteal lining, or within lenticular cavities called **lacunae.** Tiny channels known as **canaliculi,** housing slender processes of osteocytes, convey nutrients, hormones, and other necessary substances.

The organic matrix of bone is composed mainly of **type I collagen,** sulfated **glycoproteins,** and some **proteoglycans.** The matrix of collagen is calcified with **calcium hydroxyapatite** crystals, making bone one of the hardest substances in the body. The presence of these crystals makes bone the body's storehouse of calcium, phosphate, and other inorganic ions. Thus, bone is in a dynamic state of flux, continuously gaining and losing inorganic ions to maintain the body's calcium and phosphate homeostasis.

B. Cells of Bone

Osteoprogenitor cells are flattened, undifferentiated-appearing cells located in the cellular layer of the periosteum, in the endosteum, and lining the haversian canals. They give rise to osteoblasts.

Osteoblasts are cuboidal to low-columnar cells responsible for the synthesis of bone matrix. As they elaborate bone matrix, they become surrounded by the matrix and then become osteocytes. The bone matrix is calcified due to the seeding of the matrix via **matrix vesicles** derived from osteoblasts. When osteoblasts are quiescent, they lose much of their protein synthetic machinery and resemble osteoprogenitor cells.

Osteocytes are flattened, discoid cells located in **lacunae;** they are responsible for the maintenance of bone. Their cytoplasmic processes contact and form **gap junctions** with processes of other osteocytes within canaliculi; thus these cells sustain a communication network, so that a large population of osteocytes are able to respond to blood calcium levels as well as to **calcitonin** and **parathormone,** released by the thyroid and parathyroid glands, respectively. Thus these cells are responsible for the short-term calcium and phosphate homeostasis of the body.

Osteoclasts are multinucleated cells derived from monocytes; they are responsible for the resorption of bone. Cooperation between osteoclasts and osteoblasts is responsible not only for the formation, remodeling, and repair of bone but also for the long-term maintenance of calcium and phosphate homeostasis of the body.

Clinical Considerations ▨ ▨ ▪

Cartilage Degeneration

Hyaline cartilage begins to degenerate when the chondrocytes hypertrophy and die, a natural process but one that accelerates with aging. This results in decreasing mobility and joint pain.

Vitamin Deficiency

Deficiency in Vitamin A inhibits proper bone formation and growth, while an excess accelerates ossification of the epiphyseal plates producing small stature. Deficiency in vitamin D, which is essential for absorption of calcium from the intestine, results in poorly calcified (soft) bone—rickets in children and osteomalacia in adults. When in excess, bone is resorbed. Deficiency in Vitamin C, which is necessary for collagen formation, produces scurvy—resulting in poor bone growth and repair.

Hormonal Influences on Bone

Calcitonin inhibits bone-matrix resorption by altering osteoclast function, thus preventing calcium release. Parathyroid hormone activates osteoblasts to secrete osteoclast-stimulating factor, thus activating osteoclasts to increase bone resorption resulting in increased blood calcium levels. If in excess, bones become brittle and are susceptible to fracture.

Paget's Disease of Bone

Paget' disease of bone is a generalized skeletal disease that usually affects older people. Often, the disease has a familial component and its results are thickened, but softer bones of the skull and extremities. It is usually asymptomatic and is frequently discovered after radiographic examination prescribed for other reasons or as a result of blood chemistry showing elevated alkaline phosphatase levels. Calcitonin treatment may be used to slow the progression of the disease.

Osteoporosis

Osteoporosis is a decrease in bone mass arising from lack of bone formation or from increased bone resorption. It occurs commonly in old age because of decreased growth hormone and in postmenopausal women because of decreased estrogen secretion. In the latter, estrogen binding to receptors on osteoblasts stimulate the secretion of bone matrix. Without sufficient estrogen, osteoclastic activity reduces bone mass without the concomitant formation of bone, therefore making the bones more liable to fracture.

Summary of Histological Organization

I. CARTILAGE

A. Embryonic Cartilage

1. Perichondrium
The **perichondrium** is very thin and cellular.

2. Matrix
The **matrix** is scanty and smooth in appearance.

3. Cells
Numerous, small, round **chondrocytes** are housed in small spaces in the matrix. These spaces are known as **lacunae.**

B. Hyaline Cartilage

1. Perichondrium
The perichondrium has two layers, an outer **fibrous layer,** which contains collagen and fibroblasts, and an inner **chondrogenic layer,** which contains **chondrogenic cells** and **chondroblasts.**

2. Matrix
The **matrix** is smooth and basophilic in appearance. It has two regions, the **territorial (capsular) matrix,** which is darker and surrounds **lacunae,** and the **interterritorial (intercapsular) matrix,** which is lighter in color. The collagen fibrils are masked by the ground substance.

3. Cells
Either **chondrocytes** are found individually in **lacunae,** or there may be two or more chondrocytes **(isogenous group)** in a lacuna. The latter case signifies **interstitial growth. Appositional growth** occurs just deep to the perichondrium and is attributed to **chondroblasts.**

C. Elastic Cartilage

1. Perichondrium
The perichondrium is the same in elastic cartilage as in hyaline cartilage.

2. Matrix
The **matrix** contains numerous dark **elastic fibers** in addition to the **collagen fibrils.**

3. Cells
The cells are **chondrocytes, chondroblasts,** and **chondrogenic cells,** as in hyaline cartilage.

D. Fibrocartilage

1. Perichondrium
The perichondrium is usually absent.

2. Matrix
The **ground substance** of matrix is very scanty. Many thick collagen bundles are located between parallel rows of chondrocytes.

3. Cells
The **chondrocytes** in fibrocartilage are smaller than those in hyaline or elastic cartilage, and they are arranged in parallel longitudinal rows between bundles of thick collagen fibers.

II. BONE

A. Decalcified Compact Bone

1. Periosteum
The **periosteum** has two layers, an outer **fibrous layer,** containing **collagen fibers** and **fibroblasts,** and an inner **osteogenic layer,** containing **osteoprogenitor cells** and **osteoblasts.** It is anchored to bone by **Sharpey's fibers.**

2. Lamellar Systems
Lamellar organization consists of **outer** and **inner circumferential lamellae,** osteons (**haversian canal systems**), and **interstitial lamellae.**

3. Endosteum
The **endosteum** is a thin membrane that lines the **medullary cavity,** which contains **yellow** or **white bone marrow.**

4. Cells
Osteocytes are housed in small spaces called **lacunae. Osteoblasts** and **osteoprogenitor cells** are found in the osteogenic layer of the periosteum, in the endosteum, and lining haversian canals. **Osteoclasts** are located in **Howship's lacunae** along resorptive surfaces of bone. **Osteoid,** noncalcified bone matrix, is interposed between the cells of bone and the calcified tissue.

5. Vascular Supply
Blood vessels are found in the periosteum, in the marrow cavity, and in the haversian canals of osteons. Haversian canals are connected to each other by Volkmann's canals.

B. Undecalcified Compact Ground Bone

1. Lamellar Systems

The lamellar organization is clearly evident as wafer-thin layers or **lamellae** constituting bone. They are then organized as **outer** and **inner circumferential lamellae, osteons,** and **interstitial lamellae.**

Osteons are cylindrical structures composed of concentric lamellae of bone. Their **lacunae** are empty, but in living bone they contain osteocytes. **Canaliculi** radiate from **lacunae** toward the central **haversian canal,** which in living bone houses blood vessels, osteoblasts, and osteogenic cells. **Cementing lines** demarcate the peripheral extent of each osteon. **Volkmann's canals** interconnect neighboring haversian canals.

C. Decalcified Cancellous Bone

1. Lamellar Systems

Lamellar organization consists of **spicules** and **trabeculae** of bone.

2. Cells

Cells are as before, in that **osteocytes** are housed in lacunae. **Osteoblasts** line all trabeculae and spicules. Occasionally, multinuclear, large **osteoclasts** occupy **Howship's lacunae. Osteoid,** noncalcified bone matrix, is interposed between the cells of bone and the calcified tissue.

Bone marrow occupies the spaces among and between **trabeculae.**

D. Intramembranous Ossification

1. Ossification Centers

Centers of ossification are vascularized areas of **mesenchymal connective tissue** where **mesenchymal cells** probably differentiate into **osteoprogenitor cells,** which differentiate into **osteoblasts.**

2. Lamellar Systems

Lamellar organization begins when **spicules** and **trabeculae** form into primitive osteons surrounding blood vessels. The first bone formed is **primary bone (woven bone)** whose cells are larger and whose fibrillar arrangement is haphazard compared with **secondary (mature) bone.**

3. Cells

The cellular elements of intramembranous ossification are **osteoprogenitor cells, osteoblasts, osteocytes,** and **osteoclasts.** Additionally, mesenchymal and hemopoietic cells are also present.

E. Endochondral Ossification

1. Primary Ossification Center

The **perichondrium** of the **diaphysis** of the cartilage template becomes vascularized, followed by **hypertrophy** of the centrally located chondrocytes, confluence of contiguous lacunae, calcification of the cartilage remnants, and subsequent **chondrocytic death.** Concomitant with these events, the **chondrogenic cells** of the perichondrium become **osteoprogenitor cells,** which, in turn, differentiate into **osteoblasts.** The osteoblasts form the **subperiosteal bone collar,** thus converting the overlying **perichondrium** into a **periosteum.** A **periosteal bud** invades the diaphysis, entering the confluent **lacunae** left empty by the death of chondrocytes. Osteogenic cells give rise to osteoblasts, which elaborate bone on the **trabeculae of calcified cartilage.** Hemopoiesis begins in the primitive medullary cavity; **osteoclasts** (and, according to some, chondroclasts) develop, which resorb the bone-covered trabeculae of calcified cartilage as the subperiosteal bone collar becomes thicker and elongated.

2. Secondary Ossification Center

The **epiphyseal (secondary) center of ossification** is initiated somewhat after birth. It begins in the center of the epiphysis and proceeds radially from that point, leaving cartilage only at the **articular surface** and at the interface between the epiphysis and the diaphysis, the future **epiphyseal plate.**

3. Epiphyseal Plate

The **epiphyseal plate** is responsible for the future lengthening of a long bone. It is divided into five zones: 1) **zone of reserve cartilage,** a region of haphazardly arranged chondrocytes; 2) **zone of cell proliferation,** where chondrocytes are arranged in rows whose longitudinal axis parallels that of the growing bone; 3) **zone of cell maturation and hypertrophy,** where cells enlarge and the matrix between adjoining cells becomes very thin; 4) **zone of calcifying cartilage,** where lacunae become confluent and the matrix between adjacent rows of chondrocytes becomes calcified, causing subsequent chondrocytic death; and 5) **zone of provisional ossification,** where osteoblasts deposit bone on the calcified cartilage remnants between the adjacent rows. Osteoclasts (and, according to some, chondroclasts) resorb the calcified complex.

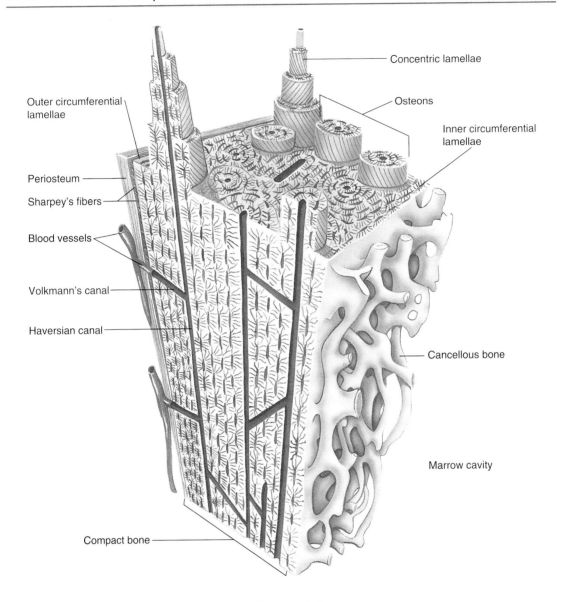

Concentric lamellae

Osteons

Inner circumferential lamellae

Outer circumferential lamellae

Periosteum

Sharpey's fibers

Blood vessels

Volkmann's canal

Haversian canal

Cancellous bone

Marrow cavity

Compact bone

Compact Bone

Compact bone is surrounded by dense irregular collagenous connective tissue, the **periosteum**, which is attached to the **outer circumferential lamellae** by **Sharpey's fibers**. Blood vessels of the periosteum enter the bone via larger nutrient canals or small **Volksmann's canals**, which not only convey blood vessels to the **Haversian canals** of **osteons** but also interconnect adjacent Haversian canals. Each osteon is composed of concentric lamellae of bone whose collagen fibers are arranged so that they are perpendicular to those of contiguous lamellae. The **inner circumferential lamellae** are lined by endosteal lined cancellous bone that protrudes into the marrow cavity.

GRAPHIC 4-2 ■ *Endochondral Bone Formation*

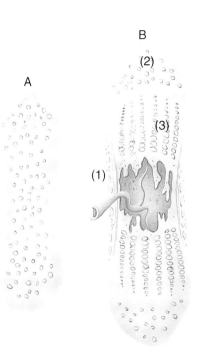

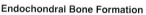

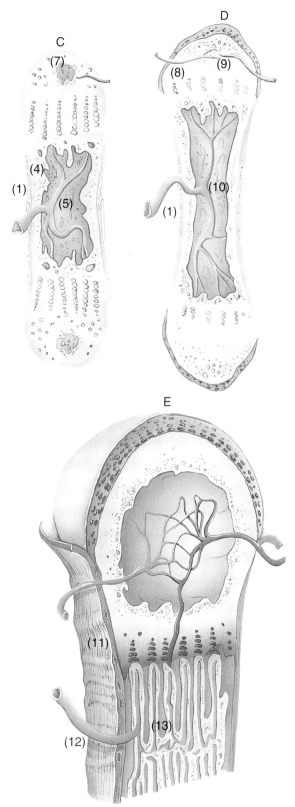

Endochondral Bone Formation

A. Endochondral bone formation requires the presence of a hyaline cartilage model.

B. Vascularization of the diaphysis perichondrium (2) results in the transformation of chondrogenic cells to osteogenic cells, resulting in the formation of a **subperiosteal bone collar** (1) (via intramembranous bone formation), which quickly becomes perforated by osteoclastic activity. Chondrocytes in the center of the cartilage hypertrophy (3), and their lacunae become confluent.

C. The subperiosteal bone collar (1) increased in length and width, the confluent lacunae are invaded by the **periosteal bud** (4), and osteoclastic activity forms a primitive marrow cavity (5) whose walls are composed of calcified cartilage-calcified bone complex. The epiphyses display the beginning of **secondary ossification centers** (7).

D and E. The subperiosteal bond collar (1) has become sufficiently large to support the developing long bone, so that much of the cartilage has been resorbed, with the exception of the **epiphyseal plate** (8) and the covering of the epiphyses (9). Ossification in the epiphyses occurs from the center (10), thus the vascular periosteum (11) does not cover the cartilaginous surface. Blood vessels (12) enter the **epiphyses**, without vascularizing the cartilage, to constitute the vascular network (13) around which spongy bone will be formed.

PLATE 4-1 ■ *Embryonic and Hyaline Cartilages*

FIGURE 1 ■ *Embryonic hyaline cartilage. Pig. Paraffin section.* × 132.

The developing hyaline cartilage is surrounded by **embryonic connective tissue** (ECT). Mesenchymal cells have participated in the formation of this cartilage. Note that the developing **perichondrium** (P), investing the cartilage, merges both with the embryonic connective tissue and with the cartilage. The chondrocytes in their lacunae are round, small cells packed closely together (arrow) with little intervening homogeneously staining matrix (arrowheads).

FIGURE 2 ■ *Hyaline cartilage. Trachea. Monkey. Paraffin section.* × 132.

The trachea is lined by **a pseudostratified ciliated columnar epithelium** (Ep). Deep to the epithelium observe the large, blood-filled **vein** (V). The lower half of the photomicrograph presents hyaline cartilage whose **chondrocytes** (C) are disposed in **isogenous groups** (IG) indicative of interstitial growth. Chondrocytes are housed in spaces known as lacunae. Note that the territorial matrix (arrow) in the vicinity of the lacunae stains darker than the interterritorial matrix (asterisk). The entire cartilage is surrounded by **a perichondrium** (P).

FIGURE 3 ■ *Hyaline cartilage. Rabbit. Paraffin section.* × 270.

The perichondrium is composed of **fibrous** (F) and **chondrogenic** (CG) layers. The former is composed of mostly collagenous fibers with a few fibroblasts, while the latter is more cellular, consisting of chondroblasts and chondrogenic cells (arrows). As chondroblasts secrete matrix they become surrounded by the intercellular substance, and are consequently known as **chondrocytes** (C). Note that chondrocytes at the periphery of the cartilage are small and elongated, while those at the center are large and ovoid to round (arrowhead). Frequently they are found in **isogenous groups** (IG).

FIGURE 4 ■ *Hyaline cartilage. Trachea. Monkey. Plastic section.* × 270.

The pseudostratified ciliated columnar epithelium displays numerous goblet cells (arrows). The cilia, appearing at the free border of the epithelium, are clearly evident. Note how the subepithelial **connective tissue** (CT) merges with the **fibrous perichondrium** (F). The **chondrogenic layer** of the perichondrium (Cg) houses chondrogenic cells and chondroblasts. As chondroblasts surround themselves with matrix, they become trapped in lacunae and are referred to as **chondrocytes** (C). At the periphery of the cartilage, the chondrocytes are flattened, while toward the interior they are round to oval. Due to the various histologic procedures, some of the chondrocytes fall out of their lacunae, which then appear as empty spaces. Although the **matrix** (M) contains many collagen fibrils, they are masked by the glycosaminoglycans; hence, the matrix appears homogeneous and smooth. The proteoglycan-rich lining of the lacunae is responsible for the more intense staining of the territorial matrix, which is particularly evident in Figures 2 and 3.

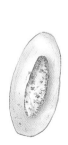
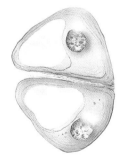

Chondroblast   Chondrocytes

■ **KEY**

C	chondrocyte	Ep	pseudostratified ciliated columnar epithelium	M	matrix
Cg	chondrogenic perichondrium			P	perichondrium
		F	fibrous perichondrium	V	vein
CT	connective tissue	IG	isogenous group		
ECT	embryonic connective tissue				

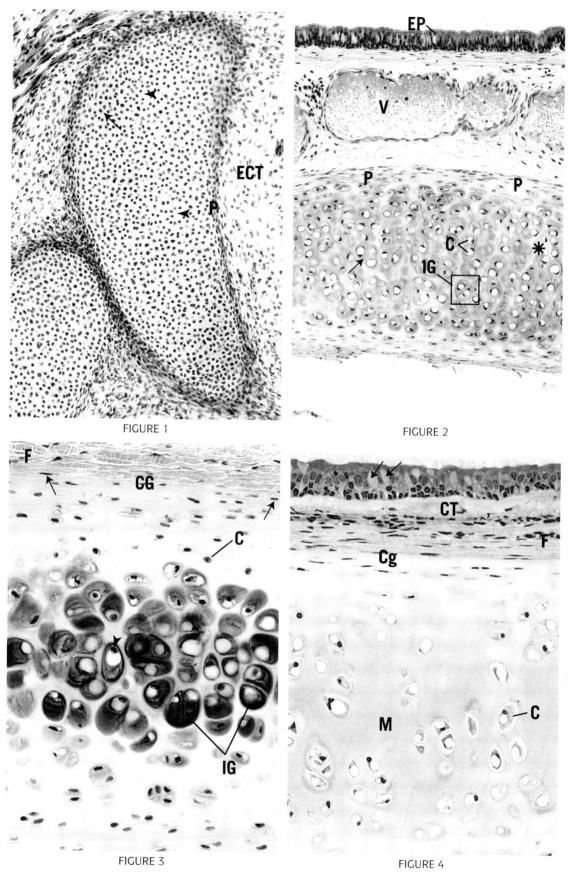

FIGURE 1

FIGURE 2

FIGURE 3

FIGURE 4

PLATE 4-2 ■ *Elastic and Fibrocartilages*

FIGURE 1 ■ *Elastic cartilage. Epiglottis. Human. Paraffin section.* × 132.

Elastic cartilage, like hyaline cartilage, is enveloped by a **perichondrium** (P). **Chondrocytes** (C), which are housed in lacunae (arrow), have shrunk away from the walls, giving the appearance of empty spaces. Occasional lacunae display two chondrocytes (asterisk), indicative of interstitial growth. The matrix has a rich **elastic fiber** (E) component that gives elastic cartilage its characteristic appearance, as well as contributing to its elasticity. The boxed area appears at a higher magnification in Figure 3.

FIGURE 2 ■ *Elastic cartilage. Epiglottis. Human. Paraffin section.* × 270.

This higher magnification of the perichondrial region of Figure 1 displays the outer **fibrous** (F) and inner **chondrogenic** (CG) regions of the perichondrium. Note that the chondrocytes (arrow) immediately deep to the chondrogenic layer are more or less flattened and smaller than those deeper in the cartilage. Additionally, the amount and coarseness of the elastic fibers increase adjacent to the large cells.

FIGURE 3 ■ *Elastic cartilage. Epiglottis. Human. Paraffin section.* × 540.

This is a high magnification of the boxed area in Figure 1. The **chondrocytes** (C) are large, oval to round cells with acentric **nuclei** (N). The cells accumulate lipids in their cytoplasm, often in the form of lipid droplets, thus imparting to the cell a "vacuolated" appearance. Note that the **elastic fibers** (E) mask the matrix in some areas, and that the fibers are of various thicknesses, especially evident in cross-sections (arrows).

FIGURE 4 ■ *Fibrocartilage. Intervertebral disc. Human. Paraffin section.* × 132.

The **chondrocytes** (C) of fibrocartilage are aligned in parallel rows, lying singly in individual lacunae. The nuclei of these chondrocytes are easily observed, while their cytoplasm is not as evident (arrow). The matrix contains thick bundles of **collagen fibers** (CF), which are arranged in a more or less regular fashion between the rows of cartilage cells. Unlike elastic and hyaline cartilages, fibrocartilage is not enveloped by a perichondrium.

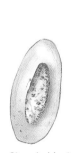 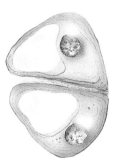

Chondroblast   Chondrocytes

■ **KEY**

C	chondrocyte	E	elastic fiber	N	nucleus
CF	collagen fiber	F	fibrous perichondrium	P	perichondrium
Cg	chondrogenic perichondrium				

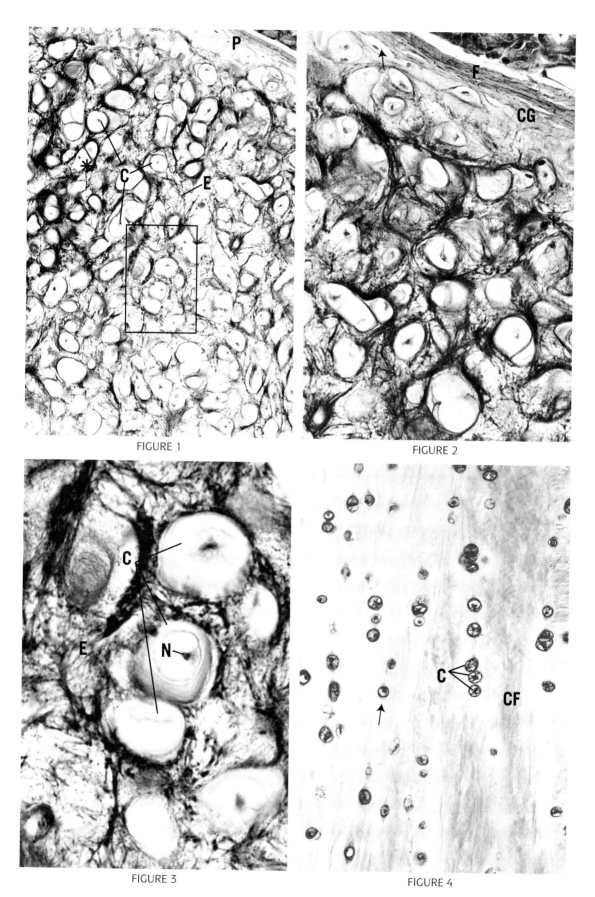

FIGURE 1

FIGURE 2

FIGURE 3

FIGURE 4

PLATE 4-3 ■ *Compact Bone*

FIGURE 1 ■ *Decalcified compact bone. Human. Paraffin section.* × 132.

Cross-section of decalcified bone, displaying **skeletal muscle** (SM) fibers that will insert a short distance from this site. The outer **fibrous periosteum** (FP) and the inner **osteogenic periosteum** (OP) are distinguishable due to the fibrous component of the former and the cellularity of the latter. Note the presence of the **inner circumferential** (IC) **lamellae, osteons** (Os), and interstitial lamellae (asterisk). Also observe the **marrow** (M) occupying the marrow cavity, as well as the endosteal lining (arrow).

FIGURE 2 ■ *Decalcified compact bone. Human. Paraffin section.* × 132.

This is a cross-section of decalcified compact bone, displaying **osteons** or **haversian canal systems** (Os), as well as **interstitial lamellae** (IL). Each osteon possesses a central **haversian canal** (HC), surrounded by several **lamellae** (L) of bone. The boundary of each osteon is visible and is referred to as a cementing line (arrowheads). Neighboring haversian canals are connected to each other by **Volkmann's canals** (VC), through which blood vessels of osteons are interconnected to each other.

FIGURE 3 ■ *Decalcified compact bone. Human. Paraffin section.* × 540.

A small osteon is delineated by its surrounding cementing line (arrowheads). The lenticular-shaped **osteocytes** (Oc) occupy flattened spaces, known as lacunae. The lacunae are lined by uncalcified osteoid matrix.

Inset. **Decalcified compact bone. Human. Paraffin section.** × 540.

A haversian canal of an osteon is shown to contain a small **blood vessel** (BV) supported by slender connective tissue elements. The canal is lined by flattened **osteoblasts** (Ob) and, perhaps, **osteogenic cells** (Op).

FIGURE 4 ■ *Undecalcified ground compact bone. x.s. Human. Paraffin section.* × 132.

This specimen was treated with India ink in order to accentuate some of the salient features of compact bone. The **haversian canals** (HC) as well as the lacunae (arrows) appear black in the figure. Note the connection between two osteons at top center, known as **Volkmann's canal** (VC). The canaliculi appear as fine, narrow lines leading to the haversian canal as they anastomose with each other and with lacunae of other osteocytes of the same osteon.

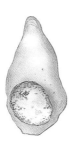
Osteoblast

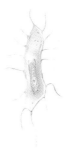
Osteocyte

■ **KEY**

BV	blood vessel	IL	interstitial lamella	Op	osteogenic cell
FP	fibrous periosteum	L	lamella	OP	osteogenic periosteum
HC	haversian canal	M	marrow	Os	osteon
IC	inner circumferential lamella	Ob	osteoblast	SM	skeletal muscle fiber
		Oc	osteocyte	VC	Volkmann's canal

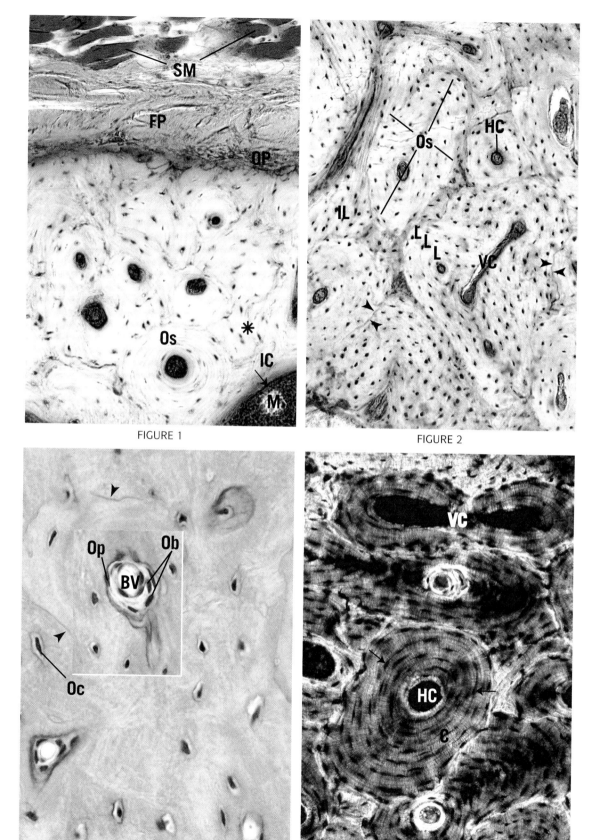

FIGURE 1

FIGURE 2

FIGURE 3

FIGURE 4

Cartilage and Bone ■ 79

PLATE 4-4 ■ *Compact Bone and Intramembranous Ossification*

FIGURE 1 ■ *Undecalcified ground bone. x.s. Human. Paraffin section.* × 270.

This transverse section of an osteon clearly displays the **lamellae** (L) of bone surrounding the **haversian canal** (HC). The cementing line acts to delineate the periphery of the osteon. Note that the **canaliculi** (C) arising from the peripheral-most lacunae usually do not extend toward other osteons. Instead, they lead toward the haversian canal. Canaliculi, which appear to anastomose with each other and with lacunae, house long osteocytic processes in the living bone.

FIGURE 2 ■ *Intramembranous ossification. Pig skull. Paraffin section.* × 132.

The anastomosing **trabeculae** (T) of forming bone appear darkly stained in a background of **embryonic connective tissue** (ECT). Observe that this connective tissue is highly vascular and that the bony trabeculae are forming primitive **osteons** (Os) surrounding large, primitive **haversian canals** (HC), whose center is occupied by **blood vessels** (BV). Observe that the **osteocytes** (Oc) are arranged somewhat haphazardly. Every trabecula is covered by **osteoblasts** (Ob).

FIGURE 3 ■ *Intramembranous ossification. Pig skull. Paraffin section.* × 270.

This photomicrograph of intramenbranous ossification is taken from the periphery of the bone-forming region. Note the developing **periosteum** (P) in the upper right-hand corner. Just deep to this primitive periosteum, **osteoblasts** (Ob) are differentiating and are elaborating **osteoid** (Ot), as yet uncalcified bone matrix. As the osteoblasts surround themselves with bone matrix, they become trapped in their lacunae and are known as **osteocytes** (Oc). These osteocytes are more numerous, larger, and more ovoid than those of mature bone, and the organization of the collagen fibers of the bony matrix is less precise than that of mature bone. Hence, this bone is referred to as immature (primary) bone, and it will be replaced by mature bone later in life.

FIGURE 4 ■ *Intramembranous ossification. Pig skull. Paraffin section.* × 540.

This photomicrograph is taken from an area similar to those of Figures 2 and 3. This trabecula demonstrates several points, namely that **osteoblasts** (Ob) cover the entire surface, and that **osteoid** (Ot) is interposed between calcified bone and the cells of bone and it appears lighter in color. Additionally, note that the osteoblast marked with the asterisk is apparently trapping itself in the matrix it is elaborating. Finally, note the large, multinuclear cells, **osteoclasts** (Ocl), which are in the process of resorbing bone. The activity of these large cells results in the formation of Howship's lacunae (arrowheads), which are shallow depressions on the bone surface. The interactions between osteoclasts and osteoblasts are very finely regulated in the normal formation and remodeling of bone.

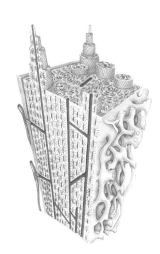

Compact bone

■ **KEY**

BV	blood vessel	L	lamella	Os	osteon
C	canaliculus	Ob	osteoblast	Ot	osteoid
ECT	embryonic connective tissue	Oc	osteocyte	P	periosteum
HC	haversian canal	Ocl	osteoclast	T	trabecula

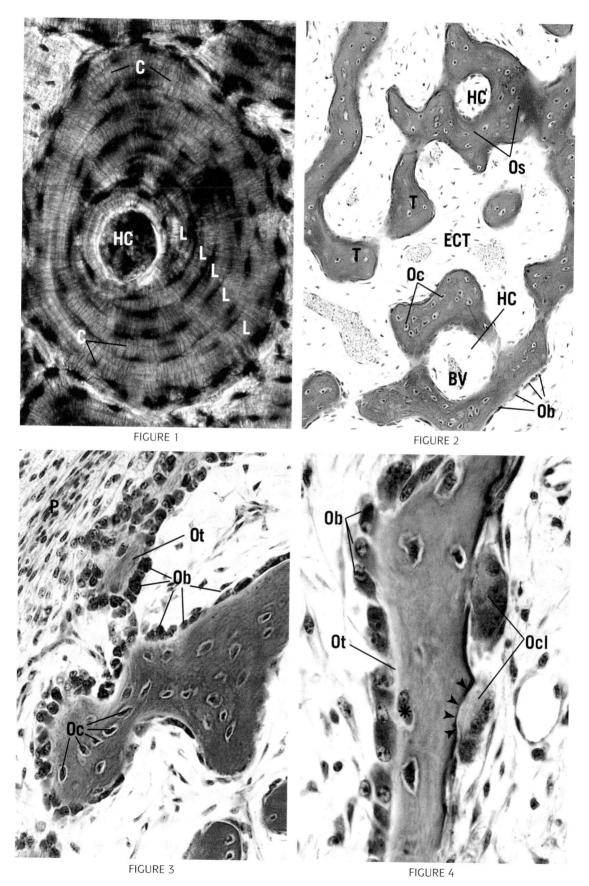

FIGURE 1

FIGURE 2

FIGURE 3

FIGURE 4

PLATE 4-5 ■ *Endochondral Ossification*

FIGURE 1 ▨ *Epiphyseal ossification center. Monkey. Paraffin section.* × 14.

Most long bones are formed by the endochondral method of ossification, which involves the replacement of a cartilage model by bone. In this low power photomicrograph, the **diaphysis** (D) of the lower phalanx has been replaced by bone, and the medullary cavity is filled with **marrow** (M). The **epiphysis** (E) of the same phalanx is undergoing ossification and is the **secondary center of ossification** (2°), thereby establishing the **epiphyseal plate** (ED). The **trabeculae** (T) are clearly evident on the diaphyseal side of the epiphyseal plate.

FIGURE 2 ■ *Endochondral ossification. l.s. Monkey. Paraffin section.* × 14.

Much of the cartilage has been replaced in the diaphysis of this forming bone. Note the numerous **trabeculae** (T) and the developing **bone marrow** (M) of the medullary cavity. Ossification is advancing toward the **epiphysis** (E), in which the secondary center of ossification has not yet appeared. Observe the **periosteum** (P), which appears as a definite line between the subperiosteal bone collar and the surrounding connective tissue. The boxed area is represented in Figure 3.

FIGURE 3 ▨ *Endochondral ossification. Monkey. Paraffin section.* × 132.

This montage is a higher magnification of the boxed area of Figure 2. The region where the periosteum and perichondrium meet is evident (arrowheads). Deep to the periosteum is the **subperiosteal bone collar** (BC), which was formed via intramembranous ossification. Endochondral ossification is evident within the cartilage template. Starting at the top of the montage, note how the chondrocytes are lined up in long columns (arrows), indicative of their intense mitotic activity at the future epiphyseal plate region. In the epiphyseal plate this will be the **zone of cell proliferation** (ZP). The chondrocytes increase in size in the **zone of cell maturation and hypertrophy** (ZH) and resorb some of their lacunar walls, enlarging them to such an extent that some of the lacunae become confluent. The chondrocytes die in the **zone of calcifying cartilage** (ZC). The presumptive medullary cavity is being populated by bone marrow, osteoclastic and osteogenic cells, and blood vessels. The osteogenic cells are actively differentiating into osteoblasts, which are elaborating bone on the calcified walls of the confluent lacunae. At the bottom of the photomicrograph observe the bone-covered trabeculae of calcified cartilage (asterisks).

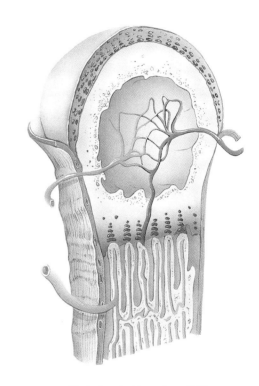

Endochondral bone formation

■ **KEY**

BC	subperiosteal bone collar	P	periosteum	ZC	zone of calcifying cartilage
D	diaphysis	2°	secondary center of ossification	ZH	zone of cell maturation and hypertrophy
E	epiphysis				
ED	epiphyseal plate	T	trabecula	ZP	zone of proliferation
M	marrow				

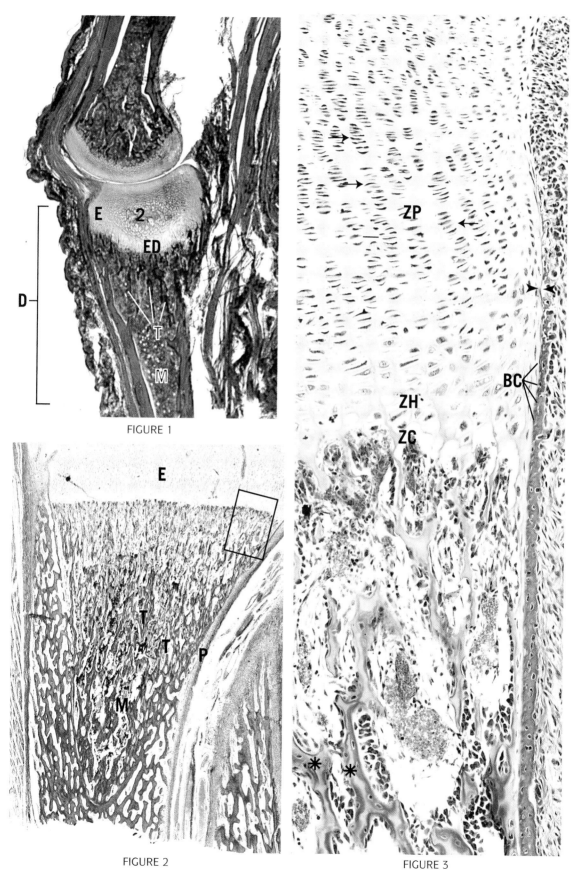

FIGURE 1

FIGURE 2

FIGURE 3

Cartilage and Bone ▪ 83

PLATE 4-6 ■ *Endochondral Ossification*

FIGURE 1 ■ *Endochondral ossification. Monkey. Paraffin section.* × 132.

This photomicrograph is a higher magnification of a region of Plate 4.5, Figure 3. Observe the multinucleated osteoclast (arrowheads) resorbing the bone-covered trabeculae of calcified cartilage. The **subperiosteal bone collar** (BC) and the **periosteum** (P) are clearly evident, as is the junction between the bone collar and the cartilage (arrows). The medullary cavity is being established and is populated by **blood vessels** (BV), osteogenic cells, osteoblasts, and hematopoietic cells.

FIGURE 2 ■ *Endochondral ossification. Monkey. Paraffin section.* × 270.

This photomicrograph is a higher magnification of the boxed area in Figure 1. Note that the trabeculae of calcified cartilage are covered by a thin layer of bone. The darker staining bone (arrow) contains osteocytes, while the lighter staining **calcified cartilage** (CC) is acellular, since the chondrocytes of this region have died, leaving behind empty lacunae that are confluent with each other. Observe that **osteoblasts** (Ob) line the trabecular complexes, and that they are separated from the calcified bone by thin intervening **osteoid** (Ot). As the subperiosteal bone collar increases in thickness, the trabeculae of bone-covered calcified cartilage will be resorbed so that the cartilage template will be replaced by bone. The only cartilage that will remain will be the epiphyseal plate and the articular covering of the epiphysis.

FIGURE 3 ■ *Endochondral ossification. x.s. Monkey. Paraffin section.* × 196.

A cross-section of the region of endochondral ossification presents many round spaces in calcified cartilage that are lined with bone (asterisks). These spaces represent confluent lacunae in the cartilage template, where the chondrocytes have hypertrophied and died. Subsequently, the cartilage calcified and the invading osteogenic cells have differentiated into osteoblasts (arrowheads) and lined the calcified cartilage with bone. Since neighboring spaces were separated from each other by calcified cartilage walls, bone was elaborated on the sides of the walls. Therefore, these trabeculae, which in longitudinal section appear to be stalactite-like structures of bone with a calcified cartilaginous core are, in fact, spaces in the cartilage template that are lined with bone. The walls between the spaces are the remnants of cartilage between lacunae that became calcified and form the substructure upon which bone was elaborated.

Observe the forming **medullary cavity** (MC), housing **blood vessels** (BV), **hematopoietic tissue** (HT), osteogenic cells, and osteoblasts (arrowheads). The **subperiosteal bone collar** (BC) is evident and is covered by a **periosteum,** whose two layers, **fibrous** (FP) and **osteogenic** (Og), are clearly discernible.

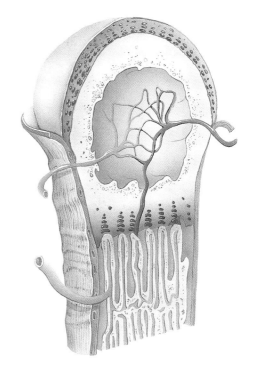

Endochondral bone formation

■ KEY

BC	subperiosteal bone collar	HT	hematopoietic tissue	Og	osteogenic periosteum
BV	blood vessel	MC	medullary cavity	Ot	osteoid
CC	calcified cartilage	Ob	osteoblast	P	periosteum
FP	fibrous periosteum				

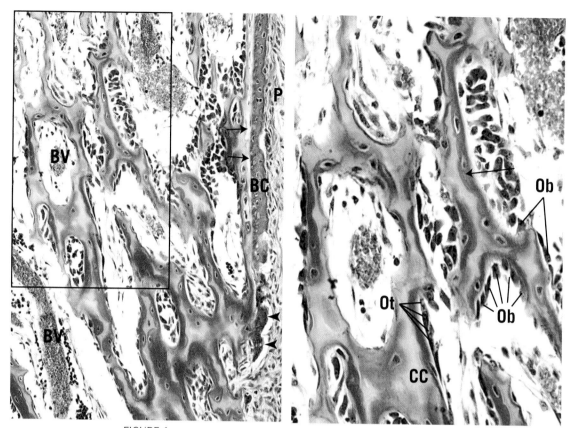

FIGURE 1

FIGURE 2

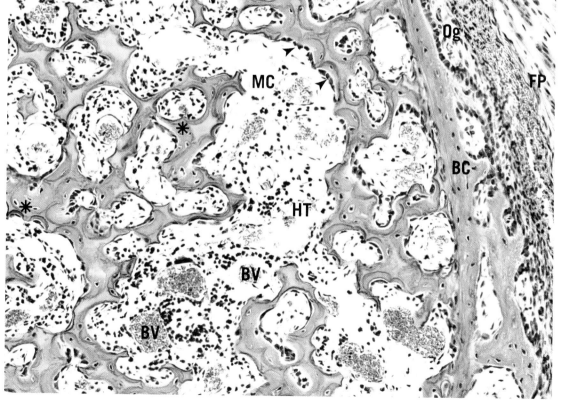

FIGURE 3

PLATE 4-7 ■ *Hyaline Cartilage, Electron Microscopy*

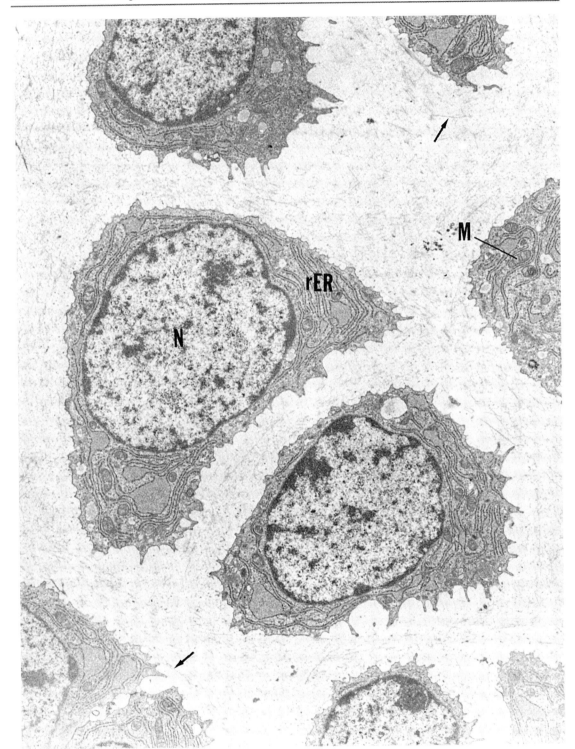

FIGURE 1 ■ *Hyaline cartilage. Mouse. Electron microscopy.* × 6120.

The hyaline cartilage of a neonatal mouse trachea presents chondrocytes, whose centrally positioned **nuclei** (N) are surrounded with a rich **rough endoplasmic retic-**ulum (rER) and numerous **mitochondria** (M). The matrix displays fine collagen fibrils (arrows). (From Seegmiller R, Ferguson C, Sheldon H: *J Ultrastruct Res* 38:288–301, 1972.)

PLATE 4-8 ■ *Osteoblasts, Electron Microscopy*

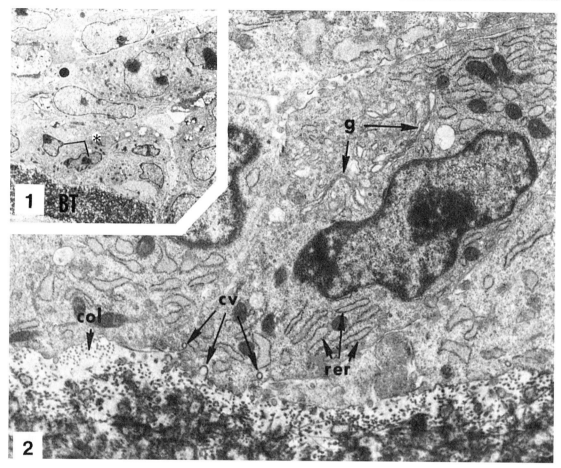

FIGURE 1 ▓ *Osteoblasts from long bone. Rat. Electron microscopy.* × 1350.

This low magnification electron micrograph displays numerous fibroblasts and osteoblasts in the vicinity of a **bony trabecula** (BT). The osteoblasts (asterisk) are presented at a higher magnification in Figure 2. (From Ryder M, Jenkins S, Horton J: *J Dent Res* 60:1349–1355, 1981.)

FIGURE 2 ▓ *Osteoblasts. Rat. Electron microscopy.* × 9450.

Osteoblasts, at higher magnification, present well-developed **Golgi apparatus** (g), extensive **rough endoplasmic reticulum** (rer), and several **coated vacuoles** (cv) at the basal cell membrane. Observe the cross-sections of **collagen fibers** (col) in the bone matrix. (From Ryder M, Jenkins S, Horton J: *J Dent Res* 60:1349–1355, 1981.)

PLATE 4-9 ■ *Osteoclast, Electron Microscopy*

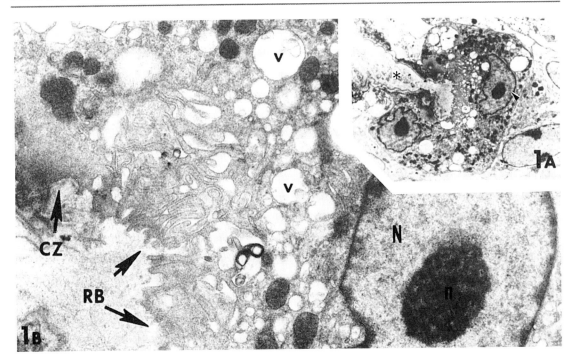

FIGURE 1A ■ *Osteoclast from long bone. Rat. Electron microscopy.* × 1800.

Two nuclei of an osteoclast are evident in this section. Observe that the cell is surrounding a bony surface (asterisk). The region of the nucleus marked by an arrowhead is presented at a higher magnification in Figure 1B.

FIGURE 1B ■ *Osteoclast. Rat. Electron microscopy.* × 10,800.

This is a higher magnification of a region of Figure 1A. Note the presence of the **nucleus** (N) and its **nucleolus** (n), as well as the **ruffled border** (RB) and **clear zone** (CZ) of the osteoclast. Numerous **vacuoles** (v) of various size may be observed throughout the cytoplasm. (From Ryder M, Jenkins S, Horton J: *J Dent Res* 60:1349–1355, 1981.)

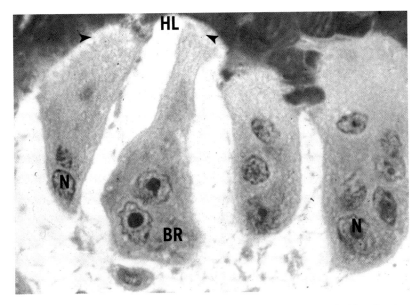

FIGURE 2 ■ *Osteoclasts. Human. Paraffin section.* × 600.

The nuclei (N) of these multinuclear cells are located in their **basal region** (BR), away from **Howship's lacunae** (HL). Note that the **ruffled border** (arrowheads) is in intimate contact with Howship's lacunae. (Courtesy of Dr. J. Hollinger.)

Blood and Hemopoiesis

The total volume of blood in an average person is approximately 5 liters; it is a **specialized type of connective tissue,** composed of cells, cell fragments, and plasma, a fluid extracellular element. Blood circulates throughout the body and is well adapted for its manifold functions in transporting nutrients, oxygen, waste products, carbon dioxide, hormones, cells, and other substances. Moreover, blood also functions in the maintenance of body temperature.

FORMED ELEMENTS OF BLOOD

The formed elements of blood are red blood cells (erythrocytes), white blood cells (leukocytes), and platelets. **Red blood cells (RBC),** the most populous, are anucleated and function entirely within the circulatory system by transporting oxygen and carbon dioxide to and from the tissues of the body. **White blood cells (WBC)** perform their functions outside the circulatory system and use the bloodstream as a mode of transportation to reach their destinations. There are two major categories of white blood cells, **agranulocytes** and **granulocytes.** Lymphocytes and monocytes compose the first group, whereas neutrophils, eosinophils, and basophils compose the latter. **Lymphocytes** are the basic cells of the immune system and, although there are three categories (**T lymphocytes, B lymphocytes,** and **null cells**), special immunocytochemical techniques are necessary for their identification. When **monocytes** leave the bloodstream and enter the connective tissue spaces, they become known as **macrophages,** cells that function in phagocytosis of particulate matter, as well as in assisting lymphocytes in their immunologic activities. **Granulocytes** are recognizable by their distinctive specific granules, whose coloration provides the classification for these cells. Granules of **neutrophils** possess very limited affinity to stains, whereas those of **eosinophils** stain a reddish-orange color and those of **basophils** stain a dark blue color with dyes used in studying blood preparations. Neutrophils function in **phagocytosis** of bacteria and because of that they are frequently referred to as microphages. Eosinophils participate in antiparasitic activities and phagocytose antigen-antibody complexes. Although the precise function of basophils is unknown, the contents of their granules are similar to those of mast cells and they also release these pharmacologic agents via degranulation. Additionally, basophils also produce and release other pharmacologic agents from the arachidonic acid in their membranes.

Circulating blood also contains cell fragments known as **platelets (thrombocytes).** These small, oval-to-round structures derived from **megakaryocytes** of the bone marrow function in hemostasis, the clotting mechanism of blood.

PLASMA

Plasma, the fluid component of blood, comprises approximately 55% of the total blood volume. It contains electrolytes and ions, such as calcium, sodium, potassium, and bicarbonate; larger molecules, namely, **albumins, globulins,** and **fibrinogen;** and organic compounds as varied as amino acids, lipids, vitamins, hormones, and cofactors. Subsequent to clotting, a straw-colored **serum** is expressed from blood. This fluid is identical to plasma but contains no fibrinogen or other components necessary for the clotting reaction.

HEMOPOIESIS

Circulating blood cells have relatively short life spans and must be replaced continuously by newly formed cells. This process of blood cell replacement is known as hemopoiesis (hematopoiesis). All blood cells develop from a single pluripotential precursor cell known as the **pluripotential hemopoietic stem cell (PHSC).** These cells undergo mitotic activity, whereby they give rise to two types of **multipotential** hemopoietic stem cells, **CFU-S** (colony-forming unit-spleen) and **CFU-Ly** (colony-forming unit-lymphocyte). Most PHSCs and other hemopoietic stem cells of adults are located in the **red bone marrow** of short and flat bones. The marrow of long bones is red in young individuals, but when it becomes infiltrated by fat in the adult, it takes on a yellow appearance and is known as yellow marrow. Although it was once believed that adipose cells accumulated the fat, it is now known that the cells actually responsible for storing fat in the marrow are the **adventitial reticular cells.** Stem cells, in response to various hemopoietic growth factors, undergo cell division and maintain the population of circulating erythrocytes, leukocytes, and platelets.

The nomenclature developed for the cells described below is based on their colorations with dyes utilized in hematology.

Erythrocytic Series

Erythrocyte development proceeds from **CFU-S,** which, in response to elevated levels of **erythropoietin,** gives rise to cells known as BFU-E, which, in response to lower erythropoietin levels, then give rise to CFU-E. Although there are several generations of

CFU-E, the later ones are recognizable histologically as **proerythroblasts.** These cells give rise to **basophilic erythroblasts,** which, in turn, undergo cell division to form **polychromatophilic erythroblasts** that will divide mitotically to form **orthochromatophilic erythroblasts (normoblasts).** Cells of this stage no longer divide, will extrude their nuclei, and differentiate into **reticulocytes** (not to be confused with reticular cells of connective tissue), which, in turn, become mature red blood cells.

Granulocytic Series

The development of the granulocytic series is initiated from the multipotential CFU-S. The first histologically distinguishable member of this series is the **myeloblast,** which gives rise mitotically to **promyelocytes,** which also undergo cell division to yield **myelocytes.** Myelocytes are the first cells of this series to possess specific granules; therefore, neutrophilic, eosinophilic, and basophilic myelocytes may be recognized. The next cells in the series are **metamyelocytes,** which no longer divide, but differentiate into **band (stab)** cells, the juvenile form, which will become mature granulocytes that enter the bloodstream (Table 5-1).

TABLE 5-1 ■ *Formed Elements of Blood*

| Element | Diameter (mm) | | No./mm^3 | % of Leukocytes | Granules | Function | Nucleus |
	Smear	Section					
Erythrocyte	7–8	6–7	5 × 10^6 (males) 4.5 × 10^6 (females)		None	Transport of O$_2$ and CO$_2$	None
Lymphocyte	8–10	7–8	1500–2500	20–25	Azurophilic only	Immunologic response	Large round acentric
Monocyte	12–15	10–12	200–800	3–8	Azurophilic only	Phagocytosis	Large, kidney-shaped
Neutrophil	9–12	8–9	3500–7000	60–70	Azurophilic and small specific (neutrophilic)	Phagocytosis	Polymorphous
Eosinophil	10–14	9–11	150–400	2–4	Azurophilic and large specific (eosinophilic)	Phagocytosis of antigen–antibody complexes and control of parasitic diseases	Bilobed (sausage-shaped)
Basophil	8–10	7–8	50–100	0.5–1	Azurophilic and large specific (basophilic) granules (heparin and histamine)	Perhaps phagocytosis	Large, S-shaped
Platelets	2–4	1–3	250,000–400,000		Granulomere	Agglutination and clotting	None

Histophysiology

I. COAGULATION

Coagulation is the result of the exquisitely controlled interaction of a number of plasma proteins and coagulation factors. The regulatory mechanisms are in place so that coagulation typically occurs only if the endothelial lining of the vessel becomes injured. The process of coagulation ensues in one of two convergent pathways, **extrinsic** and **intrinsic,** both of which lead to the final step of converting fibrinogen to fibrin. The extrinsic pathway has a faster onset and depends on the release of **tissue thromboplastin.** The intrinsic pathway is initiated slower, is dependent on contact between vessel wall collagen and platelets (or factor XII), and requires the presence of **von Willebrand's factor** and **factor VIII.** These two factors form a complex that not only binds to exposed collagen, but also attaches to receptor sites on the platelet plasmalemma, affecting platelet aggregation and adherence to the vessel wall.

II. NEUTROPHIL FUNCTION

Neutrophils possess three types of granules—specific granules, azurophilic granules, and tertiary granules. **Specific granules** contain pharmacologic agents and enzymes that permit the neutrophils to perform their antimicrobial roles. **Azurophilic granules** are lysosomes, containing the various lysosomal hydrolases, as well as myeloperoxidase, bacterial permeability increasing protein, lysozyme, and collagenase. **Tertiary granules** contain glycoproteins that are dedicated for insertion into the cell membrane, as well as gelatinase and cathepsins. These cells use the contents of the three types of granules to perform their antimicrobial function. When neutrophils arrive at their site of action, they exocytose the contents of their granules. Gelatinase increases the neutrophil's capability of migrating through the basal lamina and the glycoproteins of the tertiary granules aids in the recognition and phagocytosis of bacteria into phagosomes of the neutrophil. Azurophilic granules and specific granules fuse with and release their hydrolytic enzymes into the phagosomes, thus initiating the enzymatic degradation of the microorganisms. In addition to the enzymatic degradation, microorganisms are also destroyed by the capability of neutrophils to undergo a sudden increase in O_2 utilization, known as a respiratory burst. The O_2 is used by the cell to form superoxides, hydrogen peroxide, and hypochlorous acid, highly reactive compounds that destroy bacteria within the phagosomes. Frequently, the avid response of neutrophils results in the release of some of these highly potent compounds into the surrounding connective tissue precipitating tissue damage. The neutrophils also produce leukotrienes from plasmalemma arachidonic acids to aid in the initiation of an inflammatory response. Subsequent to the performance of these functions, the neutrophils die and become a major component of pus.

III. POSTNATAL HEMOPOIESIS

Hemopoiesis in the adult involves a single type of stem cell, the **pluripotential hemopoietic stem cell (PHSC),** which resembles a lymphocyte and is a member of the **null cell** population of lymphocytes. PHSCs are located in large numbers in the bone marrow, but they are also present in circulating blood. These cells have a high mitotic index and form more PHSCs, as well as two **multipotential hemopoietic stem cells, CFU-S** and **CFU-Ly.** Morphologically, CFU-S and CFU-Ly are identical with PHSCs, but they have a more limited potential. CFU-Ly, known as the **lymphoid stem cell,** will give rise to CFU-LyB and CFU-LyT, the progenitors of B and T lymphocytes, respectively. CFU-S is also referred to as the **myeloid stem cell,** since it will give rise to BFU-E (and/or **CFU-E**), the progenitor of erythrocytes; **CFU-Eo,** the progenitor of eosinophils; **CFU-Ba,** the progenitor of basophils; and **CFU-NM,** which will give rise to CFU-N and CFU-M, the progenitors of neutrophils and monocytes, respectively. **Stem cells** and **progenitor cells** resemble lymphocytes, whereas **precursor cells** can be recognized histologically as members of a cell population that will differentiate into a particular blood cell. Furthermore, stem cells are less committed than are progenitor cells.

Several **hemopoietic growth factors** activate and promote hemopoiesis. These act by binding to plasma membrane receptors of their target cell, controlling their mitotic rate, as well as the number of mitotic events. Additionally, they stimulate cell differentiation and enhance the survival of the progenitor cell population. The best known factors are **erythropoietin** (acts on BFU-E and CFU-E), **interleukin-3** (acts on PHSC, CFU-S, and myeloid progenitor cells), **interleukin-7** (acts on CFU-Ly), **granulocyte-macrophage colony-stimulating factor** (acts on granulocyte and monocyte progenitor cells), **granulocyte colony-stimulating factor** (acts on granulocyte progenitor cells), and **macrophage colony-stimulating factor** (acts on monocyte progenitor cells).

IV. LYMPHOCYTES

The three types of lymphocytes—B lymphocytes (B cells), T lymphocytes (T cells), and null cells—are morphologically indistinguishable. It is customary to speak of **T cells** as being responsible for the **cellularly mediated immune response** and **B cells** as functioning in the **humorally mediated immune response**. Null cells are few in number, possess no determinants on their cell membrane, and are of two types, **pluripotential hemopoietic stem cells** and **natural killer cells**.

A. T Cells

T cells not only function in the cellularly mediated immune response, but also are responsible for the formation of cytokines that facilitate the initiation of the humorally mediated immune response. They are formed in the bone marrow and migrate to the thymic cortex to become immunocompetent cells. They recognize **epitopes** (antigenic determinants) that are displayed by cells possessing **HLA** (human leukocyte antigen; also known as major histocompatibility complex molecules). There are various subtypes of T cells, each possessing a **T-cell receptor (TCR)** surface determinant and **cluster of differentiation determinants (CD molecules)**. The former recognizes the epitope, whereas the latter recognizes the type of HLA on the displaying cell surface.

The various subtypes of T cells are T helper cells (T_H1 and T_H2), cytotoxic T cells (T_C), T suppressor cells (T_S), and T memory cells.

B. B Cells

B cells bear HLA type II (also known as MHC II) surface markers and **surface immunoglobulins (SIG)** on their plasmalemma. They are formed in and become immunocompetent in the bone marrow. They are responsible for the humoral response and, under the direction of T_H2 cells and in response to an antigenic challenge, will differentiate into antibody-manufacturing **plasma cells** and **B memory cells**.

C. Natural Killer (NK) Cells

NK cells belong to the null cell population. They possess F_C receptors but no cell surface determinants and are responsible for **nonspecific cytotoxicity** against virus-infected and tumor cells. They also function in **antibody-dependent cell-mediated cytotoxicity (ADCC)**.

Clinical Considerations ▨ ▨ ■

NADPH Oxidase Deficiency
Certain individuals suffer from persistent bacterial infection due to a hereditary NADPH oxidase deficiency. The neutrophils of these individuals are unable to effect a respiratory burst and, therefore, are incapable of forming the highly reactive compounds, such as hypochlorous acid, hydrogen peroxide, and superoxide that assist in the killing of bacteria within their phagosomes.

Multiple Myeloma
Multiple myeloma is a relatively uncommon malignant neoplasm with greater incidence in males than females. Its origin is the bone marrow and is characterized by the presence of large numbers of malignant plasma cells that may also be abnormal in morphology. These cells accumulate in the bone marrow of various regions of the skeletal system. Frequently the cell proliferation is so great in the marrow that the huge number of cells place pressure on the walls of the marrow cavity causing bone pains and even fractures of bones such as the ribs. These cells also produce abnormal proteins such as Bence-Jones proteins that enter the urine where they can be detected to provide a diagnosis for multiple myeloma. Treatment includes local radiation therapy, aimed at the bones in which the patient is experiencing pain. Patients with Bence-Jones proteins in their urine are instructed to drink lots of fluids to reduce the chances of dehydration and of kidney failure. Chemotherapy has been shown to be effective in reducing the progression of the disease.

Summary of Histological Organization

I. CIRCULATING BLOOD[a]

A. Erythrocytes (RBC)

RBCs are pink, biconcave disks that are 7–8 μm in diameter. They are filled with hemoglobin and possess no nuclei.

B. Agranulocytes

1. Lymphocytes

Histologically, **lymphocytes** may be **small, medium,** or **large** (this bears no relationship to T cells, B cells, or null cells). Most lymphocytes are small (8–10 μm in diameter) and possess a dense, blue, acentrically positioned nucleus that occupies most of the cell, leaving a thin rim of light blue, peripheral cytoplasm. Azurophilic granules (lysosomes) may be evident in the cytoplasm.

2. Monocytes

Monocytes are the largest of all circulating blood cells (12–15 μm in diameter). There is a considerable amount of **grayish-blue cytoplasm** containing numerous azurophilic granules. The **nucleus** is acentric and kidney-shaped and possesses a coarse chromatin network with clear spaces. Lobes of the nucleus are superimposed on themselves, and their outlines appear to be distinctly demarcated.

C. Granulocytes

1. Neutrophils
Neutrophils, the most populous of the leukocytes, are 9–12 μm in diameter and display a **light pink cytoplasm** housing many **azurophilic** and smaller **specific granules**. The specific granules do not stain well, hence the name of these cells. The **nucleus** is dark blue, coarse, and **multilobed,** with most being two- to three-lobed with thin connecting strands.

2. Eosinophils
Eosinophils are 10–14 μm in diameter and possess numerous refractive, spherical, large, reddish-orange **specific granules**. Azurophilic granules are also present. The **nucleus,** which is brownish-black, is **bilobed,** resembling sausage links united by a thin connecting strand.

3. Basophils
Basophils, the least numerous of all leukocytes, are 8–10 μm in diameter. Frequently, their cytoplasm is so filled with dark, large, **basophilic specific granules** that they appear to press against the cell membrane, giving it an angular appearance. The specific granules usually mask the **azurophilic granules,** as well as the S-shaped, light blue nucleus.

D. Platelets

Platelets, occasionally called **thrombocytes,** are small, round (2–4 μm in diameter) cell fragments. As such, they possess no nuclei, are frequently clumped together, and present with a dark blue, central granular region, the **granulomere,** and a light blue, peripheral, clear region, the **hyalomere.**

II. HEMOPOIESIS[a]

During the maturation process, hemopoietic cells undergo clearly evident morphologic alterations. As the cells become more mature, they decrease in size. Their nuclei also become smaller, the chromatin network appears coarser, and their nucleoli (which resemble pale grayish spaces) disappear. The granulocytes first acquire azurophilic and then specific granules, and their nuclei become segmented. Cells of the erythrocytic series never display granules and eventually lose their nuclei.

A. Erythrocytic Series

1. Proerythroblast

a. Cytoplasm
Light blue to deep blue clumps in a pale grayish-blue background.

b. Nucleus
Round with a fine chromatin network; it is a rich burgundy red with 3–5 pale gray nucleoli.

2. Basophilic Erythroblast

a. Cytoplasm
Bluish clumps in a pale blue cytoplasm with a hint of grayish pink in the background.

b. Nucleus
Round, somewhat coarser than the previous stage; burgundy red. A nucleolus may be present.

---

[a] All of the colors designated in this summary are based on the Wright or Giemsa's modification of the Romanovsky-type stains as applied to blood smears.

3. Polychromatophilic Erythroblast

a. Cytoplasm

Yellowish pink with bluish tinge.

b. Nucleus

Small and round with a condensed, coarse chromatin network; dark, reddish black. No nucleoli are present.

4. Orthochromatophilic Erythroblast

a. Cytoplasm

Pinkish with a slight tinge of blue.

b. Nucleus

Dark, condensed, round structure that may be in the process of being extruded from the cell.

5. Reticulocyte

a. Cytoplasm

Appears just like a normal, circulating RBC; if stained with supravital dyes (e.g., methylene blue), however, a bluish reticulum—composed mostly of rough endoplasmic reticulum—is evident.

b. Nucleus

Not present.

B. Granulocytic Series

The first two stages of the granulocytic series, the myeloblast and promyelocyte, possess no specific granules. These make their appearance in the myelocyte stage, when the three types of myelocytes (neutrophilic, eosinophilic, and basophilic) may be distinguished. Since they only differ from each other in their specific granules, only the neutrophilic series is described in this summary, with the understanding that myelocytes, metamyelocytes, and stab (band) cells occur in these three varieties.

1. Myeloblast

a. Cytoplasm

Small blue clumps in a light blue background. No granules. Cytoplasmic blebs extend along the periphery of the cell.

b. Nucleus

Reddish-blue, round nucleus with fine chromatin network. Two or three pale gray nucleoli are evident.

2. Promyelocyte

a. Cytoplasm

The cytoplasm is bluish and displays numerous, small, dark, azurophilic granules.

b. Nucleus

Reddish-blue, round nucleus whose chromatin strands appear more coarse than in the previous stage. A nucleolus is usually present.

3. Neutrophilic Myelocyte

a. Cytoplasm

Pale blue cytoplasm containing dark azurophilic and smaller neutrophilic (specific) granules. A clear, paranuclear Golgi region is evident.

b. Nucleus

Round, usually somewhat flattened, acentric nucleus, with a somewhat coarse chromatin network. Nucleoli are not distinct.

4. Neutrophilic Metamyelocyte

a. Cytoplasm

Similar to the previous stage except that the cytoplasm is paler in color and the Golgi area is nestled in the indentation of the nucleus.

b. Nucleus

Kidney-shaped, acentric nucleus with a dense, dark chromatin network. Nucleoli are not present.

5. Neutrophilic Stab (Band) Cell

a. Cytoplasm

A little more blue than the cytoplasm of a mature neutrophil. Both azurophilic and neutrophilic (specific) granules are present.

b. Nucleus

The nucleus is horseshoe-shaped and dark blue, with a very coarse chromatin network. Nucleoli are not present.

PLATE 5-1 ■ *Circulating Blood*

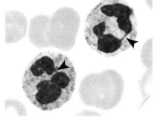

FIGURE 1 ■ *Red Blood Cells. Human.* × 1325.
Red blood cells (arrows) display a central clear region that represents the thinnest area of the biconcave disc. Note that the platelets (arrowheads) possess a central dense region, the granulomere, and a peripheral light region, the hyalomere.

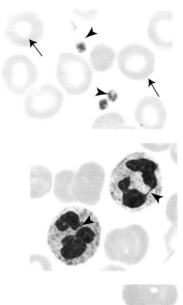

FIGURE 2 ■ *Neutrophils. Human.* × 1325.
Neutrophils display a somewhat granular cytoplasm and lobulated (arrowheads) nuclei.

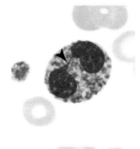

FIGURE 3 ■ *Eosinophils. Human.* × 1325.
Eosinophils are recognized by their large pink granules and their sausage-shaped nucleus. Observe the slender connecting link (arrowhead) between the two lobes of the nucleus.

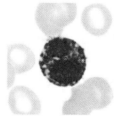

FIGURE 4 ■ *Basophils. Human.* × 1325.
Basophils are characterized by their dense, dark, large granules.

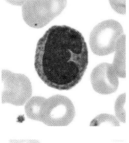

FIGURE 5 ■ *Monocytes. Human.* × 1325.
Monocytes are characterized by their large size, acentric, kidney-shaped nucleus, and lack of specific granules.

FIGURE 6 ■ *Lymphocytes. Human.* × 1325.
Lymphocytes are small cells that possess a single, large, acentrically located nucleus, and a narrow rim of light blue cytoplasm.

PLATE 5-2 ■ *Circulating Blood*

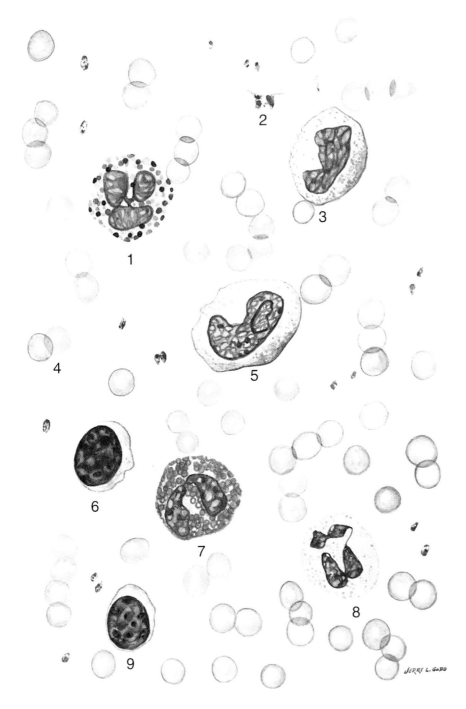

FIGURE 1

■ **KEY**

1. Basophil
2. Platelets
3. Monocyte
4. Erythrocytes
5. Monocyte
6. Lymphocyte
7. Eosinophil
8. Neutrophil
9. Lymphocyte

PLATE 5-3 ■ *Blood and Hemopoiesis*

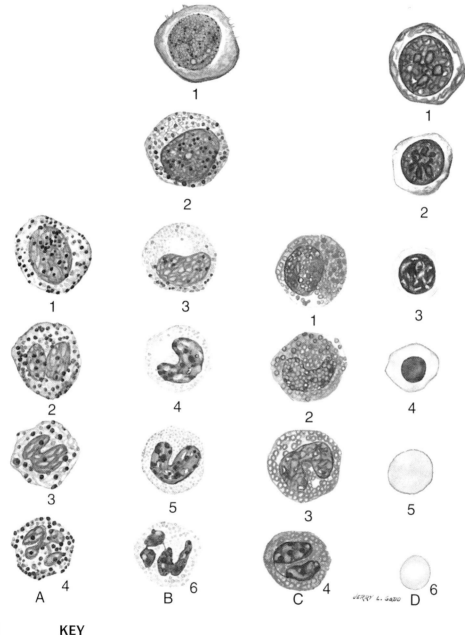

KEY

A
1. Basophilic myelocyte
2. Basophilic metamyelocyte
3. Basophil stab cell
4. Basophil

B
1. Myeloblast
2. Promyelocyte
3. Neutrophilic myelocyte
4. Neutrophilic metamyelocyte
5. Neutrophilic stab cell
6. Neutrophil

C
1. Eosinophilic myelocyte
2. Eosinophilic metamyelocyte
3. Eosinophil stab cell
4. Eosinophil

D
1. Proerythroblast
2. Basophilic erythroblast
3. Polychromatophilic erythroblast
4. Orthochromatophilic erythroblast
5. Reticulocyte
6. Erythrocyte

PLATE 5-4 ■ *Bone Marrow and Circulating Blood*

FIGURE 1 ■ *Bone marrow. Human. Paraffin section.* × 132.

This transverse section of a decalcified human rib displays the presence of **haversian canals** (H), **Volkmann's canals** (V), **osteocytes** (O) in their lacunae, and the **endosteum** (E). The marrow presents numerous **adventitial reticular cells** (A), blood vessels, and **sinusoids** (S). Moreover, the forming blood elements are also evident as small nuclei (arrows). Note the large **megakaryocytes** (M), cells that are the precursors of platelets. The boxed area is represented in Figure 2.

FIGURE 2 ■ *Bone marrow. Human. Paraffin section.* × 270.

This photomicrograph is a higher magnification of the boxed area of Figure 1. Observe the presence of **osteocytes** (O) in their lacunae, as well as the flattened cells of the **endosteum** (E). The endothelial lining of the sinusoids (arrows) are clearly evident, as are the numerous cells that are in the process of hemopoiesis. Two large **megakaryocytes** (M) are also discernible.

FIGURE 3 ■ *Blood smear. Human. Wright stain.* × 270.

This normal blood smear presents **erythrocytes** (R), **neutrophils** (N), and **platelets** (P). The apparent holes in the centers of the erythrocytes represent the thinnest areas of the biconcave discs. Note that the erythrocytes far outnumber the platelets and they, in turn, are much more numerous than the white blood cells. Since neutrophils constitute the highest percentage of white blood cells, they are the ones most frequently encountered of the white blood cell population.

FIGURE 4 ■ *Bone marrow smear. Human. Wright stain.* × 270.

This normal bone marrow smear presents forming blood cells, as well as **erythrocytes** (R) and **platelets** (P). In comparison with a normal peripheral blood smear (Figure 3), marrow possesses many more nucleated cells. Some of these are of the erythrocytic series (arrows), whereas others are of the granulocytic series (arrowheads).

■   **KEY**

A	Adventitial reticular cell	M	Megakaryocyte	R	Erythrocyte
BV	Blood vessel	N	Neutrophil	S	Sinusoid
E	Endosteum	O	Osteocyte	V	Volkmann's canal
H	Haversian canal	P	Platelet		

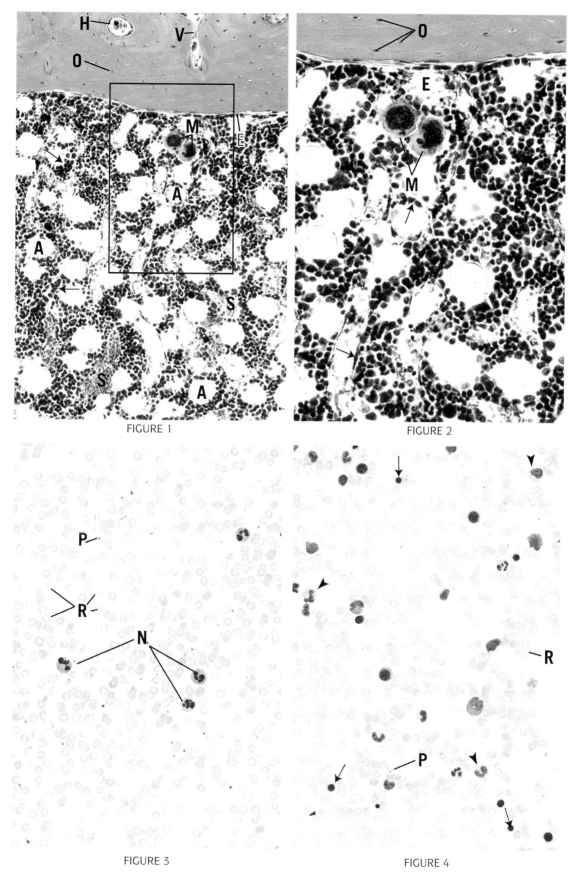

FIGURE 1

FIGURE 2

FIGURE 3

FIGURE 4

PLATE 5-5 ■ *Erythropoiesis*

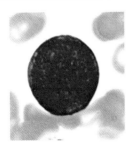

FIGURE 1 ■ *Human marrow smear.* × 1325.
Proerythroblast.

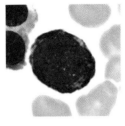

FIGURE 2 ■ *Human marrow smear.* × 1325.
Basophilic erythroblast.

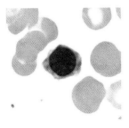

FIGURE 3 ■ *Human marrow smear.* × 1325.
Polychromatophilic erythroblast.

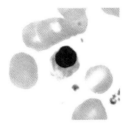

FIGURE 4 ■ *Human marrow smear.* × 1325.
Orthochromatophilic erythroblast.

FIGURE 5 ■ *Human marrow smear.* × 1325.
Reticulocyte.

FIGURE 6 ■ *Human marrow smear.* × 1325.
Erythrocyte.

PLATE 5-6 ■ *Granulocytopoiesis*

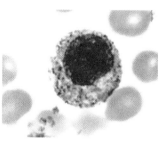

FIGURE 1 ■ *Myeloblast. Human bone marrow smear.* × 1325.

FIGURE 2 ■ *Promyelocyte. Human bone marrow smear.* × 1325.

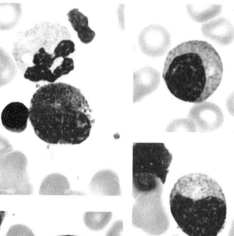

FIGURE 3B ■ *Neutrophilic myelocyte. Human bone marrow smear.* × 1325.

FIGURE 3A ■ *Eosinophilic myelocyte. Human bone marrow smear.* × 1325.

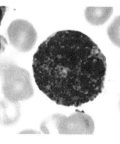

FIGURE 4B ■ *Neutrophilic metamyelocyte. Human bone marrow smear.* × 1325.

FIGURE 4A ■ *Eosinophilic metamyelocyte. Human bone marrow smear.* × 1325.

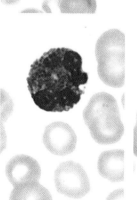

FIGURE 5B ■ *Neutrophilic stab cell. Human bone marrow smear.* × 1325.

FIGURE 5A ■ *Eosinophilic stab cell. Human bone marrow smear.* × 1325.

FIGURE 6 ■ *Neutrophil. Human bone marrow smear.* × 1325.

Muscle

The ability of animals to move is due to the presence of specific cells that have become highly differentiated, so that they function almost exclusively in contraction. The contractile process has been harnessed by the organism to permit various modes of movement and other activities for its survival. Some of these activities depend on quick contractions of short duration; others depend on long-lasting contractions without the necessity for rapid actions, whereas still others depend on powerful, rhythmic contractions that must be repeated in rapid sequences. These varied needs are accommodated by three types of muscle, namely, skeletal, smooth, and cardiac. There are basic similarities among the three muscle types. They are all **mesodermally derived** and are elongated parallel to their axis of contraction; they possess numerous mitochondria to accommodate their high energy requirements, and all contain **contractile elements** known as **myofilaments**, in the form of **actin** and **myosin**, as well as additional contractile-associated proteins. Myofilaments of skeletal and cardiac muscles are arranged in a specific ordered array that gives rise to a repeated sequence of uniform banding along their length—hence, their collective name, **striated muscle**.

Since muscle cells are much longer than they are wide, they are commonly referred to as **muscle fibers**. However, it must be appreciated that these fibers are living entities, unlike the nonliving fibers of connective tissue. Neither are they analogous to nerve fibers, which are living extensions of nerve cells. Often, certain unique terms are used to describe muscle cells; thus, the muscle cell membrane is **sarcolemma** (although earlier use of this term included the attendant basal lamina and reticular fibers), cytoplasm is **sarcoplasm**, mitochondria are **sarcosomes**, and endoplasmic reticulum is **sarcoplasmic reticulum**.

SKELETAL MUSCLE

Skeletal muscle (see Graphics 6-1 and 6-2) is invested by dense collagenous connective tissue known as the **epimysium**, which penetrates the substance of the gross muscle, separating it into fascicles. Each fascicle is surrounded by **perimysium**, a looser connective tissue. Finally, each individual muscle fiber within a fascicle is enveloped by fine reticular fibers, the **endomysium**. The vascular and nerve supplies of the muscle travel in these interrelated connective tissue compartments. Each skeletal muscle fiber is roughly cylindrical in shape, possessing numerous elongated nuclei located at the periphery of the cell, just deep to the sarcolemma. Longitudinally sectioned muscle fibers display intracellular contractile elements, which are the parallel arrays of longitudinally disposed myofibrils. This arrangement produces an overall effect of **cross-banding** of alternating light and dark bands traversing each skeletal muscle cell. The dark bands are **A bands**, and the light bands are **I bands**. Each I band is bisected by a thin dark **Z disc**, and the region of the myofibril extending from Z disc to Z disc, the **sarcomere**, is the contractile unit of skeletal muscle. The A band is bisected by a paler **H zone**, the center of which is marked by the dark **M disc**. During muscle contraction, the various transverse bands behave characteristically, in that the width of the A band remains constant, the two Z discs move closer to each other approaching the A band, and the I band and H zone become extinguished. Electron microscopy has revealed that banding is the result of interdigitation of thick and thin myofilaments. These thin filaments are attached to Z discs by α-actinin. The I band consists solely of thin filaments, while the A band, with the exception of its H and M components, consists of both thick and thin filaments. During contraction the thick and thin filaments slide past each other (sliding filament theory of contraction), and the Z discs are brought near the ends of the thick filaments. It should also be noted that the thin filaments are held in register by two molecules of the inelastic protein **nebulin**. Moreover, the thick filaments are affixed to each other at the M disc by **C proteins** and **myomesin** and are connected to the Z disc by elastic proteins called **titin**. Since titin molecules form an elastic lattice around the thick filaments they facilitate the maintenance of the spatial relationship of these thick filaments to each other, as well as to the thin filaments.

Nerve impulses, transmitted at the **myoneural junction** across the **synaptic cleft** by **acetylcholine**, cause a wave of depolarization of the sarcolemma, with the eventual result of muscle contraction. This wave of depolarization is distributed throughout the muscle fiber by transverse tubules (**T tubules**), tubular invaginations of the sarcolemma. The T tubules become closely associated with the terminal cisterns of the sarcoplasmic reticulum (SR), so that each T tubule is flanked by two of these elements of the SR, forming a triad. During depolarization the T tubules carry the impulse within the muscle fiber, thus causing the release of calcium ions from the SR. Calcium ions interact with the thin myofilaments to permit contraction to occur.

As a protective mechanism against muscle fiber tears as a result of overstretching and to provide information concerning the position of the body in three-dimensional space, tendons and muscles are equipped with specialized receptors, **Golgi tendon organs** and **muscle spindles**, respectively.

CARDIAC MUSCLE

Cardiac muscle (see Graphic 6-2) cells are also striated, but each cell usually contains only one centrally placed nucleus. These cells form specialized junctions known as **intercalated discs** as they interdigitate with each other. Heart muscle contraction is involuntary, and the cells possess an inherent rhythm, which is coordinated by **Purkinje fibers**, modified cardiac muscle cells.

SMOOTH MUSCLE

Smooth muscle (see Graphic 6-2) is also involuntary. Each fusiform smooth muscle cell houses a single, centrally placed nucleus, which becomes corkscrew shaped during contraction of the cell. Smooth muscle cells contain an apparently haphazard arrangement of thick and thin filaments, whose interdigitation during contraction is harnessed by an intermediate type of filament. These intermediate filaments form dense bodies where they cross each other and at points of attachment to the cytoplasmic aspect of the sarcolemma. Smooth muscle may be of the multiunit type, where each cell possesses its own nerve supply, or of the visceral smooth muscle type, where nerve impulses are transmitted via **nexus** (**gap junctions**) from one muscle cell to its neighbor.

Histophysiology

I. MYOFILAMENTS

Thin filaments (7 nm in diameter and 1 μm long) are composed of **F actin,** double-helical polymers of **G actin** molecules, resembling a pearl necklace twisted upon itself. Each groove of the helix houses linear **tropomyosin** molecules positioned end to end. Associated with each tropomyosin molecule is a **troponin** molecule composed of three polypeptides—**troponin T (TnT), troponin I (TnI),** and **troponin C (TnC).** TnI binds to actin, masking its active site (where it is able to interact with myosin); TnT binds to tropomyosin; and TnC (a molecule similar to **calmodulin**) has a high affinity for calcium ions. The **plus end** of each thin filament is bound to a Z disc by α-**actinin.** Additionally, two **nebulins,** inelastic proteins, entwine along the length of each thin filament and anchor it to the Z disc. The **negative end** of each thin filament extends to the junction of the A and I bands and is capped by **tropomodulin.**

Thick filaments (15 nm in diameter and 1.5 μm in length) are composed of 200–300 **myosin molecules** arranged in an antiparallel fashion. Each myosin molecule is composed of two pairs of light chains and two identical heavy chains. Each **myosin heavy chain** resembles a golf club, with a linear tail and a globular head, where the tails are wrapped around each other in a helical fashion. Digesting the myosin heavy chain with the enzyme **trypsin** cleaves it into a linear (most of the tail) segment (**light meromyosin**) and a globular segment with the remainder of the tail (**heavy meromyosin**). Another enzyme, papain, cleaves **heavy meromyosin** into a short tail region (**S2 fragment**) and a pair of globular regions (**S1 fragments**). Each pair of **myosin light chains** are associated with one of the S1 fragments. S1 fragments have **ATPase activity** but require the association with actin for this activity to be manifest. Thick filaments are anchored to Z discs by the linear, elastic protein **titin** and are linked to adjacent thick filaments, at the M line, by the proteins **myomesin** and C protein.

II. SLIDING FILAMENT MODEL OF SKELETAL MUSCLE CONTRACTION

During **contraction** the thin filaments slide past the thick filaments, penetrating deeper into the A band; thus, the sarcomere becomes shorter, whereas the myofilaments remain the same length. As a consequence of the sliding of the filaments, the I and H bands disappear, the A band remains the same width (as before contraction), the Z discs are pulled closer to each other, and the entire sarcomere is shortened in length.

Subsequent to the transmission of the impulse across the myoneural junction, the **T tubules** convey the impulse throughout the muscle cell. **Voltage-sensitive** integral proteins, **dihydropyridine-sensitive receptors (DHSR),** located in the T tubule membrane are in contact with **calcium channels (ryanodine receptors)** in the terminal cisternae of the **sarcoplasmic reticulum (SR).** This complex is visible with the electron microscope and is referred to as **junctional feet.** During depolarization of the skeletal muscle sarcolemma, the DHSRs of the T tubule undergo voltage-induced conformational change, causing the calcium channels of the terminal cisternae to open, permitting the influx of Ca^{2+} ions into the cytosol. **Troponin C** of the thin filament binds the calcium ions and changes its conformation, pressing the **tropomyosin** deeper into the grooves of the F actin filament, thus exposing the **active site** (myosin-binding site) on the **actin** molecule.

ATP, bound to the globular head (**S1 fragment**) of the myosin molecule, is **hydrolyzed,** but both **ADP** and P_i **remain attached** on the S1. The myosin molecule swivels so that the myosin head approximates the active site on the actin molecule. The P_i moiety is released, and in the presence of **calcium,** a link is formed between the **actin** and **myosin.** The bound **ADP** is freed, and the **myosin head** alters its conformation, **moving the thin filament** toward the center of the sarcomere. A new **ATP** attaches to the globular head, and the **myosin dissociates** from the active site of the **actin.** This cycle is repeated 200–300 times for complete contraction of the sarcomere.

Relaxation ensues when the **calcium pump** of the **SR** transports calcium from the cytosol into the SR cisterna, where it is bound by **calsequestrin.** The decreased cytosolic Ca^{2+} induces TnC to lose its bound calcium ions, the TnC molecule returns to its previous conformational state, the tropomyosin molecule returns to its original location, and the active site of the actin molecule is once again masked.

III. SMOOTH MUSCLE

A. Contractile Elements

Although the **thick** and **thin filaments** of smooth muscle are not arranged into myofibrils, they are organized so that they are aligned obliquely to the longitudinal axis of the cell. **Myosin molecules** of smooth muscle are unusual, since the **light meromyosin moiety** is folded in such a fashion that its free terminus binds to a "sticky region" of the globular S1 portion. The thin filaments are attached to **cytoplasmic densities,** Z disc analogs (containing α-actinin), as are the **intermediate filaments** (**desmin** in nonvascular and **vimentin** in vascular smooth muscle cells). The cytosol is rich in **calmodulin** and the enzyme **myosin light-chain kinase.**

B. Contraction

Calcium, released from caveolae, binds to calmodulin. The **Ca^{2+}-calmodulin complex** activates myosin light-chain kinase, which **phosphorylates** one of the **myosin light chains,** altering its conformation. This causes the free terminus of the light meromyosin to be released from the S1 moiety. **ATP** binds to the **S1,** and the resultant interaction between actin and myosin is similar to that of skeletal (and cardiac) muscle. As long as calcium and ATP are present, the smooth muscle cell will remain contracted. Smooth muscle contraction lasts longer but develops slower than cardiac or skeletal muscle contraction.

Clinical Considerations ■ ■ ■

Myasthenia Gravis
Myasthenia gravis is an autoimmune disease that is characterized by incremental weakening of skeletal muscles. Antibodies formed against acetylcholine receptors of skeletal muscle fibers bond to and, thus, block these receptors. The number of sites available for the initiation of depolarization of the muscle sarcolemma is decreased. The gradual weakening affects the most active muscles first (muscles of the face, eyes, and tongue), but eventually the muscles of respiration become compromised and the individual dies of respiratory insufficiency.

Duchenne's Muscular Dystrophy
Duchenne's muscular dystrophy is a muscle degenerative disease that is due to an X-linked genetic defect that strikes 1 in 30,000 males. The defect results in the absence of dystrophin molecules in the muscle cell membrane. Dystrophin is a protein that functions in the interconnection of the cytoskeleton to transmembrane proteins that interact with the extracellular matrix as well as in providing structural support for the muscle plasmalemma. Individuals afflicted with Duchenne's muscular dystrophy experience muscle weakness by the time they are seven years of age and are usually wheelchair bound by the time they are twelve years old. It is very unusual to have these patients survive into their early twenties.

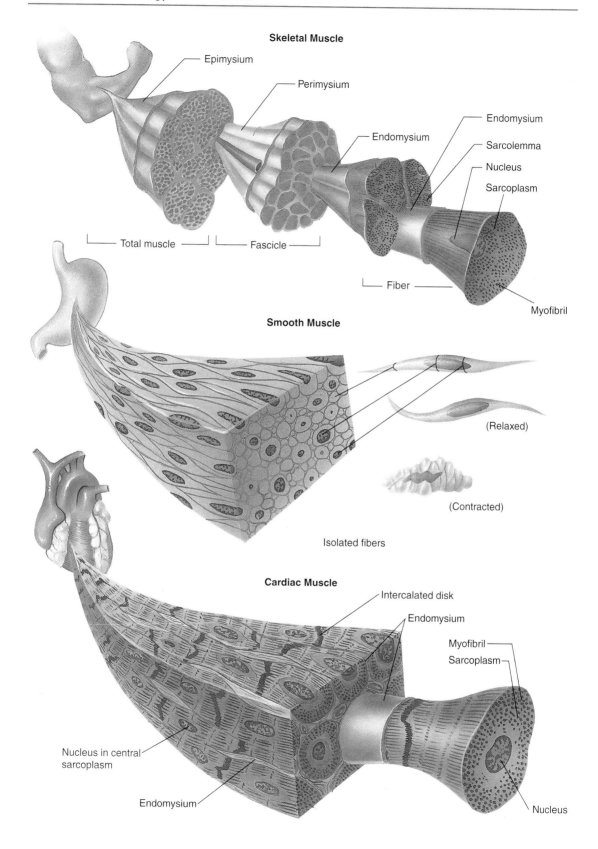

Skeletal Muscle

Epimysium

Perimysium

Endomysium

Endomysium

Sarcolemma

Nucleus

Sarcoplasm

Total muscle

Fascicle

Fiber

Myofibril

Smooth Muscle

(Relaxed)

(Contracted)

Isolated fibers

Cardiac Muscle

Intercalated disk

Endomysium

Myofibril

Sarcoplasm

Nucleus in central sarcoplasm

Endomysium

Nucleus

PLATE 6-1 ■ *Skeletal Muscle*

FIGURE 1 ■ *Skeletal muscle. l.s. Monkey. Plastic section.* × 800.

This photomicrograph displays several of the characteristics of skeletal muscle in longitudinal section. The muscle fibers are extremely long and possess a uniform diameter. Their numerous **nuclei** (N) are peripherally located. The intercellular space is occupied by endomysium, with its occasional flattened **connective tissue cells** (CT) and reticular fibers. Two types of striations are evident, longitudinal and transverse. The longitudinal striations represent **myofibrils** (M) that are arranged in almost precise register with each other. This ordered arrangement is responsible for the dark and light transverse banding that gives this type of muscle its name. Note that the **light band** (I) is bisected by a narrow dark line, the **Z disc** (Z). The **dark band** (A) is also bisected by the clear **H zone** (H). The center of the H zone is occupied by the M disc, appearing as a faintly discernible dark line in a few regions. The basic contractile unit of skeletal muscle is the **sarcomere** (S), extending from one Z disc to its neighboring Z disc. During muscle contraction the myofilaments of each sarcomere slide past one another, pulling Z discs closer to each other, thus shortening the length of each sarcomere. During this movement, the width of the A band remains constant, while the I band and H zone disappear.

FIGURE 2 ■ *Skeletal muscle. x.s. Monkey. Paraffin section.* × 132.

Portions of a few fascicles are presented in this photomicrograph. Each fascicle is composed of numerous **muscle fibers** (F) that are surrounded by connective tissue elements, known as the **perimysium** (P), which house nerves and blood vessels supplying the fascicles. The nuclei of endothelial, Schwann, and connective tissue cells are evident as black dots in the perimysium. The peripherally placed **nuclei** (N) of the skeletal muscle fibers appear as black dots; however, they are all within the muscle cell. Nuclei of satellite cells are also present, just external to the muscle fibers, but their identification at low magnification is questionable. The boxed area is presented at a higher magnification in Figure 3.

FIGURE 3 ■ *Skeletal muscle. x.s. Monkey. Paraffin section.* × 540.

This is a higher magnification of the boxed area of Figure 2. Transverse sections of several muscle fibers demonstrate that these cells appear to be polyhedral, that they possess peripherally placed **nuclei** (N), and that their **endomysia** (E) house numerous **capillaries** (C). Many of the capillaries are difficult to see because they are collapsed in a resting muscle. The pale sarcoplasm occasionally appears granular, due to the transversely sectioned myofibrils. Occasionally, nuclei which appear to belong to **satellite cells** (SC) may be observed, but definite identification cannot be expected. Moreover, the well-defined outline of each fiber was believed to be due to the sarcolemma, but now it is known to be due more to the adherent basal lamina and endomysium.

Skeletal muscle

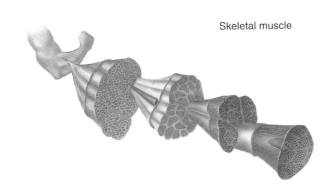

■ **KEY**

A	A band	F	muscle fiber	P	perimysium
C	capillary	H	H zone	S	sarcomere
CT	connective tissue	I	I band	SC	satellite cell
E	endomysium	N	nucleus	Z	Z disc

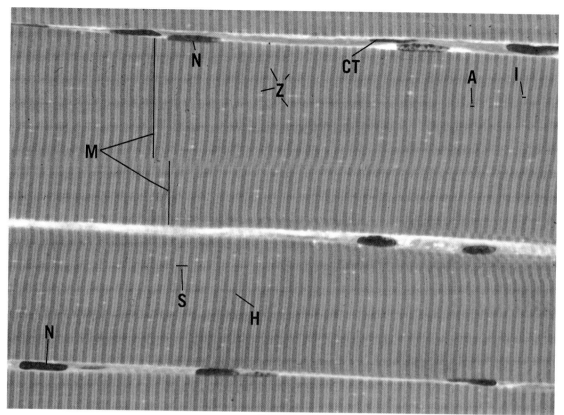

FIGURE 1

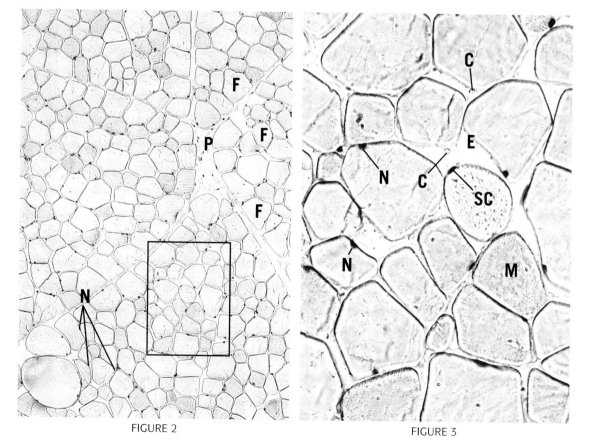

FIGURE 2

FIGURE 3

PLATE 6-2 ■ *Skeletal Muscle, Electron Microscopy*

FIGURE 1 ■ *Skeletal muscle. l.s. Rat. Electron microscopy.* × 17,100.

This moderately low power electron micrograph of skeletal muscle was sectioned longitudinally. Perpendicular to its longitudinal axis, note the dark and light cross-bandings. The **A band** (A) in this view extends from the upper left-hand corner to the lower right-hand corner and is bordered by an **I band** (I) on either side. Each I band is traversed by a **Z disc** (Z). Observe that the Z disc has the appearance of a dashed line, since individual myofibrils are separated from each other by sarcoplasm. Note that the extent of a **sarcomere** (S) is from Z disc to Z disc, and that an almost precise alignment of individual myofibrils assures the specific orientation of the various bands within the sarcomere. The **H zone** (H) and the **M disc** (MD) are clearly defined in this electron micrograph. Mitochondria are preferentially located in mammalian skeletal muscle, occupying the region at the level of the I band as they wrap around the periphery of the myofibril. Several sarcomeres are presented at a higher magnification in Figure 2. (Courtesy of Dr. J. Strum.)

FIGURE 2 ■ *Skeletal muscle. l.s. Rat. Electron microscopy.* × 28,800.

This is a higher power electron micrograph presenting several sarcomeres. Note that the **Z discs** (Z) possess projections (arrows) to which the **thin myofilaments** (tM) are attached. The **I band** (I) is composed only of thin filaments. **Thick myofilaments** (TM) interdigitate with the thin filaments from either end of the sarcomere, resulting in the **A band** (A). However, the thin filaments in a relaxed muscle do not extend all the way to the center of the A band; therefore, the **H zone** (H) is composed only of thick filaments. The center of each thick filament appears to be attached to its neighboring thick filament, resulting in localized thickenings, collectively comprising the **M disc** (MD). During muscle contraction, the thick and thin filaments slide past each other, thus pulling the Z discs toward the center of the sarcomere. Due to the resultant overlapping of thick and thin filaments, the I bands and H zones disappear, but the A bands maintain their width. The sarcoplasm houses **mitochondria** (m) preferentially located, glycogen granules (arrowhead), as well as a specialized system of sarcoplasmic reticulum and T tubules, forming **triads** (T). In mammalian skeletal muscle, triads are positioned at the junction of the I and A bands. (Courtesy of Dr. J. Strum.)

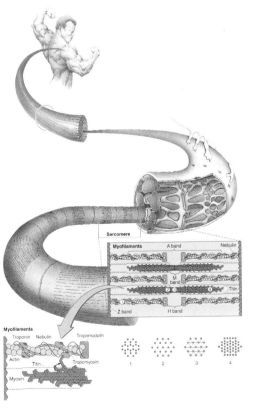

Molecular structure of skeletal muscle

■ KEY

A	A band	MD	M disc	TM	thick myofilament
H	H zone	S	sarcomere	Z	Z disc
I	I band	T	triad		
m	mitochondrion	tM	thin myofilament		

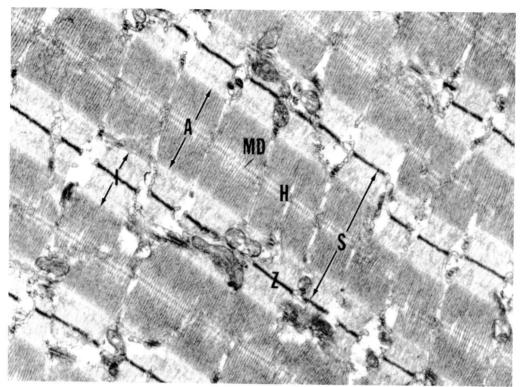

FIGURE 1

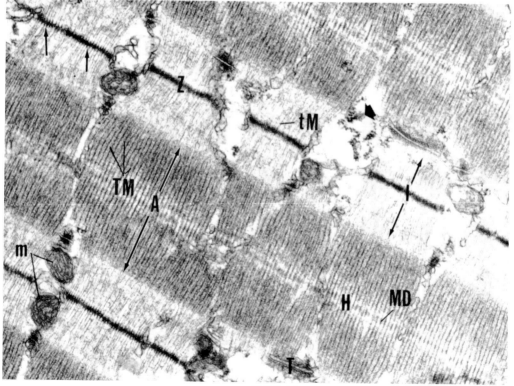

FIGURE 2

PLATE 6-3 ■ *Myoneural Junction, Light and Electron Microscopy*

FIGURE 1 ■ *Myoneural junction. Lateral view. Paraffin section.* × 540.

This view of the myoneural junction clearly displays the **myelinated nerve fiber** (MN) approaching the **skeletal muscle fiber** (SM). The **A bands** (A) and **I bands** (I) are well delineated, but the Z discs are not observable in this preparation. As the axon nears the muscle cell, it loses its myelin sheath and continues on as a **nonmyelinated axon** (nMN), but retains its Schwann cell envelope. As the axon reaches the muscle cell, it terminates as a **motor end plate** (MEP), overlying the sarcolemma of the muscle fiber. Although the sarcolemma is not visible in light micrographs, such as this one, its location is clearly approximated due to its associated basal lamina and reticular fibers.

FIGURE 2 ■ *Myoneural junction. Surface view. Paraffin section.* × 540.

This view of the myoneural junction demonstrates, as in the previous figure, that as the axon reaches the vicinity of the **skeletal muscle fiber** (SM), it loses its myelin sheath. The axon terminates, forming a **motor end plate** (MEP), composed of a few clusters of numerous small swellings (arrowhead) on the sarcolemma of the skeletal muscle fiber. Although it is not apparent in this light micrograph, the motor end plate is located in a slight depression on the skeletal muscle fiber, and the plasma membranes of the two structures do not contact each other. Figure 3 clearly demonstrates the morphology of such a synapse.

FIGURE 3 ■ *Myoneural junction. Rat. Electron microscopy.* × 15,353.

This electron micrograph is of a myoneural junction taken from the diaphragm muscle of a rat. Observe that the **axon** (ax) loses its myelin sheath, but the **Schwann cell** (sc) continues, providing a protective cover for the nonsynaptic surface of the **end foot** or **nerve terminal** (nt). The myelinated sheath ends in typical paranodal loops at the terminal heminode. The nerve terminal possesses **mitochondria** (m) and numerous clear synaptic vesicles. The margins of the 50-nm primary synaptic cleft are indicated by arrowheads. Postsynaptically, the **junctional folds** (j), many **mitochondria** (m), and portions of a **nucleus** (n) and **sarcomere** (s) are apparent in the skeletal muscle fiber. (Courtesy of Dr. C. S. Hudson.)

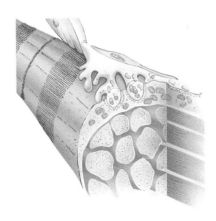

Myoneural junction

■ **KEY**

A	A band	MEP	motor end plate	s	sarcomere
ax	Axon	MN	myelinated nerve fiber	sc	Schwann cell
I	I band	n	nucleus	SM	skeletal muscle fiber
j	junctional fold	nMN	nonmyelinated axon		
m	mitochondria	nt	nerve terminal		

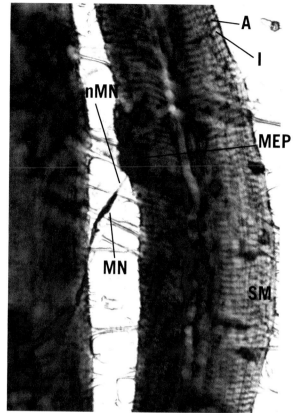

FIGURE 1

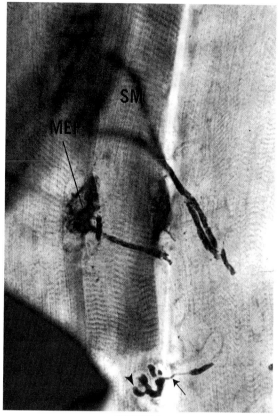

FIGURE 2

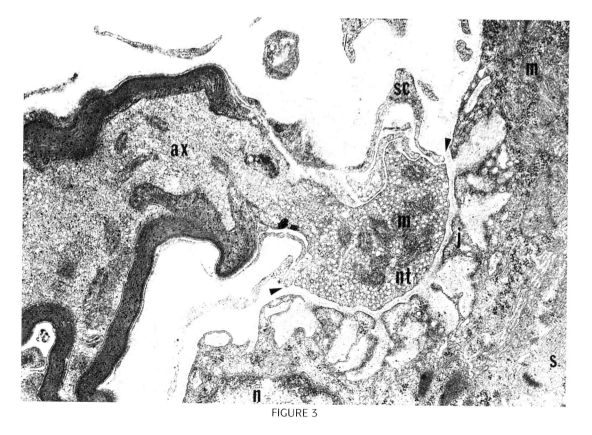

FIGURE 3

PLATE 6-4 ■ *Myoneural Junction, Scanning Electron Microscopy*

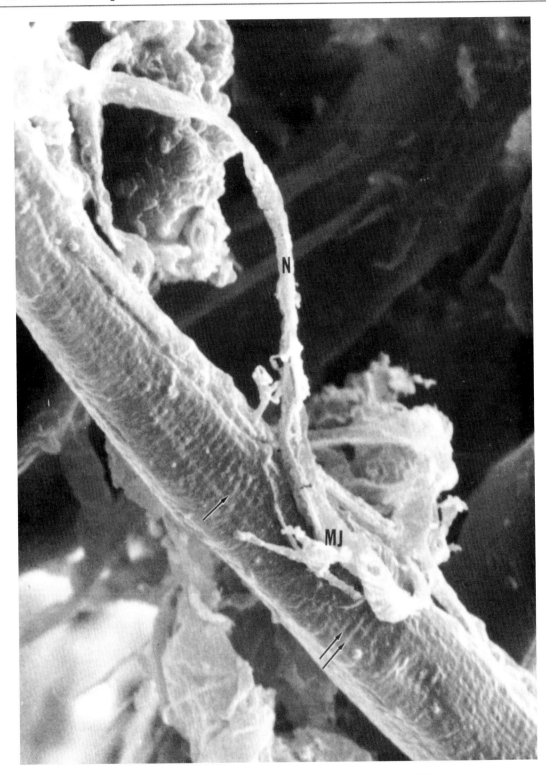

FIGURE 1 ■ *Myoneural junction. Tongue. Cat. Scanning electron microscopy.* × 2610.

The striations (arrows) of an isolated skeletal muscle fiber are clearly evident in this scanning electron micrograph. Note the **nerve** "twig" (N), which loops up and makes contact with the muscle at the **myoneural junction** (MJ). (Courtesy of Dr. L. Litke.)

PLATE 6-5 ■ *Muscle Spindle, Light and Electron Microscopy*

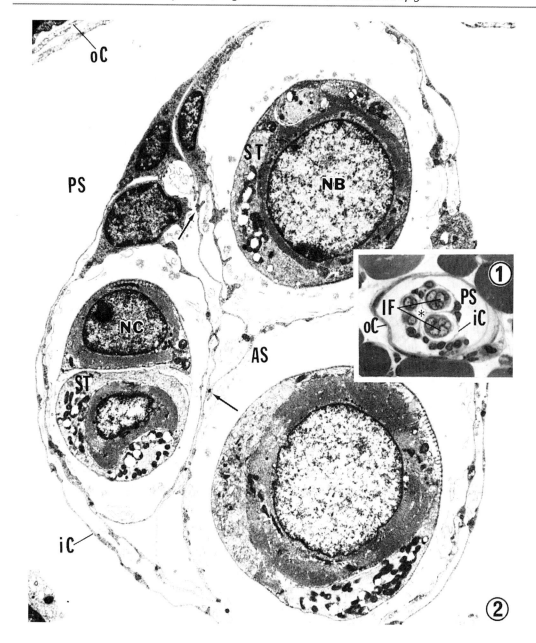

FIGURE 1 ■ *Muscle spindle. Mouse. Plastic section.* × 436.

Observe that the **outer** (oC) and **inner** (iC) **capsules** of the muscle spindle define the outer **peraxial space** (PS) and the inner **axial space** (asterisk). The inner capsule forms an envelope around the **intrafusal fibers** (IF). (From Ovalle W, Dow P: *Am J Anat* 166:343–357, 1983.)

FIGURE 2 ■ *Muscle spindle. Mouse. Electron microscopy.* × 6300.

Parts of the **outer capsule** (oC) may be observed at the corners of this electron micrograph. The **periaxial space** (PS) surrounds the slender **inner capsule** (iC) whose component cells form attenuated branches, subdividing the **axial space** (AS) into several compartments for the **nuclear chain** (NC) and **nuclear bag** (NB) intrafusal fibers and their corresponding **sensory terminals** (ST). Note that the attenuated processes of the inner capsule cells establish contact with each other (arrows). (From Ovalle W, Dow P: *Am J Anat* 166:343–357, 1983.)

PLATE 6-6 ■ *Smooth Muscle*

FIGURE 1 ■ *Smooth muscle. l.s. Monkey. Plastic section.* × 270.

The longitudinal section of smooth muscle in this photomicrograph displays long fusiform **smooth muscle cells** (sM) with centrally located, elongated **nuclei** (N). Since the muscle fibers are arranged in staggered arrays, they can be packed very closely, with only a limited amount of intervening **connective tissue** (CT). Using hematoxylin and eosin, the nuclei appear bluish, while the cytoplasm stains a light pink. Each smooth muscle cell is surrounded by a basal lamina and reticular fibers, neither of which is evident in this figure. Capillaries are housed in the connective tissue separating bundles of smooth muscle fibers. The boxed area is presented at a higher magnification in Figure 2.

FIGURE 2 ■ *Smooth muscle. l.s. Monkey. Plastic section.* × 540.

This photomicrograph is a higher magnification of the boxed area of Figure 1. Observe that the **nuclei** (N) of the smooth muscle fibers are long, tapered structures located in the center of the cell. The widest girth of the nucleus is almost as wide as the muscle fiber. However, the length of the fiber is much greater than that of the nucleus. Note also that any line drawn perpendicular to the direction of the fibers will intersect only a few of the nuclei. Observe the difference between the **connective tissue** (CT) and **smooth muscle** (sM). The smooth muscle cytoplasm stains darker and appears smooth relative to the paleness and rough-appearing texture of the connective tissue. Observe **capillaries** (C) located in the connective tissue elements between bundles of muscle fibers.

Inset. **Smooth muscle. Contracted. l.s. Monkey. Plastic section.** × 540.

This longitudinal section of smooth muscle during contraction displays the characteristic corkscrew-shaped **nuclei** (N) of these cells.

FIGURE 3 ■ *Smooth muscle. Uterine myometrium. x.s. Monkey. Plastic section.* × 270.

The myometrium of the uterus consists of interlacing bundles of smooth muscle fibers, surrounded by **connective tissue** (CT) elements. Note that some of these bundles are cut in longitudinal section (1), others are sectioned transversely (2), and still others are cut obliquely (3). At low magnifications, such as in this photomicrograph, the transverse sections present a haphazard arrangement of dark **nuclei** (N) in a lightly staining region. With practice, it will become apparent that these nuclei are intracellular and that the pale circular regions represent smooth muscle fibers sectioned transversely. Note the numerous **blood vessels** (BV) traveling in the connective tissue between the smooth muscle bundles.

FIGURE 4A ■ *Smooth muscle. x.s. Monkey. Plastic section.* × 540.

In order to understand the three-dimensional morphology of smooth muscle as it appears in two dimensions, refer to Figure 2 directly above this photomicrograph. Once again note that the muscle fibers are much longer than their nuclei and that both structures are spindle-shaped, being tapered at both ends. Recall also that at its greatest girth, the nucleus is almost as wide as the cell. In transverse section this would appear as a round nucleus surrounded by a rim of cytoplasm (asterisk). If the nucleus is sectioned at its tapered end, merely a small dot of it would be present in the center of a large muscle fiber (double asterisks). Sectioned anywhere between these two points, the nucleus would have varied diameters in the center of a large muscle cell. Additionally, the cell may be sectioned in a region away from its nucleus, where only the sarcoplasm of the large muscle cell would be evident (triple asterisks). Moreover, if the cell is sectioned at its tapered end, only a small circular profile of sarcoplasm is distinguishable (arrowhead). Therefore, in transverse sections of smooth muscle one would expect to find only few cells containing nuclei of various diameters. Most of the field will be closely packed profiles of sarcoplasm containing no nuclei.

FIGURE 4B ■ *Smooth muscle. Duodenum. Monkey. Plastic section.* × 132.

This photomicrograph of the duodenum demonstrates the **glandular portion** (G) with its underlying **connective tissue** (CT). Deep to the connective tissue, note the two smooth, muscle layers, one of which is sectioned longitudinally (1) and the other transversely (2).

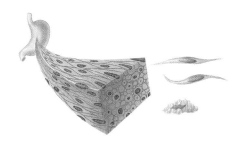

Smooth muscle

■ KEY

BV	blood vessel	CT	connective tissue	N	nucleus
C	capillary	G	glandular portion	sM	smooth muscle cell

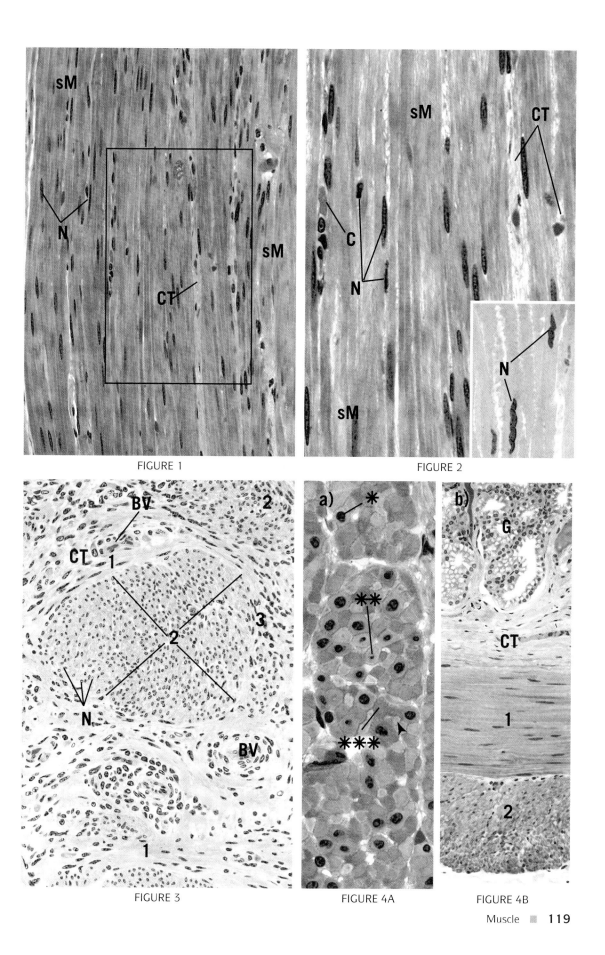

FIGURE 1

FIGURE 2

FIGURE 3

FIGURE 4A

FIGURE 4B

Muscle ▓ **119**

PLATE 6-7 ■ *Smooth Muscle, Electron Microscopy*

FIGURE 1 ■ *Smooth muscle. l.s. Mouse. Electron microscopy.* × 15,120.

Smooth muscle does not display cross-bandings, transverse tubular systems, or the regularly arranged array of myofilaments characteristic of striated muscle. However, smooth muscle does possess myofilaments that, along with a system of intermediate filaments, are responsible for its contractile capabilities. Moreover, the plasma membrane appears to possess the functional, if not the structural, aspects of the T tubule. Observe that each smooth muscle is surrounded by an **external lamina** (EL), which is similar in appearance to basal lamina of epithelial cells. The **sarcolemma** (SL) displays the presence of numerous pinocytotic-like invaginations, the **caveolae** (Ca), that are believed to act as T tubules of striated muscles in conducting impulses into the interior of the fiber.

Some suggest that they may also act in concert with the sarcoplasmic reticulum in modulating the availability of calcium ions. The cytoplasmic aspect of the sarcolemma also displays the presence of **dense bodies** (DB), which are indicative of the attachment of **intermediate microfilaments** (IM) at that point. Dense bodies, composed of β-actinin (Z disc protein found in striated muscle), are also present in the sarcoplasm (arrows). The **nucleus** (N) is centrally located and, at its pole, **mitochondria** (m) are evident. Actin and myosin are also present in smooth muscle, but cannot be identified with certainty in longitudinal sections. Parts of a second smooth muscle fiber may be observed to the left of the cell described. A small **capillary** (C) is evident in the lower right-hand corner. Note the **adherens junctions** (AJ) between the two epithelial cells, one of which presents a part of its **nucleus** (N).

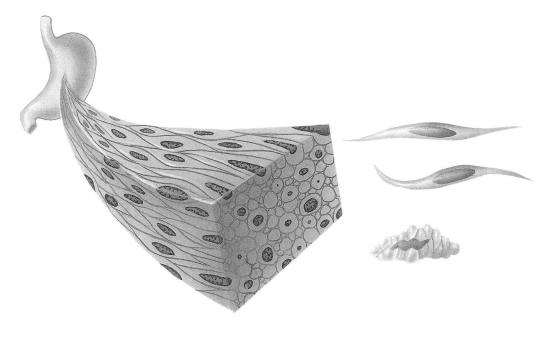

Smooth muscle

■ KEY

AJ	adherens junction	DB	dense body	m	mitochondrion
C	capillary	EL	external lamina	N	nucleus
Ca	caveola	IM	intermediate filament	SL	sarcolemma

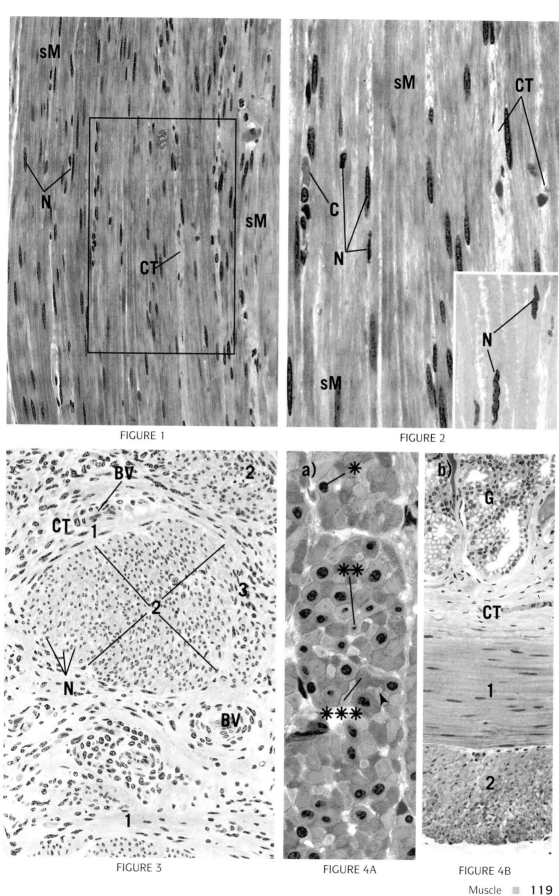

FIGURE 1

FIGURE 2

FIGURE 3

FIGURE 4A

FIGURE 4B

PLATE 6-7 ■ *Smooth Muscle, Electron Microscopy*

FIGURE 1 ■ *Smooth muscle. l.s. Mouse. Electron microscopy.* × 15,120.

Smooth muscle does not display cross-bandings, transverse tubular systems, or the regularly arranged array of myofilaments characteristic of striated muscle. However, smooth muscle does possess myofilaments that, along with a system of intermediate filaments, are responsible for its contractile capabilities. Moreover, the plasma membrane appears to possess the functional, if not the structural, aspects of the T tubule. Observe that each smooth muscle is surrounded by an **external lamina** (EL), which is similar in appearance to basal lamina of epithelial cells. The **sarcolemma** (SL) displays the presence of numerous pinocytotic-like invaginations, the **caveolae** (Ca), that are believed to act as T tubules of striated muscles in conducting impulses into the interior of the fiber.

Some suggest that they may also act in concert with the sarcoplasmic reticulum in modulating the availability of calcium ions. The cytoplasmic aspect of the sarcolemma also displays the presence of **dense bodies** (DB), which are indicative of the attachment of **intermediate microfilaments** (IM) at that point. Dense bodies, composed of β-actinin (Z disc protein found in striated muscle), are also present in the sarcoplasm (arrows). The **nucleus** (N) is centrally located and, at its pole, **mitochondria** (m) are evident. Actin and myosin are also present in smooth muscle, but cannot be identified with certainty in longitudinal sections. Parts of a second smooth muscle fiber may be observed to the left of the cell described. A small **capillary** (C) is evident in the lower right-hand corner. Note the **adherens junctions** (AJ) between the two epithelial cells, one of which presents a part of its **nucleus** (N).

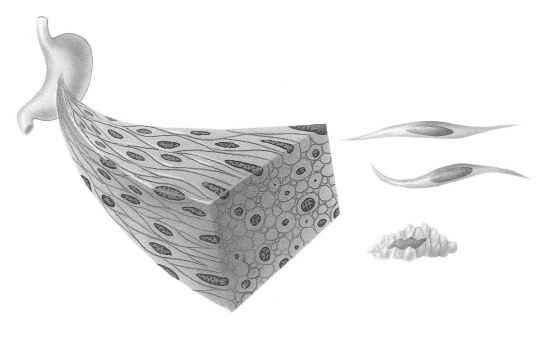

Smooth muscle

■ **KEY**

AJ	adherens junction	DB	dense body	m	mitochondrion
C	capillary	EL	external lamina	N	nucleus
Ca	caveola	IM	intermediate filament	SL	sarcolemma

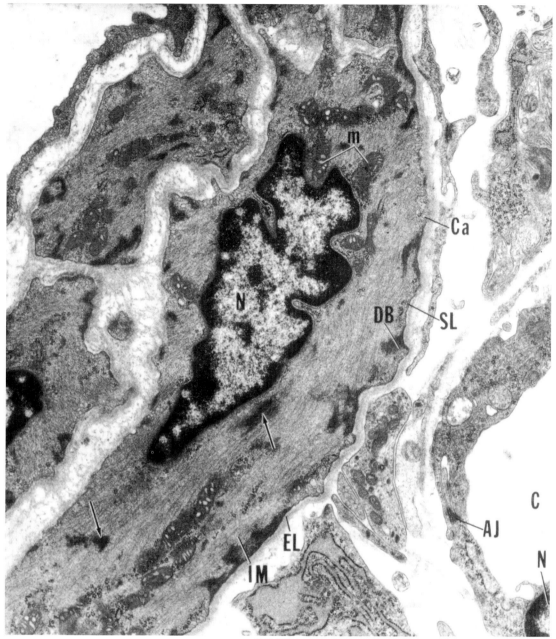

FIGURE 1

PLATE 6-8 ■ *Cardiac Muscle*

FIGURE 1 ■ *Cardiac muscle. l.s. Human. Plastic section.* × 270.

This low magnification of longitudinally sectioned cardiac muscle displays many of the characteristics of this muscle type. The branching (arrow) of the fibers is readily apparent, as are the dark and light bands (arrowheads) running transversely along the length of the fibers. Each muscle cell possesses a large, centrally located, oval **nucleus** (N), although occasional muscle cells may possess two nuclei. The **intercalated discs** (ID), indicating intercellular junctions between two cardiac muscle cells, clearly delineated in this photomicrograph, are not easily demonstrable in sections stained with hematoxylin and eosin. The intercellular spaces of cardiac muscle are richly endowed by blood vessels, especially capillaries. Recall that, in contrast to cardiac muscle, the long skeletal muscle fibers do not branch, their myofilaments parallel one another, their many nuclei are peripherally located, and they possess no intercalated discs. The boxed area appears at a higher magnification in Figure 2.

FIGURE 2 ■ *Cardiac muscle. l.s. Human. Plastic section.* × 540.

This is a higher magnification of the boxed area of Figure 1. The branching of the fibers (arrows) is evident, and the cross-striations, I and A bands (arrowheads) are clearly distinguishable. The presence of **myofibrils** (M) within each cell is well displayed in this photomicrograph, as is the "step-like" appearance of the **intercalated discs** (ID). The oval, centrally located **nucleus** (N) is surrounded by a clear area usually occupied by mitochondria. The intercellular areas are richly supplied by **capillaries** (C) supported by slender connective tissue elements.

FIGURE 3 ■ *Cardiac muscle. x.s. Human. Plastic section.* × 270.

Cross-sections of cardiac muscle demonstrate polygon-shaped areas of **cardiac muscle fibers** (CM) with relatively large intercellular spaces whose rich **vascular supply** (BV) is readily evident. Note that the **nucleus** (N) of each muscle cell is located in the center, but not all cells display a nucleus. The clear areas in the center of some cells (arrows) represent the perinuclear regions at the poles of the nucleus. These regions are rich in sarcoplasmic reticulum, glycogen, lipid droplets, and an occasional Golgi apparatus. The numerous smaller nuclei in the intercellular areas belong to endothelial and connective tissue cells. In contrast to cardiac muscle, cross-sections of skeletal muscle fibers display a homogeneous appearance with peripherally positioned nuclei. The connective tissue spaces between skeletal muscle fibers display numerous (frequently collapsed) capillaries.

FIGURE 4 ■ *Cardiac muscle. x.s. Human. Plastic section.* × 540.

At high magnifications of cardiac muscle in cross-section, several aspects of this tissue become quite apparent. Numerous **capillaries** (C) and larger **blood vessels** (BV) abound in the connective tissue spaces. Note the **endothelial nuclei** (EN) of these vessels, as well as the **white blood cells** (WBC) within the venule in the upper right-hand corner. **Nuclei** (N) of the muscle cells are centrally located, and the perinuclear clear areas (arrow) housing mitochondria are quite evident. The central clear zones at the nuclear poles are denoted by asterisks. Cross-sections of myofibrils (arrowheads) are recognizable as numerous small dots of varying diameters within the sarcoplasm.

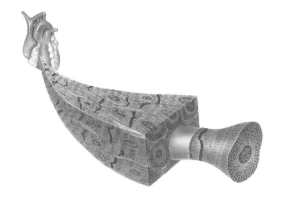

Cardiac muscle

■ **KEY**

BV	blood vessel	EN	endothelial nucleus	N	nucleus
C	capillary	ID	intercalated disc	WBC	white blood cell
CM	cardiac muscle fiber	M	myofibril		

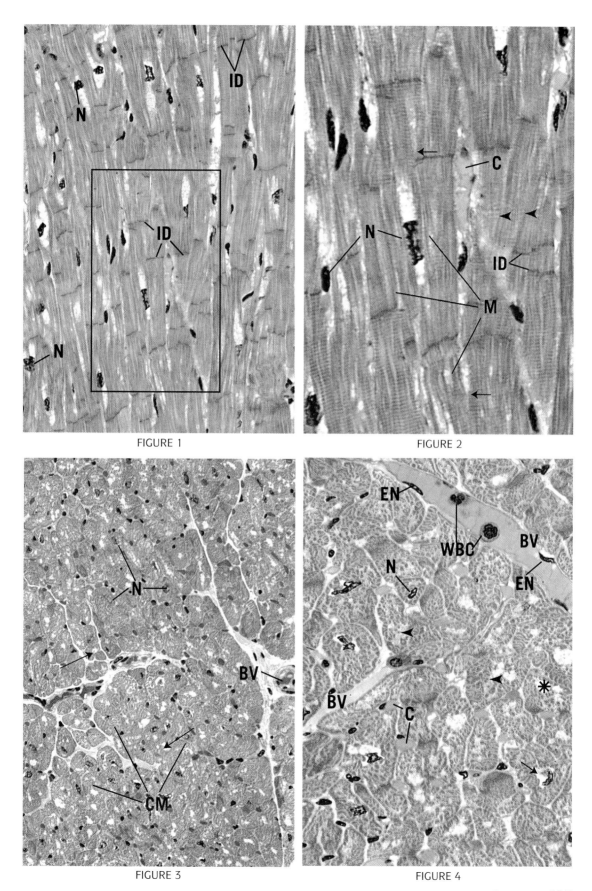

FIGURE 1

FIGURE 2

FIGURE 3

FIGURE 4

PLATE 6-9 ■ *Cardiac Muscle, Electron Microscopy*

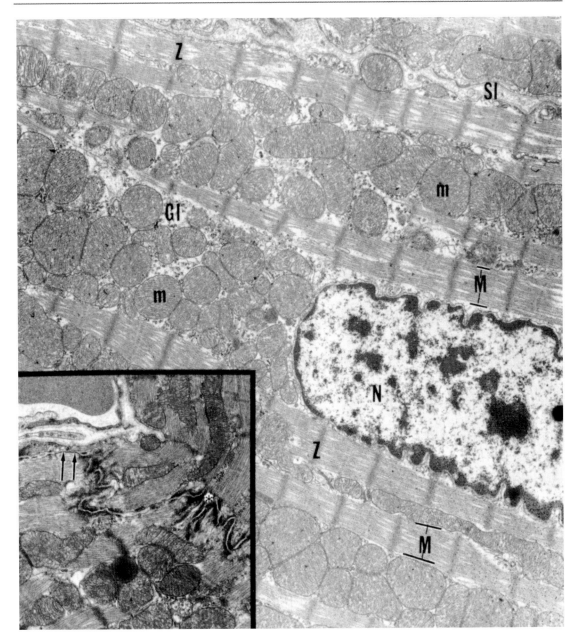

FIGURE 1 ■ *Cardiac muscle, l.s. Mouse. Electron microscopy.* × 11,700.

The **nucleus** (N) of cardiac muscle cells is located in the center of the cell, as is evident from the location of the **sarcolemma** (Sl) in the upper part of the photomicrograph. The sarcoplasm is well endowed with **mitochondria** (m) and **glycogen** (Gl) deposits. Since this muscle cell is contracted, the I bands are not visible. However, the **Z discs** (Z) are clearly evident, as are the individual **myofibrils** (M).

Inset. **Cardiac muscle. l.s. Mouse. Electron microscopy.** × 20,700.

An intercalated disc is presented in this electron micrograph. Note that this intercellular junction has two zones, the transverse portion (asterisk) composed mostly of desmosome-like junctions, and a longitudinal portion that displays extensive gap junctions (arrows).

Nervous Tissue

Nervous tissue is one of the four basic tissues of the body and it specializes in receiving information from the external and internal milieu. The information is processed, integrated, and compared with stored experiences and/or predetermined (reflex) responses, to select and effect an appropriate reaction. The reception of information is the function of the sensory component of the **peripheral nervous system** (**PNS**). The processes of integration, analysis, and response are performed by the brain and spinal cord comprising the **central nervous system** (**CNS**) with its gray and white matter. The transmission of the response to the effector organ is relegated to the motor component of the PNS. Therefore, it should be appreciated that the PNS is merely a physical extension of the CNS, and the separation of the two should not imply a strict dichotomy.

The nervous system may also be divided functionally into somatic and autonomic nervous systems. The **somatic nervous system** exercises conscious control over voluntary functions, while the **autonomic nervous system** controls involuntary functions. The autonomic nervous system is a motor system, acting on smooth muscle, cardiac muscle, and some glands. Its two components, **sympathetic** and **parasympathetic nervous systems,** usually act in concert to maintain homeostasis. The sympathetic nervous system prepares the body for action as in a "fight or flight" mode, whereas the parasympathetic system functions to calm the body and provides secretomotor innervation to most exocrine glands.

The CNS is protected by a bony housing, consisting of the skull and vertebral column, and the **meninges,** a triple-layered connective tissue sheath. The outermost meninx is the thick fibrous **dura mater.** Deep to the dura mater is the **arachnoid,** a nonvascular connective tissue membrane. The innermost, vascular **pia mater** is the most intimate investment of the CNS. Located between the latter two meninges is the **cerebrospinal fluid** (**CSF**).

NEURONS AND SUPPORTING CELLS

The structural and functional unit of the nervous system is the **neuron,** a cell that is highly specialized to perform its two major functions of irritability and conductivity. Each neuron is composed of a **cell body** (**soma, perikaryon**) and processes of varied lengths, known as **axons** and **dendrites** located on opposite sides of the cell body (see Graphic 7-2). A neuron possesses only a single axon. However, depending on the number of dendrites a neuron possesses, it may be **unipolar** (a single process but no dendrites–rare in vertebrates, but see below), **bipolar** (an axon and one dendrite), or the more common **multipolar** (an axon and several dendrites). An additional category exists where the single dendrite and the axon fuse during embryonic development, giving the false appearance of a unipolar neuron; therefore, it is known as a **pseudounipolar neuron,** although recently neuroanatomists began to refer to this neuron type as a **unipolar neuron.**

Neurons also may be classified according to their function. **Sensory neurons** receive stimuli from either the internal or external environment then transmit these impulses toward the CNS for processing. **Interneurons** act as connectors between neurons in a chain or typically between sensory and motor neurons within the CNS. **Motor neurons** conduct impulses from the CNS to the targets cells (muscles, glands, and other neurons).

Information is transferred from one neuron to another across an intercellular space or gap, the **synapse.** Depending on the regions of the neurons participating in the formation of the synapse, it could be axodendritic, axosomatic, axoaxonic, or dendrodendritic. Most synapses are axodendritic and involve one of many **neurotransmitter substances** (such as **acetylcholine**) that is released by the axon of the first neuron into the synaptic cleft. The chemical momentarily destabilizes the plasma membrane of the dendrite, and a wave of depolarization passes along the second neuron, which will cause the release of a neurotransmitter substance at the terminus of its axon. This type of a chemical synapse is an **excitatory synapse,** which results in the transmission of an impulse. Another type of synapse may stop the transmission of an impulse by stabilizing the plasma membrane of the second neuron; it is called an **inhibitory synapse.**

Neuroglial cells function in the metabolism and the support neurons. To prevent spontaneous or accidental depolarization of the neuron's cell membrane, specialized neuroglial cells provide a physical covering over its entire surface. In the CNS these cells are known as **astrocytes** and oligodendroglia, while in the PNS they are capsule and Schwann cells. **Oligodendroglia** and **Schwann cells** have the capability of forming **myelin sheaths** around axons (Graphic 7-2), which increases the conduction velocity of the impulse along the axon. The region where the myelin sheath of one Schwann cell (or oligodendroglion) ends and the next one begins is referred to as the **node of Ranvier.** Additionally, the CNS possesses **microglia, macrophages** derived from monocytes, and **ependymal cells,** which line brain ventricles and the central canal of the spinal cord.

Certain terms must be defined to facilitate understanding of the nervous system. A **ganglion** is a collection of nerve cell bodies in the PNS, while a similar collection of soma in the CNS is called a **nucleus.** A bundle of axons traveling together in the CNS is known as a **tract (fasciculus, column),** whereas the same bundle in the PNS is known as a **peripheral nerve** (nerve).

PERIPHERAL NERVES

Peripheral nerves are composed of numerous nerve fibers collected into several fascicles (bundles). These bundles possess a thick connective tissue sheath, the **epineurium** (see Graphic 7-1). Each fascicle within the epineurium is surrounded by a **perineurium** consisting of an outer connective tissue layer and an inner layer of flattened epithelioid cells. Each nerve fiber and associated Schwann cell has its own slender connective tissue sheath, the **endoneurium,** whose components include fibroblasts, an occasional macrophage, and collagenous and reticular fibers.

Histophysiology

I. MEMBRANE RESTING POTENTIAL

The normal concentration of K^+ is about 20 times greater inside the cell than outside, whereas the concentration of Na^+ is 10 times greater outside the cell than inside, in part because of the action of a Na^+-K^+ pump. The **resting potential** across the neuron cell membrane is maintained by the presence of **potassium leak channels** in the plasmalemma. It is through these channels that K^+ ions diffuse from inside the cell to the outside, thus establishing a **positive charge on the outer** aspect and a **negative (less positive) charge on the internal** aspect of the cell membrane, with a total differential of about 40 to 100 mV.

II. ACTION POTENTIAL

The **action potential** is an electrical activity where charges move along the membrane surface. It is an **all-or-none response** whose duration and amplitude are constant. Some axons are capable of sustaining up to 1000 impulses/sec.

Generation of an action potential begins when a region of the plasma membrane is **depolarized.** As the resting potential diminishes, a **threshold level** is reached, voltage-gated Na^+ channels open, Na^+ rushes into the cell, and at that point the **resting potential is reversed,** so that the inside becomes positive with respect to the outside. In response to this reversal of the resting potential, the Na^+ channel closes and for the next 1–2 msec cannot be opened (the **refractory period**). Depolarization also causes the **opening** of voltage-gated K^+ channels through which potassium ions exit the cell, thus repolarizing the membrane and ending not only the refractory period of the Na^+ channel but also the closure of the voltage-gated potassium channel.

The movement of Na^+ ions that enter the cell causes depolarization of the cell membrane toward the axon terminal (**orthodromic spread**). Although sodium ions also move away from the axon terminal (**antidromic spread**), they are unable to affect sodium channels in the antidromic direction, since those channels are in their refractory period.

III. MYONEURAL JUNCTION

Mitochondria, synaptic vesicles, and elements of smooth endoplasmic reticulum are present in the axon terminal. The axolemma involved in the formation of the synapse is known as the **presynaptic membrane,** whereas the sarcolemmal counterpart is known as the **postsynaptic membrane.** The presynaptic membrane has **sodium channels, voltage-gated calcium channels,** and **carrier proteins** for the cotransport of Na^+ and choline. The postsynaptic membrane has **acetylcholine receptors,** as well as slight invaginations known as **junctional folds.** A basal lamina containing the enzyme **acetylcholinesterase** is also associated with the postsynaptic membrane. As the impulse reaches the end-foot, sodium channels open, and the presynaptic membrane becomes depolarized, resulting in the opening of the voltage-gated calcium channels and the influx of Ca^+ into the end-foot. The high intracellular calcium concentration causes the synaptic vesicles, containing **acetylcholine,** proteoglycans, and ATP, to fuse with the presynaptic membrane and release their contents into the synaptic cleft. This excess membrane will be recycled via the formation of clathrin-coated vesicles, thus maintaining the morphology and requisite surface area of the presynaptic membrane. The released acetylcholine binds to **acetylcholine receptors** of the sarcolemma, thus opening **sodium channels,** resulting in sodium influx into the muscle cell, depolarization of the postsynaptic membrane, and the subsequent generation of an action potential and muscle cell contraction. **Acetylcholinesterase** of the basal lamina cleaves acetylcholine into **choline** and acetate, ensuring that a single release of the neurotransmitter substance will not continue to generate excess action potentials. The choline is returned to the end-foot via carrier proteins that are powered by a sodium gradient, where it is combined with activated acetate (derived from mitochondria), a reaction catalyzed by **acetylcholine transferase,** to form acetylcholine. The newly formed acetylcholine is transported into forming synaptic vesicles by a proton pump-driven, antiport carrier protein.

IV. NEUROTRANSMITTER SUBSTANCES

Neurotransmitter substances are signaling molecules (chemical messengers) that are released at the presynaptic membrane and effect a response by binding to receptor molecules (integral proteins) of the postsynaptic membrane. Neurotransmitter substances are varied in chemical composition and are categorized according to their chemical construction as cholinergic, monoaminergic, peptidergic, non-peptidergic, GABAergic, glutamatergic, and glycinergic.

V. BLOOD-BRAIN BARRIER

The selective barrier that exists between the neural tissues of the CNS and many blood-borne substances is termed the **blood-brain barrier**. This barrier is formed by the fasciae occludentes of contiguous endothelial cells lining the continuous capillaries that course through the neural tissues. Certain substances (i.e., O_2, H_2O, CO_2, and selected small lipid-soluble substances and some drugs) can penetrate the barrier. However, others, including glucose, certain vitamins, amino acids, and drugs, among others, access passage only by **receptor-mediated transport** and/or **facilitated diffusion**. Certain ions are also transported via **active transport**. It is also believed that some of the perivascular neuroglia may play a minor role in the maintenance of the blood-brain barrier.

Clinical Considerations ▨ ▨ ▪

Huntington's Chorea
Huntington's chorea is a hereditary condition that becomes evident in the third and fourth decade of life. Initially, this condition affects only the joints but later is responsible for motor dysfunction and dementia. It is thought to be caused by the loss of neurons of the CNS that produce the neurotransmitter **GABA**. The advent of dementia is thought to be related to the loss of acetylcholine-secreting cells.

Parkinson's Disease
Parkinson's disease is related to the loss of the neurotransmitter **dopamine** in the brain. This crippling disease causes muscular rigidity, tremor, slow movement, and progressively difficult voluntary movement. L-dopa can be administered but its beneficial effects are only temporary. Transplanted fetal adrenal gland tissue provides some relief but it is also of short duration.

Therapeutic Circumvention of the Blood-Brain Barrier
Therapeutic circumvention of the blood-brain barrier: The selective nature of the blood-brain barrier prevents certain therapeutic drugs and neurotransmitters conveyed by the bloodstream from entering the CNS. For example, the perfusion of **mannitol** into the blood stream changes the capillary permeability by altering the tight junctions, thus permitting administration of therapeutic drugs. Other therapeutic drugs can be attached to antibodies developed against **transferrin receptors** located on the luminal aspect of the plasma membranes of these endothelial cells that will permit transport into the CNS.

Guillain-Barré Syndrome
Guillain-Barré Syndrome is a form of immune-mediated condition resulting in rapidly progressing weakness with possible paralysis of the extremities and occasionally, even of the respiratory and facial muscles. This demyelinating disease is often associated with a recent respiratory or gastrointestinal infection; the muscle weakness reaches its greatest point within three weeks of the initial symptoms and 5% of the afflicted individuals die of the disease. Early recognition of the disease is imperative for complete (or nearly complete) recovery. Treatment includes immediate hospitalization and monitoring for need for respirator therapy. Monitoring for bedsores and physical therapy are also indicated. Plasmapheresis and administration of autoimmune globulin are treatments of choice.

Summary of Histological Organization

I. SPINAL CORD

A. Gray Matter

The **gray matter,** centrally located and more or less in the shape of an H, has two **dorsal horns** and two **ventral horns.** Ventral horns display numerous **multipolar (motor) cell bodies.** The perikaryon possesses a large, clear **nucleus** and a dense **nucleolus.** Its cytoplasm is filled with clumps of basophilic **Nissl substance** (rough endoplasmic reticulum) that extends into **dendrites** but not into the **axon.** The origin of the axon is indicated by the **axon hillock** of the **soma.** Numerous small nuclei abound in the gray matter; they belong to the various **neuroglia.** The nerve fibers and neuroglial processes in the gray matter are referred to as the **neuropil.** The right and left halves of the gray matter are connected to each other by the **gray commissure,** which houses the **central canal** lined by simple cuboidal **ependymal cells.**

B. White Matter

The **white matter** of the spinal cord is peripherally located and consists of **ascending** and **descending fibers.** These fibers are mostly **myelinated** (by **oligodendroglia**), accounting for the coloration in live tissue. **Nuclei** noted in white matter belong to the various **neuroglia.**

C. Meninges

The **meninges** of the spinal cord form three layers. The most intimate layer is the **pia mater,** surrounded by the **arachnoid,** which, in turn, is invested by the thick, collagenous **dura mater.**

II. CEREBELLUM

A. Cortex

The **cortex** of the cerebellum consists of an outer **molecular layer** and an inner **granular layer** with a single layer of **Purkinje cells** interposed between them. The **perikaryons** of the molecular layer are small and relatively few in number. Most of the fibers are unmyelinated. **Purkinje cells** are easily distinguished by their location, large size, and extensive **dendritic arborization.** The **granular layer** displays crowded arrays of nuclei belonging to **granule cells**

and intervening clear regions known as **glomeruli** (or **cerebellar islands**). These mainly represent areas of synapses on granule cell dendrites.

B. Medullary Substance

The **medullary substance** (internal white mass) is the region of **white matter** deep to the granular layer of the cerebellum, composed mostly of myelinated fibers and associated **neuroglial cells.**

III. CEREBRUM

A. Cortex

The **cerebral cortex** is composed of **gray matter,** mostly subdivided into six layers, with each housing neurons whose morphology is characteristic of that particular layer. The major neuronal types are **pyramidal cells, stellate (granule) cells, horizontal cells,** and **inverted (Martinotti) cells.** The following description refers to the **neocortex** and is presented from superficial to deep order. The first layer is just deep to the pia mater, while the sixth level is the deepest cortical layer, bordering the central white matter of the cerebrum.

1. Molecular Layer
Composed of **horizontal cells** and cell processes.

2. External Granular Layer
Consists mostly of **granule (stellate) cells,** tightly packed.

3. External Pyramidal Layer
Large **pyramidal cells** and **granule (stellate) cells.**

4. Internal Granular Layer
Closely packed **granule (stellate) cells,** most of which are small, although some are larger.

5. Internal Pyramidal Layer
Medium and large **pyramidal cells** constitute this layer.

6. Multiform Layer
Consisting of various cell shapes, many of which are fusiform. This layer also houses **Martinotti cells.**

B. White Matter

Deep to the cerebral cortex is the **subcortical white matter** composed mostly of myelinated fibers and associated **neuroglial cells.**

IV. CHOROID PLEXUS

The **choroid plexus** consists of tufts of small vascular elements (derived from the pia-arachnoid) that are covered by **modified ependymal cells** (simple cuboidal in shape). These structures, located in the ventricles of the brain, are responsible for the formation of the **cerebrospinal fluid** (CSF).

V. DORSAL ROOT GANGLION (DRG)

A. Neurons

The **somata** of these cells are **pseudounipolar**, with large nuclei and nucleoli. Surrounding each soma are **capsule cells,** recognized by their small, round nuclei. **Fibroblasts** (satellite cells) are also evident. Synapses do not occur in the DRG.

B. Fibers

Fibers are mostly myelinated and travel in bundles through the DRG.

C. Connective Tissue

The DRG is surrounded by collagenous **connective tissue** whose septa penetrate the substance of the ganglion.

VI. PERIPHERAL NERVE

A. Longitudinal Section

The parallel fibers stain a pale pink with hematoxylin and eosin, although **Schwann cell** and occasional **fibroblast nuclei** are clearly evident. The most characteristic feature is the apparent wavy, zigzag course of the nerve fibers. At low magnification the **perineurium** is clearly distinguishable, while at high magnification the **nodes of Ranvier** may be recognizable.

B. Transverse Section

The most characteristic feature of transverse sections of nerve fibers is the numerous, small, irregular circles with a centrally located dot. Thin spokes appear to traverse the empty-looking space between the dot and the circumference of the circle. These represent the **neurolemma**, the extracted **myelin** (**neurokeratin**), and the central **axon.** Occasionally, crescent-shaped nuclei hug the myelin; these belong to **Schwann cells.** The **endoneurium** may show evidence of **nuclei** of **fibroblasts** also. At lower magnification the **perineuria** of several fascicles of nerve fibers are clearly distinguishable. When stained with OsO_4, the **myelin sheath** stands out as dark, round structures with lightly staining centers.

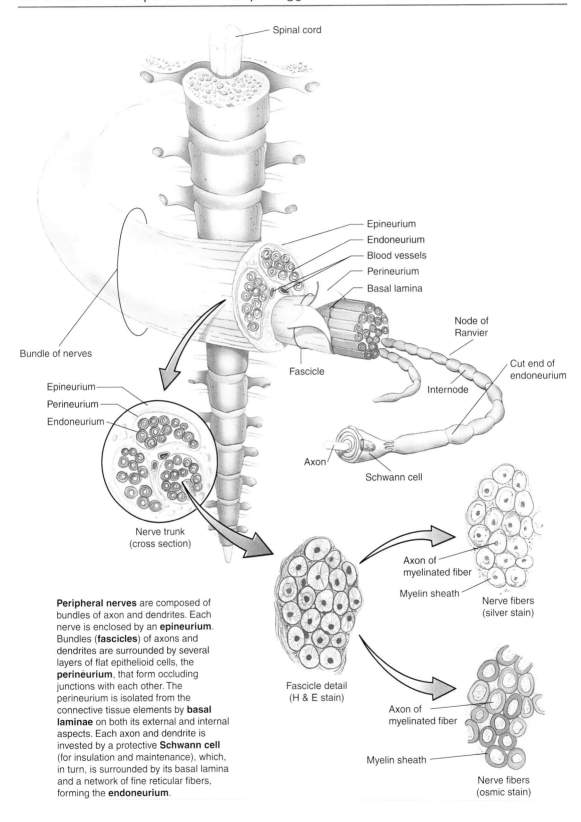

Spinal cord

Epineurium
Endoneurium
Blood vessels
Perineurium
Basal lamina

Node of Ranvier

Cut end of endoneurium

Internode

Bundle of nerves

Fascicle

Epineurium
Perineurium
Endoneurium

Axon

Schwann cell

Nerve trunk (cross section)

Axon of myelinated fiber

Myelin sheath

Nerve fibers (silver stain)

Fascicle detail (H & E stain)

Axon of myelinated fiber

Myelin sheath

Nerve fibers (osmic stain)

Peripheral nerves are composed of bundles of axon and dendrites. Each nerve is enclosed by an **epineurium**. Bundles (**fascicles**) of axons and dendrites are surrounded by several layers of flat epithelioid cells, the **perineurium**, that form occluding junctions with each other. The perineurium is isolated from the connective tissue elements by **basal laminae** on both its external and internal aspects. Each axon and dendrite is invested by a protective **Schwann cell** (for insulation and maintenance), which, in turn, is surrounded by its basal lamina and a network of fine reticular fibers, forming the **endoneurium**.

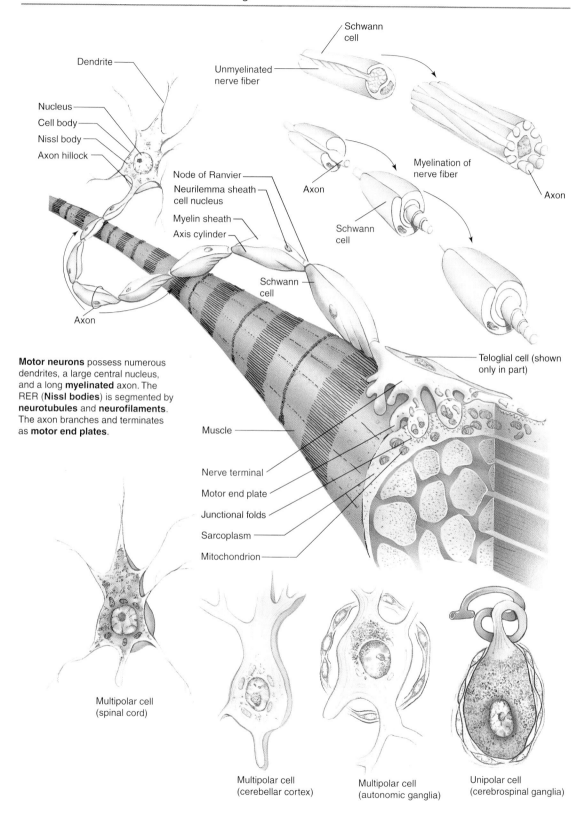

Schwann cell

Unmyelinated nerve fiber

Dendrite

Nucleus

Cell body

Nissl body

Axon hillock

Myelination of nerve fiber

Axon

Node of Ranvier

Neurilemma sheath cell nucleus

Myelin sheath

Axis cylinder

Schwann cell

Schwann cell

Axon

Axon

Axon

Motor neurons possess numerous dendrites, a large central nucleus, and a long **myelinated** axon. The RER (**Nissl bodies**) is segmented by **neurotubules** and **neurofilaments**. The axon branches and terminates as **motor end plates**.

Teloglial cell (shown only in part)

Muscle

Nerve terminal

Motor end plate

Junctional folds

Sarcoplasm

Mitochondrion

Multipolar cell (spinal cord)

Multipolar cell (cerebellar cortex)

Multipolar cell (autonomic ganglia)

Unipolar cell (cerebrospinal ganglia)

PLATE 7-1 ■ *Spinal Cord*

FIGURE 1 ■ *Spinal cord. x.s. Cat. Silver stain. Paraffin section.* × 21.

The spinal cord is invested by a protective coating, the three-layered meninges. Its outermost fibrous layer, the **dura mater** (DM), is surrounded by epidural fat, not present in this photomicrograph. Deep to the dura is the **arachnoid** (A) with its **subarachnoid space** (SS), which is closely applied to the most intimate layer of the meninges, the vascular **pia mater** (PM). The spinal cord itself is organized into **white matter** (W) and **gray matter** (G). The former, which is peripherally located and does not contain nerve cell bodies, is composed of nerve fibers, most of which are myelinated, that travel up and down the cord. It is cellular, however, since it houses various types of glial cells. The centrally positioned gray matter contains the cell bodies of the neurons, as well as the initial and terminal ends of their processes, many of which are not usually myelinated. These nerve cell processes and those of the numerous glial cells form an intertwined network of fibers that is referred to as the neuropil. The gray matter is subdivided into regions, namely the **dorsal horn** (DH), the **ventral horn** (VH), and the **gray commissure** (Gc). The **central canal** (CC) of the spinal cord passes through the gray commissure, dividing it into dorsal and ventral components. Processes of neurons leave and enter the spinal cord as **ventral** (VR) and **dorsal** (DR) **roots**, respectively. A region similar to the boxed area is represented in Figure 2.

FIGURE 2 ■ *Spinal cord. x.s. White and gray matter. Human. Paraffin section.* × 132.

This photomicrograph represents the boxed region of Figure 1. Observe that the interface between **white matter** (W) and **gray matter** (G) is readily evident (asterisks). The numerous nuclei (arrowheads) present in white matter belong to the various neuroglia, which support the axons and dendrites traveling up and down the spinal cord. The large **nerve cell bodies** (CB) in the ventral horn of the gray matter possess vesicular-appearing nuclei with dense, dark nucleoli. **Blood vessels** (BV), which penetrate deep into the gray matter, are surrounded by processes of neuroglial cells, forming the blood-brain barrier, not visible in this photomicrograph. Small nuclei (arrows) in gray matter belong to the neuroglial cells, whose cytoplasm and cellular processes are not evident.

FIGURE 3 ■ *Spinal cord. x.s. Ventral horn. Human. Paraffin section.* × 270.

The multipolar neurons and their various processes (arrows) are clearly evident in this photomicrograph of the ventral horn. Note the large **nucleus** (N) and dense **nucleolus** (n), both of which are characteristic of neurons. Observe the clumps of basophilic material, **Nissl bodies** (NB), that electron microscopy has demonstrated to be rough endoplasmic reticulum. The small nuclei belong to the various **neuroglial cells** (Ng), which, along with their processes and processes of the neurons, compose the **neuropil** (Np), the matted-appearing background substance of gray matter. The white spaces (asterisks) surrounding the soma and blood vessels are due to shrinkage artifacts.

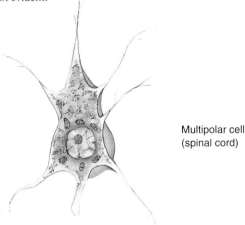

Multipolar cell
(spinal cord)

KEY

A	arachnoid	G	gray matter	Np	neuropil
BV	blood vessel	Gc	gray commissure	PM	pia mater
CB	nerve cell body	N	nucleus	SS	subarachnoid space
CC	central canal	n	nucleolus	VH	ventral horn
DH	dorsal horn	NB	Nissl body	VR	ventral root
DM	dura mater	Ng	neuroglial cell	W	white matter
DR	dorsal root				

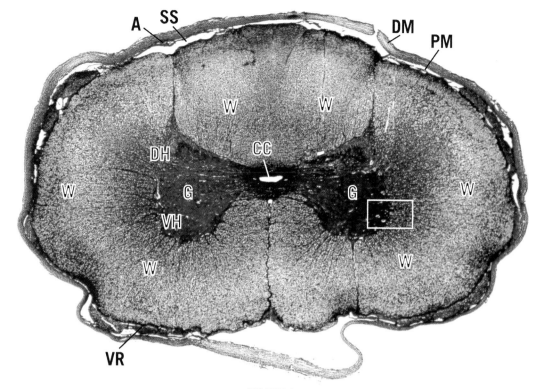

FIGURE 1

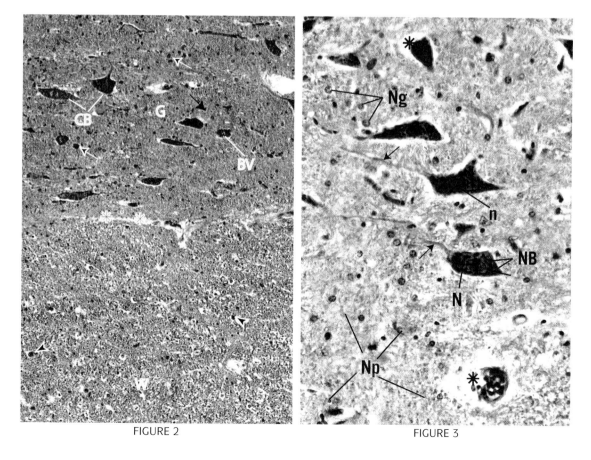

FIGURE 2

FIGURE 3

PLATE 7-2 ■ *Cerebellum, Synapse, Electron Microscopy*

FIGURE 1 ■ *Cerebellum. Human. Paraffin section.* × 14.

The cerebellum, in contrast to the spinal cord, consists of a core of **white matter** (W) and the superficially located **gray matter** (G). Although it is difficult to tell from this low-magnification photomicrograph, the gray matter is subdivided into three layers, the outer **molecular layer** (ML), a middle **Purkinje cell layer** (PL), and the inner **granular layer** (GL). The less dense appearance of the molecular layer is due to the sparse arrangement of nerve cell bodies, while the darker appearance of the granular layer is a function of the great number of darkly staining nuclei packed closely together. A region similar to the boxed area is represented in Figure 2.

FIGURE 2 ■ *Cerebellum. Human. Paraffin section.* × 132.

This photomicrograph is taken from a region similar to the area boxed in Figure 1. The **granular layer** (GL) is composed of closely packed **granule cells** (GC), which, at first glance, resemble lymphocytes due to their dark round nuclei. Interspersed among these cells are clear spaces, called glomeruli or **cerebellar islands** (CI), where synapses occur between axons entering the cerebellum from outside and dendrites of granule cells. The **Purkinje cells** (PC) send their axons into the granular layer, while their dendrites arborize in the **molecular layer** (ML). This layer also contains unmyelinated fibers from the granular layer, as well as two types of cells, **basket cells** (BC) and the more superficially located **stellate cells** (SC). The surface of the cerebellum is invested by **pia matter** (PM), just barely evident in this photomicrograph. The boxed area is presented at a higher magnification in Figure 3.

FIGURE 3 ■ *Purkinje cell. Human cerebellum. Paraffin section.* × 540.

This is a higher magnification of the boxed area of Figure 2. The **granular layer** (GL) of the cerebellum is composed of two cell types, the smaller **granule cells** (GC) and larger **Golgi type II cells** (G2). The flask-shaped **Purkinje cell** (PC) displays its large **nucleus** (N) and **dendritic tree** (D). Nuclei of numerous **basket cells** (BC) of the **molecular layer** (ML), as well as the **unmyelinated fibers** (UF) of the granule cells, are well defined in this photomicrograph. These fibers make synaptic contact (arrows) with the dendritic processes of the Purkinje cells.

Inset. **Astrocyte. Human cerebellum. Golgi stain. Paraffin section.** × 132.

Note the numerous processes of this **fibrous astrocyte** (A) in the white matter of the cerebellum.

FIGURE 4 ■ *Synapse. Afferent terminals. Electron microscopy.* × 16,200.

The lateral descending nucleus of the fifth cranial nerve displays a **primary afferent terminal** (AT) that is forming multiple synapses with **dendrites** (D) and **axons** (Ax). Observe the presence of **synaptic vesicles** (SV) in the postsynaptic axon terminals, as well as the thickening of the membrane of the primary afferent terminal (arrows). This terminal also houses **mitochondria** (m), as well as **cisternae** (Ci) for the synaptic vesicles. (From Meszler RM: *J Comp Neurol* 220:299–309, 1983.)

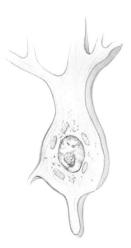

Multipolar cell
(cerebellar cortex)

KEY

A	fibrous astrocyte	G	gray matter	PC	Purkinje cell
AT	primary afferent terminal	G2	Golgi type II cell	PL	Purkinje cell layer
Ax	axons	GC	granule cell	PM	pia mater
BC	basket cell	GL	granular layer	SC	stellate cell
CI	cerebellar island	m	mitochondrion	SV	synaptic vesicle
Ci	cistern	ML	molecular layer	UF	unmyelinated fiber
D	dendrite	N	nucleus	W	white matter

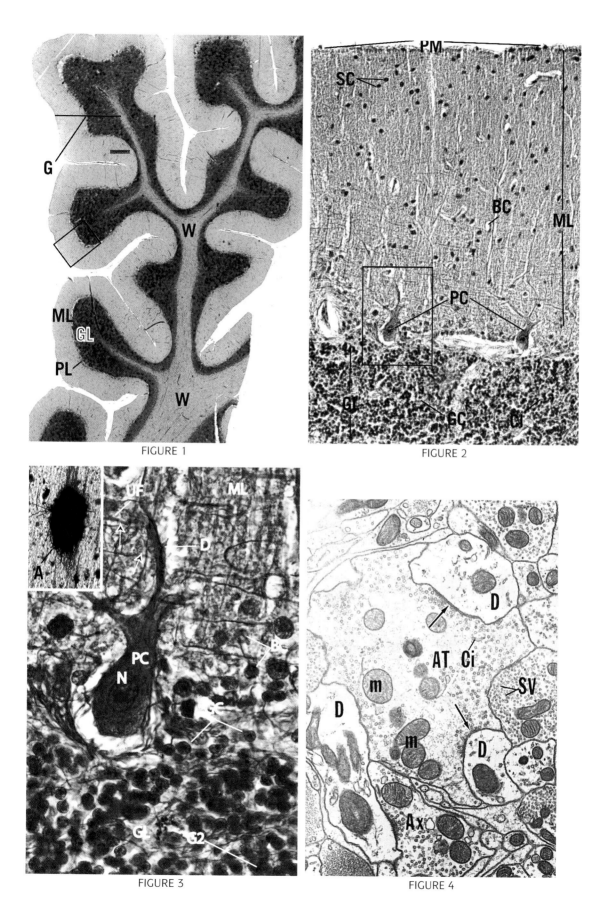

FIGURE 1

FIGURE 2

FIGURE 3

FIGURE 4

PLATE 7-3 ■ *Cerebrum, Neuroglial Cells*

FIGURES 1 AND 2 ■ *Cerebrum. Human. Paraffin section.* × 132.

These figures represent a montage of the entire human cerebral cortex, and some of the underlying **white matter** (W) at a low magnification. Observe that the numerous **blood vessels** (BV) that penetrate the entire cortex are surrounded by a clear area (arrow), which is due to shrinkage artifact. The six layers of the cortex are not clearly defined, but are approximated by brackets. The **pia mater** (PM), covering the surface of the cortex, is a vascular tissue that provides larger blood vessels, as well as **capillaries** (Ca) that penetrate the brain tissue. Layer one of the cortex is known as the **molecular layer** (1), which contains numerous fibers and only a few neuron cell bodies. It is difficult to distinguish these soma from the neuroglial cells at this magnification. The second, **external granular layer** (2), is composed of small **granule cells** (GC), as well as many **neuroglial cells** (Ng). The third layer is known as the **external pyramidal layer** (3), which is the thickest layer in this section of the cerebral cortex. It consists of **pyramidal cells** (Py), and some granule cells (GC) as well as numerous **neuroglia** (Ng) interspersed among the soma and fibers. The fourth layer, the **internal granular layer** (4), is a relatively narrow band whose cell population consists mostly of small and a few large **granule cells** (GC) and the ever present **neuroglial cells** (Ng). The **internal pyramidal layer** (5) houses medium and large **pyramidal cells** (Py) as well as the ubiquitous **neuroglia** (Ng), whose nuclei appear as small dots. Although not evident in this preparation, nerve fibers of the internal band of Baillarger pass horizontally through this layer, while those of the external band of Baillarger traverse the internal granular layer. The deepest layer of the cerebral cortex is the **multiform layer** (6), which contains cells of various shapes, many of which are fusiform in morphology. Neuroglial cells and Martinotti cells are also present in this layer, but cannot be distinguished from each other at this magnification. The **white matter** (W) appears very cellular, due to the nuclei of the numerous neuroglial cells supporting the cell processes derived from and traveling to the cortex.

FIGURE 3 ■ *Astrocytes. Silver stain. Paraffin section.* × 132.

This photomicrograph of the white matter of the cerebrum presents a matted appearance due to the interweaving of various nerve cell and glial cell processes. Note also the presence of two **blood vessels** (BV) passing horizontally across the field. The long processes of the **fibrous astrocytes** (FA) approach the blood vessels (arrows) and assist in the formation of the blood-brain barrier.

FIGURE 4 ■ *Microglia. Silver stain. Paraffin section.* × 540.

This photomicrograph is of a section of the cerebral cortex, demonstrating **nuclei** (N) of nerve cells, as well as the presence of **microglia** (Mi). Note that microglia are very small and possess a dense **nucleus** (N), as well as numerous cell processes (arrows).

■ **KEY**

BV	blood vessel	Ng	neurological cell	3	external pyramidal layer
Ca	capillary	PM	pia mater	4	internal granular layer
FA	fibrous astrocyte	Py	pyramidal cell	5	internal pyramidal layer
GC	granule cell	W	white matter	6	multiform layer
Mi	microglia	1	molecular layer		
N	nucleus	2	external granular layer		

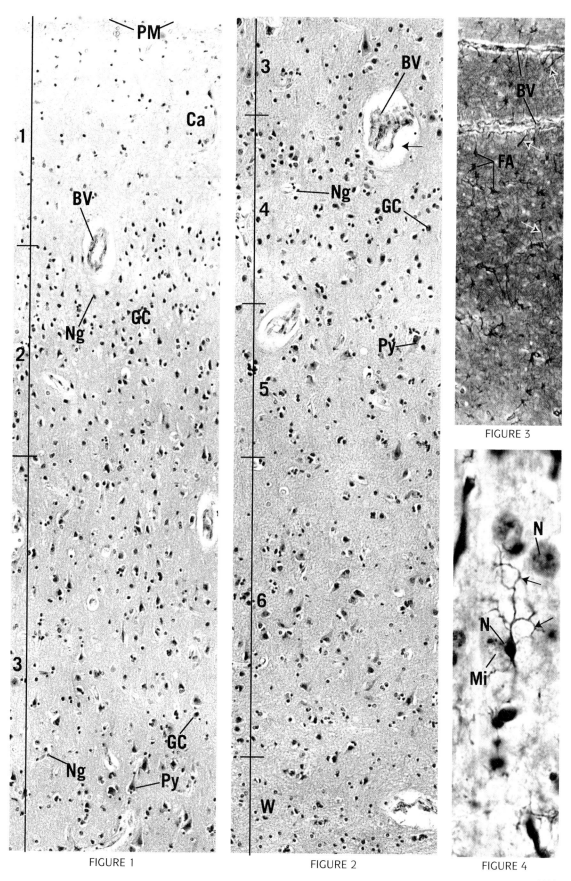

FIGURE 1

FIGURE 2

FIGURE 3

FIGURE 4

PLATE 7-4 ■ *Sympathetic Ganglia, Sensory Ganglia*

FIGURE 1 ■ *Sympathetic ganglion. l.s. Paraffin section.* × 132.

Sympathetic ganglia are structures that receive axons of presynaptic cells, whose soma are within the CNS. Located within the ganglion are soma of postsynaptic neurons upon which the presynaptic cell axons synapse. These ganglia are enveloped by a collagenous connective tissue **capsule** (C), which sends **septa** (S) containing **blood vessels** (BV) within the substance of the ganglion. The arrangement of the cell bodies of the **multipolar neurons** (MN) within the ganglion appears to be haphazard. This very vascular structure contains numerous nuclei which belong to **endothelial cells** (E), intravascular **leukocytes** (L), **fibroblasts** (F), **Schwann cells** (ScC), and those of the **supporting cells** (SS) surrounding the nerve cell bodies. A region similar to the boxed area is presented in Figure 2.

FIGURE 2 ■ *Sympathetic ganglion. l.s. Paraffin section.* × 540.

This photomicrograph presents a higher magnification of a region similar to the boxed area of Figure 1. Although neurons of the sympathetic ganglion are multipolar, their processes are not evident in this specimen stained with hematoxylin and eosin. The **nucleus** (N) with its prominent **nucleolus** (n) is clearly visible. The cytoplasm contains **lipofuscin** (Li), a yellowish pigment that is very prevalent in neurons of older individuals. The clear space between the soma and the **supporting cells** (SS) is a shrinkage artifact. Note the numerous **blood vessels** (BV) containing red blood cells (arrows) and a **neutrophil** (Ne).

FIGURE 3 ■ *Sensory ganglion. l.s. Human. Paraffin section.* × 132.

The dorsal root ganglion provides a good representative example of a sensory ganglion. It possesses a **vascular** (BV) connective tissue **capsule** (C), which also envelops its sensory root. The neurons of the dorsal root ganglion are pseudounipolar in morphology; therefore, their **somata** (So) appear spherical in shape. The **fibers** (f), many of which are myelinated, alternate with rows of cell bodies. Note that some somata are large (arrow), while others are small (arrowhead). Each soma is surrounded by neuroectodermally derived **capsule cells** (Cc). A region similar to the boxed area is presented at a high magnification in Figure 4.

FIGURE 4 ■ *Sensory ganglion. l.s. Human. Paraffin section.* × 270.

This photomicrograph is a higher magnification of a region similar to the boxed area of Figure 3. The spherical cell bodies display their centrally located **nuclei** (N) and **nucleoli** (n). Observe that both small (arrowheads) and large (arrows) somata are present in the field, and that the nuclei are not always in the plane of section. Hematoxylin and eosin stains the somata a more or less homogeneous pink, so that organelles such as Nissl substance are not visible. However, the nuclei and cytoplasm of **capsule cells** (Cc) are clearly evident. Moreover, the small, elongated, densely staining nuclei of **fibroblasts** (F) are also noted to surround somata, just peripheral to the capsule cells. **Axons** (Ax) of myelinated nerve fibers belong to the large pseudounipolar neurons.

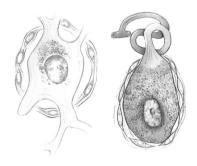

Multipolar cell (autonomic ganglia)
Unipolar cell (pseudounipolar cell
from dorsal root ganglion)

■ **KEY**

Ax	axon	f	nerve fiber	Ne	neutrophil
BV	blood vessel	L	leukocyte	S	septum
C	capsule	Li	lipofuscin	ScC	Schwann cell
Cc	capsule cell	n	nucleolus	So	soma
E	endothelial cell	MN	multipolar neuron	SS	supporting cell
F	fibroblast	N	nucleus		

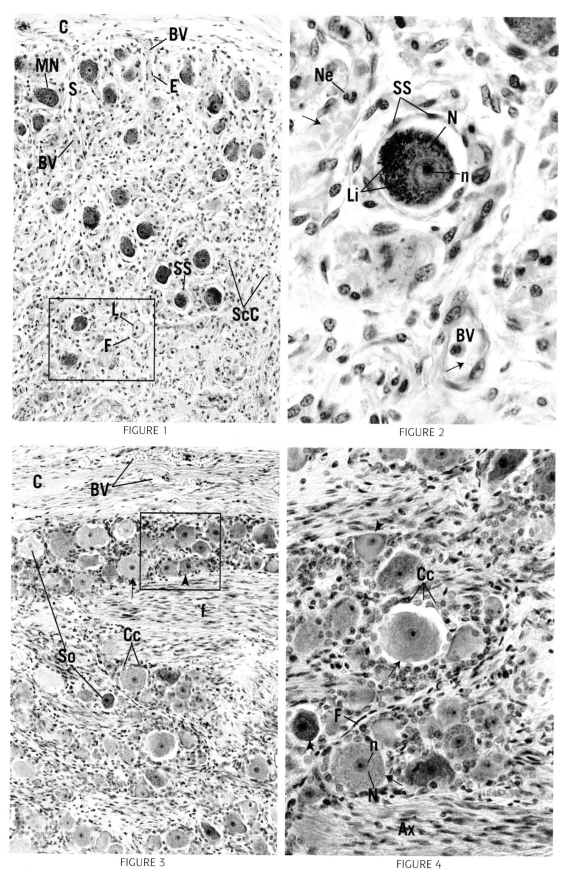

FIGURE 1

FIGURE 2

FIGURE 3

FIGURE 4

PLATE 7-5 ■ *Peripheral Nerve, Choroid Plexus*

FIGURE 1A ■ *Peripheral nerve. l.s. Monkey. Plastic section.* × 132.

The longitudinal section of the peripheral nerve fascicle presented in this photomicrograph is enveloped by its **perineurium** (P), composed of an outer **connective tissue layer** (CT) and an inner layer of flattened **epithelioid cells** (E). The perineurium conducts small **blood vessels** (BV), which are branches of larger vessels traveling in the surrounding epineurium, a structure composed of loose connective tissue with numerous fat cells. The peripheral nerve is composed of numerous nonmyelinated and myelinated nerve fibers, an example of which is presented in Figure 1b. The dense nuclei (arrows) within the nerve fascicle belong to Schwann cells and endoneurial cells. A region similar to the boxed area is presented in Figure 2.

FIGURE 1B ■ *Teased, myelinated nerve fiber. Paraffin section. l.s.* × 540.

This longitudinal section of a single myelinated nerve fiber displays its **axon** (Ax) and the neurokeratin network, the remnants of the dissolved **myelin** (M). Note the **node of Ranvier** (NR), a region where two Schwann cells meet. It is here, where the axon is not covered by myelin, that saltatory conduction of impulses occur. Observe that **Schmidt-Lanterman incisures** (SL) are clearly evident. These are regions where the cytoplasm of Schwann cells is trapped in the myelin sheath.

FIGURE 3 ■ *Peripheral nerve. x.s. Paraffin section.* × 132.

This transverse section presents portions of two fascicles, each surrounded by **perineurium** (P). The intervening loose connective tissue of the **epineurium** (Ep) with its **blood vessels** (BV) is clearly evident. The perineurium forms a **septum** (S), which subdivides this fascicle into two compartments. Note that the **axon.s** (Ax) are in the center of the **myelin sheath** (MS) and occasionally a crescent-shaped nucleus of a **Schwann cell** (ScC) is evident. The denser, smaller nuclei (arrows) belong to endoneurial cells.

Inset. **Peripheral nerve. x.s. Silver stain. Paraffin section.** × 540.

Silver-stained sections of myelinated nerve fibers have the large clear spaces (arrow) that indicate the dissolved myelin. The **axons** (Ax) stain well as dark, dense structures, and the delicate **endoneurium** (En) is also evident.

FIGURE 2 ■ *Peripheral nerve. l.s. Paraffin section.* × 270.

This is a higher magnification of a region similar to the boxed area of Figure 1a. A distinguishing characteristic of longitudinal sections of peripheral nerves is that they appear to follow a ziz-zag course, particularly evident in this photomicrograph. The sinuous course of these fibers is accentuated by the presence of nuclei of **Schwann cells** (ScC), **fibroblasts** (F), and endothelial cells of capillaries belonging to the endoneurium. Many of these nerve fibers are **myelinated** (M) as corroborated by the presence of the **nodes of Ranvier** (NR) and neurokeratin around the **axons** (Ax).

FIGURE 4 ■ *Choroid plexus. Paraffin section.* × 270.

The choroid plexus, located within the ventricles of the brain, is responsible for the formation of cerebrospinal fluid. This structure is composed of tufts of **capillaries** (Ca) whose tortuous course is followed by **villi** (Vi) of the simple cuboidal **choroid plexus epithelium** (cp). The **connective tissue core** (CT) of the choroid plexus is contributed by pia-arachnoid, while the simple cuboidal epithelium is modified ependymal lining of the ventricle. The clear spaces surrounding the choroid plexus belong to the ventricle of the brain.

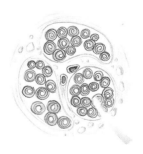

Nerve trunk (cross section)

■ **KEY**

Ax	axon	En	endoneurium	P	perineurium
BV	blood vessel	Ep	epineurium	S	septum
Ca	capillary	F	fibroblast	ScC	Schwann cell
cp	choroid plexus epithelium	M	myelin	SL	Schmidt-Lanterman incisure
CT	connective tissue	MS	myelin sheath		
E	epithelioid cell	NR	node of Ranvier	Vi	villus

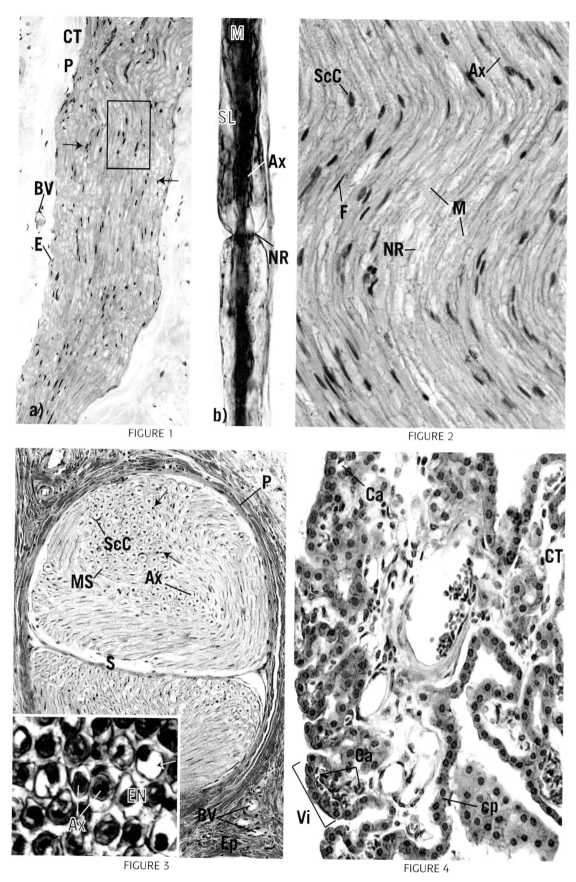

FIGURE 1

FIGURE 2

FIGURE 3

FIGURE 4

PLATE 7-6 ■ *Peripheral Nerve, Electron Microscopy*

FIGURE 1 ■ *Peripheral nerve. x.s. Mouse. Electron microscopy.* × 33,300.

This electron micrograph presents a cross-section of three myelinated and several unmyelinated nerve fibers. Note that the **axons** (Ax) (although they may be the afferent fibers of pseudounipolar neurons) are surrounded by a thick **myelin sheath** (MS), peripheral to which is the bulk of the **Schwann cell cytoplasm** (ScC) housing **mitochondria** (m), **rough endoplasmic reticulum** (rER), and **pinocytotic vesicles** (PV). The Schwann cell is surrounded by a **basal lamina** (BL) isolating this cell from the **endoneurial connective tissue** (CT). The myelin sheath is derived from the plasma membrane of the Schwann cell, which presumably wraps spirally around the axon, resulting in the formation of an **external** (EM) and **internal** (IM) **mesaxon**. The **axolemma** (Al) is separated from the Schwann cell membrane by a narrow cleft, the periaxonal space. The axoplasm houses

mitochondria (m), as well as **neurofilaments** (Nf) and **neurotubules** (Nt). Occasionally, the myelin wrapping is surrounded by Schwann cell cytoplasm on its outer and inner aspects, as in the nerve fiber in the upper right-hand corner. The **unmyelinated nerve fibers** (f) in the top of this electron micrograph display their relationship to the **Schwann cell** (ScC). The fibers are positioned in such a fashion that each lies in a complicated membrane-lined groove within the Schwann cell. Some fibers are situated superficially, while others are positioned more deeply within the grooves. However, a periaxonal (or peridendritic) space (arrows) is always present. **Mitochondria** (m), **neurofilaments** (Nf), and **neurotubules** (Nt) are also present. Note that the entire structure is surrounded by a **basal lamina** (BL), which covers but does not extend into the grooves (arrowheads) housing the nerve fibers. (Courtesy of Dr. J. Strum.)

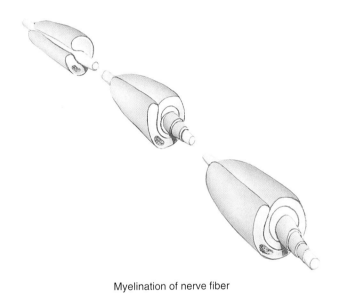

Myelination of nerve fiber

■ **KEY**

Al	axolemma	EM	external mesaxon	Nf	neurofilament
Ax	axon	f	nerve fiber	Nt	neurotubule
BL	basal lamina	IM	internal mesaxon	PV	pinocytotic vesicle
CT	endoneurial connective tissue	m	mitochondrion	rER	rough ER
		MS	myelin sheath	ScC	Schwann cell cytoplasm

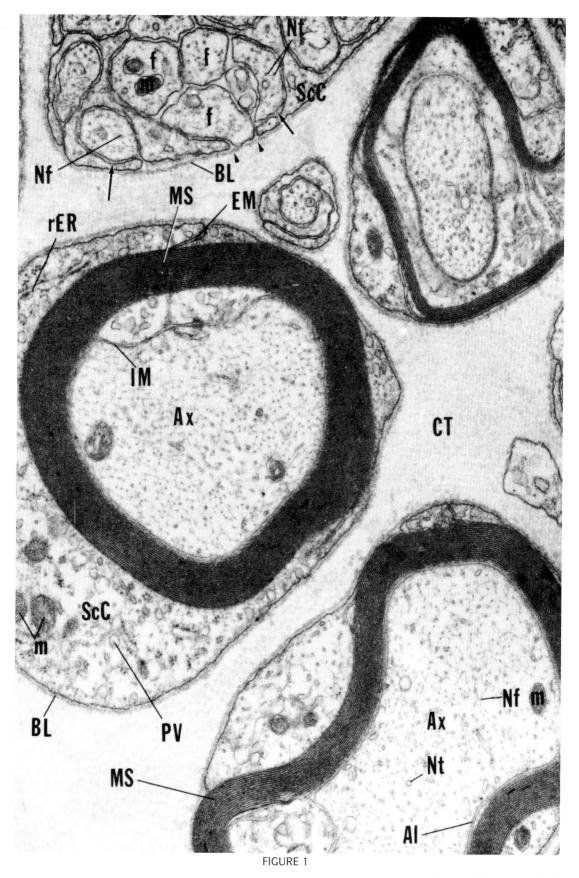

FIGURE 1

PLATE 7-7 ■ *Neuron Cell Body, Electron Microscopy*

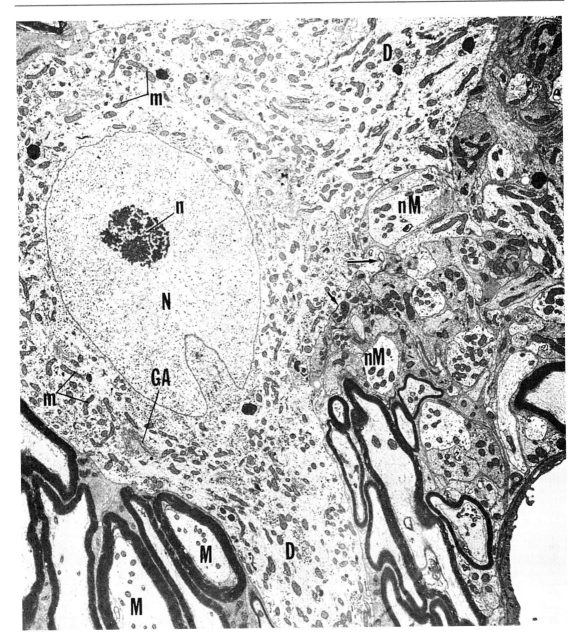

FIGURE 1 ▨ *Neuron. Lateral descending nucleus. Electron microscopy.* × 3589.

The soma of this neuron presents a typical appearance. Note the large **nucleus** (N) and **nucleolus** (n) surrounded by a considerable amount of cytoplasm rich in organelles. Observe the extensive **Golgi apparatus** (GA), numerous **mitochondria** (m), and elements of rough endoplasmic reticulum, which extend into the **dendrites** (D). **Myelinated** (M) and **nonmyelinated** (nM) fibers are also present, as are synapses (arrows) along the cell surface. (From Meszler R, Auker C, Carpenter D: *J Comp Neurol* 196:571–584, 1981.)

8

Circulatory System

The circulatory system is composed of two separate but connected components: the blood vascular system (cardiovascular system) that transports blood and the lymphatic vascular system that collects and returns excess extracellular fluid (lymph) to the blood vascular system. Lymphoid tissue is presented in Chapter 9.

BLOOD VASCULAR SYSTEM

The **blood vascular system,** consisting of the heart and blood vessels, functions in propelling and transporting blood and its various constituents throughout the body. The heart, acting as a pump, forces blood at high pressure into large, elastic arteries that carry the blood away from the heart. These arteries give way to increasingly smaller muscular arteries. Eventually, blood reaches extremely thin walled vessels, capillaries and small venules, where exchange of materials occurs. It is mostly here that certain cells, oxygen, nutrients, hormones, certain proteins, and additional materials leave the blood stream, whereas carbon dioxide, waste products, certain cells, and certain secretory products enter the bloodstream. **Capillary beds** are drained by the venous components of the circulatory system, which return blood to the heart. The blood vascular system is subdivided into the pulmonary and systemic circuits, which originate from the right and left sides of the heart, respectively. The **pulmonary circuit** takes oxygen-poor blood to the lungs to become oxygenated and returns it to the left side of the heart. The oxygen-rich blood is propelled via the **systemic circuit** to the remainder of the body to be returned to the right side of the heart, completing the cycle.

HEART

The heart is a four-chambered organ composed of two atria and two ventricles. The atria, subsequent to receiving blood from the pulmonary veins, venae

cavae, and coronary sinus, discharge it into the ventricles. Contractions of the ventricles then propel the blood either from the right ventricle into the pulmonary trunk for distribution to the lungs or from the left ventricle into the aorta for distribution to the remainder of the body. Although the walls of the ventricles are thicker than those of the atria, these chambers possess common characteristics, in that they are composed of three layers: epicardium, myocardium, and endocardium. **Epicardium,** the outermost layer, is covered by a simple squamous mesothelium deep to which is fibroelastic connective tissue. The deepest aspect of the epicardium is composed of adipose tissue that houses nerves and the coronary vessels. Most of the wall of the heart is composed of **myocardium,** consisting of bundles of cardiac muscle that are attached to the thick collagenous connective tissue skeleton of the heart. The **endocardium** forms the lining of the atria and ventricles and is composed of a simple squamous endothelium, as well as a subendothelial fibroelastic connective tissue. The endocardium participates in the formation of the heart valves, which control the direction of blood flow through the heart. Additionally, some cardiac muscle fibers are specialized to regulate the sequence of atrial and ventricular contractions. These are the sinoatrial and atrioventricular nodes, as well as the bundle of His and Purkinje fibers. The **sinoatrial node (SA node),** the pacemaker of the heart, is located at the junction of the superior vena cava and the right atrium. Impulses generated at this point are conducted to the **atrioventricular node (AV node),** which is located on the medial wall of the right ventricle near the tricuspid valve, as well as to the atrial myocardium. Arising from the AV node is the **bundle of His,** which bifurcates in the septum membranaceum to serve both ventricles. As these fibers reach the subendocardium, they ramify and are known as **Purkinje fibers,** which eventually merge with and become indistinguishable from cells of the myocardium. The inherent rhythm of the SA node is modulated by the autonomic nervous system, in that parasympathetic fibers derived from the vagus nerve decrease the rate of the heartbeat, whereas fibers derived from sympathetic ganglia increase it.

ARTERIES

Arteries, which conduct blood away from the heart, may be classified into three categories: elastic (conducting or large), muscular (distributing or medium), and arterioles (see Graphic 8-1). **Elastic arteries,** such as the aorta, receive blood directly from the heart and, consequently, are the largest of the arteries. **Muscular arteries** distribute blood to various organs, whereas **arterioles** regulate blood pressure and the distribution of blood to capillary beds via vasoconstriction and vasodilatation of vessel walls.

Blood vessels, including all arteries, are composed of three concentric layers: tunica intima, tunica media, and tunica adventitia. The **tunica intima** is composed of simple squamous endothelial cells lining the lumen and of various amounts of subendothelial connective tissue. The **tunica media,** usually the thickest of the three layers, is composed of circularly arranged smooth muscle cells and fibroelastic connective tissue, whose elastic content increases greatly with the size of the vessel. The **tunica adventitia** is the outermost layer of the vessel wall, consisting of fibroelastic connective tissue. In larger vessels, the tunica adventitia houses **vasa vasorum,** small blood vessels that supply the tunica adventitia and media of that vessel.

VEINS

Veins conduct blood away from body tissues and back to the heart (see Graphic 8-1). Generally, the diameters of veins are larger than those of corresponding arteries; however, veins are thinner walled, since they do not bear high blood pressures. Veins also possess three concentric, more or less definite layers: **tunica intima, tunica media,** and **tunica adventitia.** Furthermore, veins have fewer layers of smooth muscle cells in their tunica media than do arteries. Finally, many veins possess valves that act to prevent regurgitation of blood. Three categories of veins exist: small, medium, and large. The smallest veins, frequently referred to as venules, are also responsible for the exchange of materials. Moreover, **vasodilator substances,** such as **serotonin** and **histamine,** appear to act on small venules, causing them to become "leaky" by increasing the intercellular distances between the membranes of contiguous endothelial cells. Most such intercellular gaps occur in small venules rather than in capillaries.

CAPILLARIES

Capillaries usually form thin-walled networks that are supplied by arterioles and metarterioles and drained by venules (see Graphic 8-2). Frequently, capillary networks may be circumvented by specialized vessels called **arteriovenous anastomoses,** interposed between the arterial and venous systems. Capillaries are composed of highly attenuated **endothelial cells** that form narrow vascular channels 8–10 μm in diameter and are usually less than 1 mm long. Associated with capillaries are **basal laminae** and **pericytes,** but the capillary possesses no smooth muscle cells. Therefore, capillaries do not exhibit vasomotor activities. Control of blood flow into a capillary bed is established at the sites where individual capillaries arise from **terminal arterioles** or **metarterioles** and is accomplished by smooth muscle cells known as **precapillary sphincters.** The presence of **metarterioles** and **thoroughfare channels** permits the maintenance of an adequate blood supply during reduced flow through a capillary bed. Based on fine structural characteristics, three types of capillaries are recognized: fenestrated, continuous, and discontinuous. **Fenestrated capillaries** possess numerous pores, usually bridged by diaphragms, through which material may enter or leave the capillary lumen. **Continuous capillaries** are devoid of pores, and material must traverse the endothelial cell either via pinocytotic vesicles or between endothelial cell junctions. In certain areas of the body (brain, thymus, testes), however, fasciae occludentes formed by contiguous endothelial cells prevent the escape or entry of material through intercellular spaces. **Discontinuous capillaries (sinusoids)** are tortuous and possess large lumina. Their endothelial cells present large fenestrae and intercellular spaces. Moreover, their basal lamina is not continuous. Frequently, macrophages are associated with discontinuous capillaries. Some authors recognize sinusoids, venous sinusoids, and sinusoidal capillaries in place of discontinuous capillaries.

LYMPH VASCULAR SYSTEM

Excess extracellular fluid, which does not enter the venous return system at the level of the capillary bed or venule, gains entry into **lymphatic capillaries,** blindly ending thin vessels of the lymph vascular system. Subsequent to passing through chains of lymph nodes and larger lymph vessels, the fluid, known as lymph, enters the blood vascular system at the root of the neck.

Histophysiology

I. HEART

The **heart** is a muscular pump that propels blood at high pressure, via elastic arteries, to the lungs (**pulmonary circuit**) for oxygenation, and via the aorta (**systemic circuit**) for distribution of oxygenated blood to the tissues of the body.

A. Generation and Conduction of Impulse

The **sinoatrial node** (**SA node**) of the heart generates impulses, which results in the contraction of the atrial muscles, and blood from the atria enter the ventricles. The impulse is then transmitted to the **atrioventricular node** (**AV node**).

The **atrioventricular bundle** (**of His**) arises from the AV node and travels in the interventricular septum, where it subdivides to form the Purkinje fibers. The **Purkinje fibers** deliver the impulse to the cardiac muscle cells of the ventricles that contract to pump the blood from the right ventricle into the pulmonary trunk and from the left ventricle into the aorta.

B. Valves

Atrioventricular valves between the atria and ventricles prevent regurgitation of blood into the atria. Similarly, **semilunar valves** located in the pulmonary trunk and the aorta prevent regurgitation of blood from these vessels back into their respective ventricles. The closing of these valves is responsible for the sounds associated with the heart beat.

II. ARTERIES

Arteries are classified into three types: elastic, muscular, and arterioles. Capillaries arise from the terminal ends of arterioles and their walls have no smooth muscle tunic.

A. Elastic Arteries

Elastic arteries are the largest of the arteries. Since they arise directly from the heart, they are subject to cyclic changes of blood pressure, high as the ventricles pump blood into their lumina and low between the emptying of these chambers. In order to compensate for these intermittent pressure alterations, an abundance of elastic fibers are located in the walls of these vessels. These elastic fibers not only provide structural stability and permit distention of the elastic arteries, but they also assist in the maintenance of blood pressure in between heart beats.

B. Muscular Arteries

Muscular arteries comprise most of the named arteries of the body. Their tunica media is composed mostly of many layers of smooth muscle cells. Both elastic and muscular arteries are supplied by **vasa vasorum** and nerve fibers.

C. Arterioles

Arterioles are the smallest arteries and are responsible for regulating blood pressure. **Metarterioles** are the terminal ends of the arterioles, and they are characterized by the presence of incomplete rings of smooth muscle cells (**precapillary sphincters**) that encircle the origins of the capillaries. Metarterioles form the arterial (proximal) end of a **central channel,** and they are responsible for delivering blood into the capillary bed. The venous (distal) end of the central channel, known as a **thoroughfare channel,** is responsible for draining blood from the capillary bed and delivering it into venules. Contraction of precapillary sphincters of the metarteriole shunts the blood into the **thoroughfare channel,** and from there into the venule; this way, the blood bypasses the capillary bed. **Arteriovenous anastomoses** are direct connections between arteries and venules and they also function in having blood bypass the capillary bed. These shunts function in **thermoregulation** and blood pressure control.

D. Vasoconstriction and Vasodilation

Vasoconstriction is due to the action of sympathetic nerve fibers that act on the smooth muscles of the tunica media. This is especially important in the arterioles, which are responsible for the regulation of blood pressure.

Vasodilation is accomplished by parasympathetic nerve fibers in an indirect fashion. Instead of acting on smooth muscle cells, acetylcholine, released by the nerve end-foot, is bound to receptors on the endothelial cells, inducing them to release **nitric oxide (NO)**, previously known as endothelial-derived releasing factor (EDRF). Nitric oxide acts on the cGMP system of the smooth muscle cells, causing their relaxation.

III. CAPILLARIES

Capillaries are very small vessels that consist of a single layer of endothelial cells surrounded by a basal lamina and occasional **pericytes.** These vessels exhibit **selective permeability** and they, along with venules, are responsible for the exchange of gases, metabolites, and other substances between the blood stream and the tissues of the body. There are three types of capillaries, continuous, fenestrated, and sinusoidal.

A. Capillary Types

Continuous capillaries lack fenestrae, display only occasional pinocytotic vesicles, and possess a continuous basal lamina. They are present in regions such as peripheral nerve fibers, skeletal muscle, lungs, and thymus.

The endothelial cells of **fenestrated capillaries** are penetrated by relatively large diaphragm-covered pores. These cells also possess pinocytic vesicles and are enveloped by a continuous basal lamina. Fenestrated capillaries are located in endocrine glands, pancreas, and lamina propria of the intestines, and they also constitute the glomeruli of the kidneys, although their fenestrae are not covered by a diaphragm.

Sinusoidal capillaries are much larger than their fenestrated or continuous counterparts. They are enveloped by a discontinuous basal lamina, and their endothelial cells do not possess pinocytic vesicles. The intercellular junctions of their endothelial cells display gaps, thus permitting leakage of material into and out of these vessels. Sinusoidal capillaries are located in the liver, spleen, lymph nodes, bone marrow, and the suprarenal cortex.

B. Capillary Permeability

Capillary permeability is dependent not only on the endothelial cells comprising the capillary but also on the [physico]-chemical characteristics, such as size, charge, and shape, of the traversing substance. Some molecules, such as H_2O diffuse through, whereas others are actively transported by carrier proteins across the endothelial cell plasma membrane.

Still others move through fenestrae or through gaps in the intercellular junctions. Certain pharmacological agents, such as **bradykinin** and **histamine**, have the ability to alter capillary permeability. Leukocytes leave the bloodstream by passing through intercellular junctions of the endothelial cells (**diapedesis**) to enter the extracellular spaces of tissues and organs.

C. Metabolic Functions of Capillaries

Capillary endothelial cells possess the capacity to **deactivate substances,** such as prostaglandins, serotonin, and bradykinin; **catabolize** lipoproteins into triglycerides, fatty acids, and monoglycerides; **convert** angiotensin I to angiotensin II; **release prostacyclins** to inhibit the aggregation of platelets; promote **fibrinolysis** by producing activators of plasminogens; express **binding sites** for certain clotting factors; and, if injured, **release tissue factors** that initiate the clotting response.

IV. VEINS

Veins, unlike arteries, are low pressure vessels that conduct blood from the tissues of the body back to the heart. Generally, they have larger lumina and thinner walls with fewer layers of smooth muscle cells than their companion arteries. Also, many veins contain valves in the lumen that prevent retrograde blood flow.

V. LYMPHATIC VASCULAR SYSTEM

Lymphatic capillaries begin as blind-ending vessels. Excess extracellular fluid enters these capillaries, becomes known as lymph; this fluid is delivered into lymphatic vessels of larger and larger diameters. Interspersed among these vessels are a series of lymph nodes that filter the lymph. The lymphatic vessels eventually deliver their contents into the **thoracic** and **right lymphatic ducts** that empty the lymph into large veins in the root of the neck. Large lymphatic vessels are similar in structure to small veins, except that they possess valves, have larger lumina, and have thinner walls.

Clinical Considerations ▨ ▨ ▨

Valve Defects

Children who have had rheumatic fever may develop valve defects. These valve defects may be related to improper closing (**incompetency**) or improper opening (**stenosis**). Fortunately, most of these defects can be repaired surgically.

Aneurysm

A damaged vessel wall may, over time, become weakened and begin to enlarge and form a bulging defect known as an aneurysm. This condition occurs most often in large vessels such as the aorta. If undetected or left untreated, it may rupture without warning and cause internal bleeding with fatal consequences. Surgical repair is possible depending upon the health of the individual.

Atherosclerosis

Atherosclerosis, the deposition of plaque within the walls of large- and medium-sized arteries, results in reduced blood flow within that vessel. If this condition involves the coronary arteries, the decreased blood flow to the myocardium causes coronary heart disease. The consequences of this disease may be angina pectoris, myocardial infarct, chronic ischemic cardiopathy, or even sudden death.

Raynaud's Disease

Raynaud's disease is an idiopathic condition where the arterioles of the fingers and toes go into sudden spasms lasting minutes to hours, cutting off blood supply to the digits with a resultant cyanosis and loss of sensation. This condition, affecting mostly younger women, is believed to be due to exposure to cold as well as to the patient's emotional state. Other causes include atherosclerosis, scleroderma, injury, as well as a reaction to certain medications. The treatment of choice is limiting exposure to cold, prescribing mild sedatives, and discontinuing the use of tobacco products. Occasionally, the practicing of relaxation therapy may also control the condition.

Summary of Histological Organization

I. ELASTIC ARTERY (CONDUCTING ARTERY)

Among these are the **aorta, common carotid,** and **subclavian arteries.**

A. Tunica Intima

Lined by short, polygonal **endothelial cells.** The **subendothelial connective tissue** is fibroelastic and houses some longitudinally disposed smooth muscle cells. **Internal elastic lamina** is not clearly defined.

B. Tunica Media

Characterized by numerous **fenestrated membranes** (spiral to concentric sheets of fenestrated elastic membranes). Enmeshed among the elastic material are circularly disposed **smooth muscle cells** and associated **collagenous, reticular,** and **elastic fibers.**

C. Tunica Adventitia

Thin, **collagenous connective tissue** containing some **elastic fibers** and a few longitudinally oriented **smooth muscle cells. Vasa vasorum** (vessels of vessels) are also present.

II. MUSCULAR ARTERY (DISTRIBUTING ARTERY)

Among these are the named arteries, with the exception of the elastic arteries.

A. Tunica Intima

These are lined by polygonal-shaped flattened **endothelial cells** that bulge into the lumen during vasoconstriction. The **subendothelial connective tissue** houses fine **collagenous fibers** and few longitudinally disposed **smooth muscle cells.** The **internal elastic lamina,** clearly evident, is frequently split into two membranes.

B. Tunica Media

Characterized by many layers of circularly disposed **smooth muscle cells,** with some **elastic, reticular,** and **collagenous fibers** among the muscle cells. The **external elastic lamina** is well defined.

C. Tunica Adventitia

Usually a very thick **collagenous** and **elastic tissue,** with some longitudinally oriented **smooth muscle fibers. Vasa vasorum** are also present.

III. ARTERIOLES

These are arterial vessels whose diameter is less than 100 μm.

A. Tunica Intima

Endothelium and a variable amount of **subendothelial connective tissue** are always present. The **internal elastic lamina** is present in larger arterioles, but absent in smaller arterioles.

B. Tunica Media

The spirally arranged **smooth muscle fibers** may be up to three layers thick. An **external elastic lamina** is present in larger arterioles, but absent in smaller arterioles.

C. Tunica Adventitia

This is composed of **collagenous** and **elastic connective tissues,** whose thickness approaches that of the tunica media.

IV. CAPILLARIES

Most **capillaries** in cross section appear as thin, circular profiles 8–10 μm in diameter. Occasionally, a fortuitous section will display an **endothelial cell nucleus,** a red blood cell, or, very infrequently, a white blood cell. Frequently, capillaries will be collapsed and not evident with the light microscope. **Pericytes** are usually associated with capillaries.

V. VENULES

Venules possess much larger lumina and thinner walls than corresponding arterioles.

A. Tunica Intima

Endothelium lies on a very thin **subendothelial connective tissue** layer, which increases with the size of the vessel. **Pericytes** are frequently associated with smaller venules.

B. Tunica Media

Absent in smaller venules, while in larger venules one or two layers of **smooth muscle cells** may be observed.

C. Tunica Adventitia

Consists of **collagenous connective tissue** with **fibroblasts** and some **elastic fibers.**

VI. MEDIUM-SIZED VEINS

A. Tunica Intima

The **endothelium** and a scant amount of **subendothelial connective tissue** are always present. Occasionally, a thin **internal elastic lamina** is observed. **Valves** may be evident.

B. Tunica Media

Much thinner than that of the corresponding artery, but does possess a few layers of **smooth muscle cells.** Occasionally, some of the muscle fibers, instead of being circularly disposed, are longitudinally disposed. Bundles of **collagen fibers** interspersed with a few **elastic fibers** are also present.

C. Tunica Adventitia

Composed of **collagen** and some **elastic fibers,** which constitute the bulk of the vessel wall. Occasionally, longitudinally oriented **smooth muscle cells** may be present. **Vasa vasorum** are noted to penetrate even the **tunica media.**

VII. LARGE VEINS

A. Tunica Intima

Same as that of medium-sized veins, but displays thicker **subendothelial connective tissue.** Some large veins have well-defined **valves.**

B. Tunica Media

Not very well defined, although it may present some **smooth muscle cells** interspersed among **collagenous** and **elastic fibers.**

C. Tunica Adventitia

Thickest of the three layers and accounts for most of the vessel wall. May contain longitudinally oriented **smooth muscle fiber bundles** among the thick layers of **collagen** and **elastic fibers. Vasa vasorum** are commonly present.

VIII. HEART

An extremely thick, muscular organ composed of three layers: **endocardium, myocardium,** and **epicardium.** The presence of **cardiac muscle** is characteristic of this organ. Additional structural parameters may include **Purkinje fibers,** thick **valves, atrioventricular** and **sinoatrial nodes,** as well as the **chordae tendineae** and the thick, connective tissue **cardiac skeleton.**

IX. LYMPHATIC VESSELS

Lymphatic vessels are either collapsed and, therefore, not discernible, or they are filled with lymph. In the latter case, they present the appearance of a clear, endothelial-lined space resembling a blood vessel. However, the lumina contain no **red blood cells,** though **lymphocytes** may be present. The **endothelium** may display **valves.**

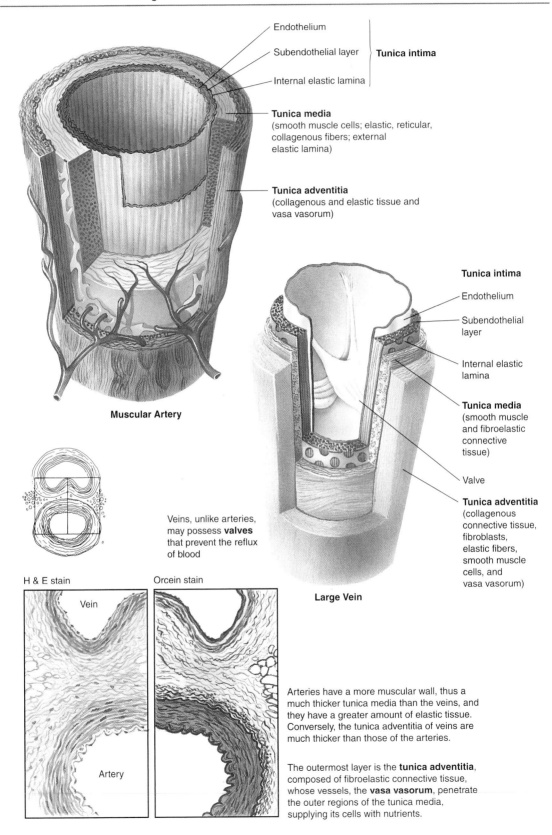

Endothelium

Subendothelial layer

Internal elastic lamina

Tunica intima

Tunica media
(smooth muscle cells; elastic, reticular, collagenous fibers; external elastic lamina)

Tunica adventitia
(collagenous and elastic tissue and vasa vasorum)

Muscular Artery

Tunica intima

Endothelium

Subendothelial layer

Internal elastic lamina

Tunica media
(smooth muscle and fibroelastic connective tissue)

Valve

Tunica adventitia
(collagenous connective tissue, fibroblasts, elastic fibers, smooth muscle cells, and vasa vasorum)

Veins, unlike arteries, may possess **valves** that prevent the reflux of blood

Large Vein

H & E stain

Vein

Orcein stain

Artery

Arteries have a more muscular wall, thus a much thicker tunica media than the veins, and they have a greater amount of elastic tissue. Conversely, the tunica adventitia of veins are much thicker than those of the arteries.

The outermost layer is the **tunica adventitia**, composed of fibroelastic connective tissue, whose vessels, the **vasa vasorum**, penetrate the outer regions of the tunica media, supplying its cells with nutrients.

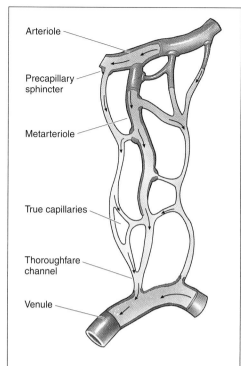

Arteriole

Precapillary
sphincter

Metarteriole

True capillaries

Thoroughfare
channel

Venule

Some capillary beds, such as those of the skin, are designed so that they may be bypassed under certain circumstances. One method whereby blood flow may be controlled is the use of **central channels** that convey blood from and arteriole to a venule. The proximal half of the central channel is a **metarteriole**, a vessel with an incomplete smooth muscle coat. Flow of blood into each capillary that arises from the metarteriole is controlled by a smooth muscle cell, the **precapillary sphincter**. The distal half of the central channel is the **thoroughfare channel**, which possesses no smooth muscle cells and accepts blood from the capillary bed. If the capillary bed is to be bypassed, the precapillary sphincters contract, preventing blood flow into the capillary bed, and the blood goes directly into the venule.

Capillaries consists of a simple squamous epithelium rolled into a narrow cylinder 8–10 μm in diameter. **Continuous (somatic) capillaries** have no fenestrae; material transverses the endothelial cell in either direction via **pinocytotic vesicles**. **Fenestrated (visceral) capillaries** are characterized by the presence of perforations, **fenestrae**, 60–80 μm in diameter, which may or may not be bridged by a diaphragm. **Sinusoidal capillaries** have a large lumen (30–40 μm in diameter), possess numerous fenestrae, have discontinuous basal lamina, and lack pinocytotic vesicles. Frequently, adjacent endothelial cells of sinusoidal capillaries overlap one another in an incomplete fashion.

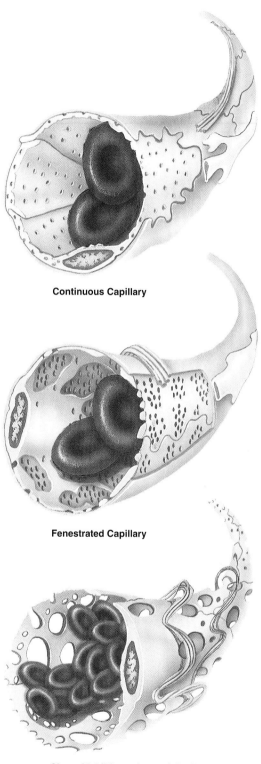

Continuous Capillary

Fenestrated Capillary

Sinusoidal (Discontinuous) Capillary

PLATE 8-1 ■ *Elastic Artery*

FIGURE 1 ▧ *Elastic artery. l.s. Aorta. Monkey. Plastic section.* × 132.

This low magnification photomicrograph displays almost the entire thickness of the wall of the aorta, the largest artery of the body. The **tunica intima** (TI) is lined by a simple squamous epithelium whose nuclei (arrowheads) bulge into the lumen of the vessel. The lines, which appear pale at this magnification, are elastic fibers and laminae, while the nuclei belong to smooth muscle cells and connective tissue cells. The internal elastic lamina is not readily identifiable, because the intima is rich in elastic fibers. The **tunica media** (TM) is composed of smooth muscle cells whose **nuclei** (N) are clearly evident. These smooth muscle cells lie in the spaces between the concentrically layered **fenestrated membranes** (FM), composed of elastic tissue. The **external elastic lamina** (xEL) is that portion of the media that adjoins the adventitia. The outermost coat of the aorta, the **tunica adventitia** (TA), is composed of collagenous and elastic fibers interspersed with connective tissue cells and blood vessels, the **vasa vasorum** (VV). Regions similar to the boxed areas are presented in Figures 2 and 3.

FIGURE 2 ▧ *Elastic artery. x.s. Monkey. Plastic section.* × 540.

This is a higher magnification of a region of the tunica intima, similar to the boxed area of Figure 1. The endothelial lining of the blood vessel presents **nuclei** (arrowhead), which bulge into the **lumen** (L). The numerous **elastic fibers** (EF) form an incomplete elastic lamina. Note that the interstices of the tunica intima house many **smooth muscle cells** (SM), whose nuclei are corkscrew-shaped (arrows), indicative of muscle contraction. Although most of the cellular elements are smooth muscle cells, it has been suggested that fibroblasts and macrophages may also be present; however, it is believed that the elastic fibers and the amorphous intercellular substances are synthesized by the smooth muscle cells.

FIGURE 3 ▧ *Elastic artery. x.s. Monkey. Plastic section.* × 540.

This is a higher magnification of the tunica adventitia similar to the boxed region of Figure 1. The outermost region of the **tunica media** (TM) is demarcated by the **external elastic lamina** (xEL). The **tunica adventitia** (TA) is composed of thick bundles of **collagen fibers** (CF) interspersed with elastic fibers. Observe the nuclei of **fibroblasts** (F) located in the interstitial spaces among the collagen fiber bundles. Since the vessel wall is very thick, nutrients diffusing from the lumen cannot serve the entire vessel; therefore, the adventitia is supplied by small vessels known as **vasa vasorum** (VV). Vasa vasorum provide circulation not only for the tunica adventitia but also for the outer portion of the tunica media. Moreover, lymphatic vessels (not observed here) are also present in the adventitia.

FIGURE 4 ▧ *Elastic artery. x.s. Human. Elastic stain. Paraffin section.* × 132.

The use of a special stain to demonstrate the presence of concentric elastic sheets, known as **fenestrated membranes** (FM), displays the highly elastic quality of the aorta. The number of fenestrated membranes, as well as the thickness of each membrane, increase with age, so that the adult will possess almost twice as many of these structures as an infant. These membranes are called fenestrated, since they possess spaces (arrows) through which nutrients and waste materials diffuse. The interstices between the fenestrated membranes are occupied by smooth muscle cells, whose **nuclei** (N) are evident, as well as amorphous intercellular materials, collagen, and fine elastic fibers. The **tunica adventitia** (TA) is composed mostly of **collagenous fiber bundles** (CF) and some **elastic fibers** (EF). Numerous **fibroblasts** (F) and other connective tissue cells occupy the adventitia.

■ **KEY**

CF	collagen fiber	L	lumen	TI	tunica intima
EF	elastic fiber	N	nucleus	TM	tunica media
F	fibroblast	SM	smooth muscle cell	VV	vasa vasorum
FM	fenestrated membrane	TA	tunica adventitia	xEL	external elastic lamina

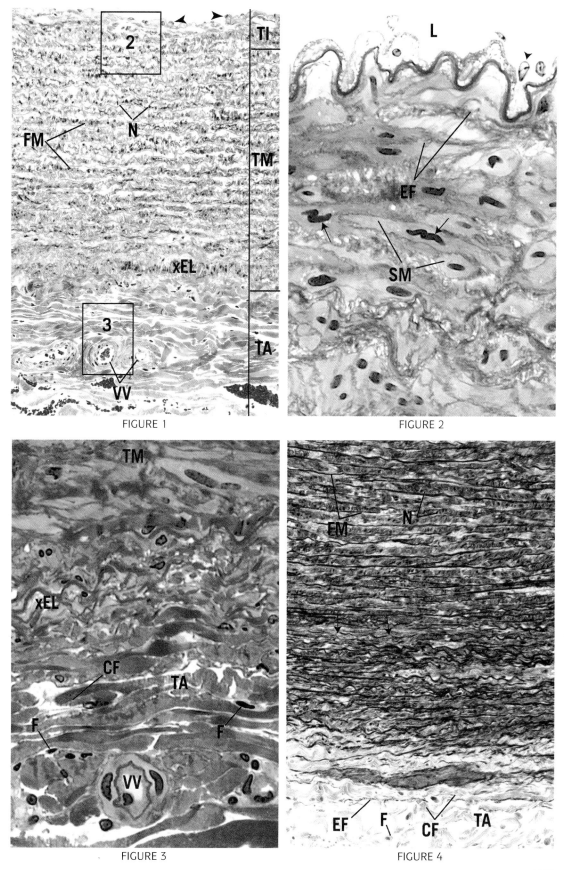

FIGURE 1

FIGURE 2

FIGURE 3

FIGURE 4

PLATE 8-2 ■ *Muscular Artery, Vein*

FIGURE 1 ■ *Artery and vein. x.s. Monkey. Plastic section.* × 132.

This low magnification photomicrograph presents a **muscular artery** (MA) and corresponding **vein** (V). Observe that the wall of the artery is much thicker than that of the vein and contains considerably more muscle fibers. The three concentric tunicae of the artery are evident. The **tunica intima** (TI) with its **endothelial layer** (En) and **internal elastic lamina** (iEL) is readily apparent. The thick **tunica media** (TM) is identified by the circularly or spirally displayed **smooth muscle cells** (SM) that are embedded in an elastic type of intercellular material. These elastic fibers, as well as the external elastic lamina—the outermost layer of the tunica media—are not apparent with hematoxylin and eosin stain. The **tunica adventitia** (TA), almost as thick as the media, contains no smooth muscle cells. It is composed chiefly of **collagen** (CF) and **elastic** (EF) fibers, as well as fibroblasts and other connective tissue cells. The wall of the companion vein presents the same three tunicae: **intima** (TI), **media** (TM), and **adventitia** (TA); however, all three (but especially the media) are reduced in thickness.

FIGURE 2 ■ *Artery and vein. x.s. Elastic stain. Paraffin section.* × 132.

The elastic stain used in this transverse section of a **muscular artery** (MA) and corresponding **vein** (V) clearly demonstrates the differences between arteries and veins. The **tunica intima** (TI) of the artery stains dark, due to the thick internal elastic lamina, while that of the vein does not stain nearly as intensely. The thick **tunica media** (TM) of the artery is composed of numerous layers of circularly or spirally disposed **smooth muscle cells** (SM) with many elastic fibers ramifying through this tunic. The **tunica media** (TM) of the vein has only a few smooth muscle cell layers with little intervening elastic fibers. The **external elastic lamina** (xEL) of the artery is much better developed than that of the vein. Finally, the **tunica adventitia** (TA) constitutes the bulk of the wall of the vein and is composed of **collagenous** (CF) and **elastic** (EF) fibers. The **tunica adventitia** (TA) of the artery is also thick, but it comprises only about half the thickness of its wall. It is also composed of collagenous and elastic fibers. Both vessels possess their own **vasa vasorum** (VV) in their tunicae adventitia. A region similar to the boxed area is presented at a higher magnification in Figure 3.

FIGURE 3 ■ *Artery. x.s. Elastic stain. Paraffin section.* × 132.

This photomicrograph is a higher magnification of a region similar to the boxed area of Figure 2. The **endothelium** (En), subendothelial connective tissue (arrow), and the highly contracted **internal elastic lamina** (iEL) are readily evident. These three structures constitute the tunica intima of the muscular artery. The **tunica media** (TM) is very thick and consists of many layers of spirally or circularly disposed **smooth muscle cells** (SM), whose **nuclei** (N) are readily identifiable with this stain. Numerous **elastic fibers** (EF) ramify through the intercellular spaces between smooth muscle cells. The **external elastic lamina** (xEL), which comprises the outermost layer of the tunica media, is seen to advantage in this preparation. Finally, note the **collagenous** (CF) and **elastic** (EF) fibers of the **tunica adventitia** (TA), as well as the nuclei (arrowhead) of the various connective tissue cells.

FIGURE 4 ■ *Large vein. x.s. Human. Paraffin section.* × 270.

Large veins, as the inferior vena cava in this photomicrograph, are very different from the medium-sized veins of Figures 1 and 2. The **tunica intima** (TI) is composed of **endothelium** (EN) and some subendothelial connective tissue, whereas the **tunica media** (TM) is greatly reduced in thickness and contains only occasional smooth muscle cells. The bulk of the wall of the vena cava is composed of the greatly thickened **tunica adventitia** (TA), consisting of three concentric regions. The innermost layer (1) displays thick collagen bundles (arrows) arrayed in a spiral configuration, which permits it to become elongated or shortened, with respiratory excursion of the diaphragm. The middle layer (2) presents smooth muscle (or cardiac muscle) cells, longitudinally disposed. The outer layer (3) is characterized by thick bundles of **collagen fibers** (CF) interspersed with elastic fibers. This region contains **vasa vasorum** (VV), which supply nourishment to the wall of the vena cava.

■ **KEY**

CF	collagen fiber	N	nucleus	TM	tunica media
EF	elastic fiber	SM	smooth muscle cell	V	vein
En	endothelial layer	TA	tunica adventitia	VV	vasa vasorum
iEL	internal elastic lamina	TI	tunica intima	xEL	external elastic lamina
MA	muscular artery				

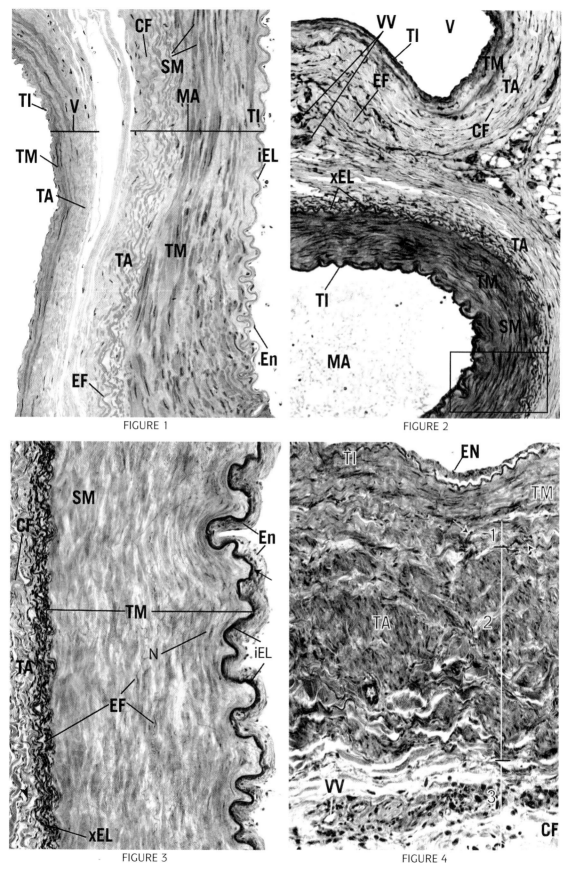

FIGURE 1

FIGURE 2

FIGURE 3

FIGURE 4

PLATE 8-3 ■ *Arterioles, Venules, Capillaries, Lymph Vessels*

FIGURE 1 ■ *Arteriole and venule. l.s. Monkey. Plastic section.* × 270.

This longitudinal section of a large **arteriole** (A) and companion **venule** (Ve) from the connective tissue septum of a monkey submandibular gland displays a **duct** (D) of the gland between the two vessels. Observe that the thickness of the arteriole wall approximates the diameter of the **lumen** (L). The endothelial cell **nuclei** (N) are readily evident in both vessels, as are the **smooth muscle cells** (SM) of the tunica media. The arteriole also presents an **internal elastic lamina** (iEL) between the tunica media and the endothelial cells. The **tunica adventitia** (TA) of the arteriole displays nuclei of fibroblasts, while those of the venule merge imperceptibly with the surrounding connective tissue. Glandular acini are evident in this field as are **serous units** (SU) and **serous demilunes** (SD).

FIGURE 2 ■ *Arteriole and venule. x.s. Monkey. Plastic section.* × 540.

This small **arteriole** (A) and its companion **venule** (Ve) are from the submucosa of the fundic region of a monkey stomach. Observe the obvious difference between the diameters of the **lumina** (L) of the two vessels, as well as the thickness of their walls. Due to the greater muscularity of the **tunica media** (TM) of the arteriole, the **nuclei** (N) of its endothelial cells bulge into its round lumen. The **tunica media** (TM) of the venule is much reduced, while the **tunica adventitia** (TA) is well developed and is composed of **collagenous connective tissue** (CT) interspersed with elastic fibers (not evident in this hematoxylin and eosin section).

FIGURE 3 ■ *Capillary. l.s. Monkey. Plastic section.* × 540.

In this photomicrograph of the monkey cerebellum, the molecular layer displays longitudinal sections of a capillary. Note that the endothelial cell **nuclei** (N) are occasionally in the field of view. The **cytoplasm** (Cy) of the highly attenuated endothelial cells is visible as thin, dark lines, bordering the **lumina** (L) of the capillary. Red blood cells (arrows) are noted to be distorted as they pass through the narrow lumina of the vessel.

Inset. Capillary. x.s. Monkey. Plastic section. × 540.

The connective tissue represented in this photomicrograph displays bundles of **collagen fibers** (CF), nuclei of connective tissue cells (arrow), as well as a cross section of a **capillary** (C), whose endothelial cell **nucleus** (N) is clearly evident.

FIGURE 4 ■ *Lymphatic vessel. l.s. Monkey. Plastic section.* × 270.

This photomicrograph presents a villus from monkey duodenum. Note the simple columnar **epithelium** (E) interspersed with occasional **goblet cells** (GC). The connective tissue lamina propria displays numerous **plasma cells** (PC), **mast cells** (MC), **lymphocytes** (Ly), and **smooth muscle fibers** (SM). The longitudinal section of the **lumen** (L) lined with **endothelium** (En) is a lacteal, a blindly ending lymphatic channel. Since lymph vessels do not transport red blood cells, the lacteal appears to be empty, but in fact it contains lymph. Subsequent to a fatty meal, lacteals contain chylomicrons. Observe that the wall of the lacteal is very flimsy in relation to the diameter of the vessel.

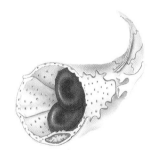

Continuous capillary

■ **KEY**

A	arteriole	En	endothelium	PC	plasma cell
C	capillary	GC	goblet cell	SD	serous demilune
CF	collagen fiber	iEL	internal elastic lamina	SM	smooth muscle cell
CT	collagenous connective tissue	L	lumen	SU	serous unit
Cy	cytoplasm	Ly	lymphocyte	TA	tunica adventitia
D	duct	MC	mast cell	TM	tunica media
E	epithelium	N	nucleus	Ve	venule

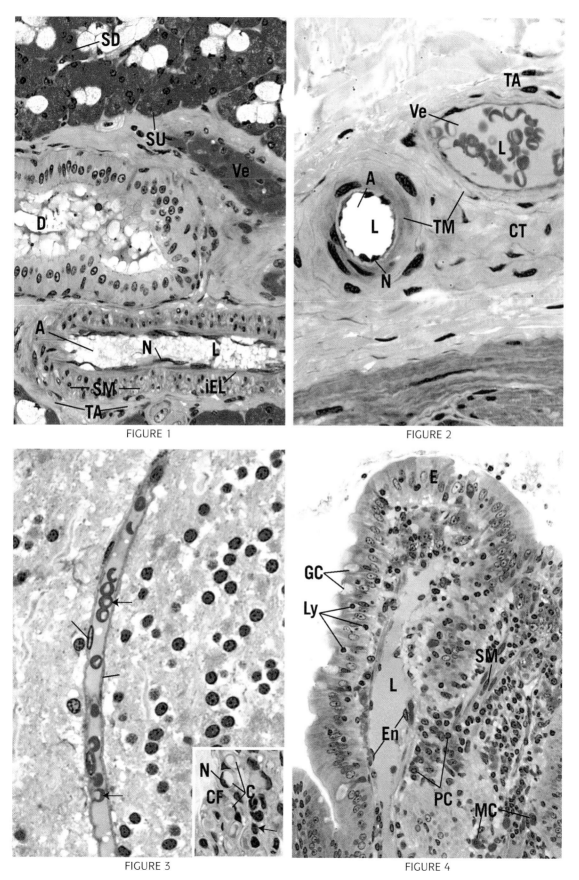

FIGURE 1

FIGURE 2

FIGURE 3

FIGURE 4

PLATE 8-4 ■ *Heart*

FIGURE 1 ■ *Endocardium. Human. Paraffin section.* × 132.

The endocardium, the innermost layer of the heart, is lined by a simple squamous epithelium that is continuous with the endothelial of the various blood vessels entering or exiting the heart. The endocardium is composed of three layers, the innermost of which consists of the **endothelium** (En) and the subendothelial **connective tissue** (CT), whose collagenous fibers and connective tissue cell **nuclei** (N) are readily evident. The middle layer of the endocardium, although composed of dense collagenous and elastic fibers and some smooth muscle cells, is occupied in this photomicrograph by branches of the conducting system of the heart, the **Purkinje fibers** (PF). The third layer of the endocardium borders the thick **myocardium** (My) and is composed of looser connective tissue elements housing blood vessels, occasional adipocytes, and additional connective tissue cells.

FIGURE 2 ■ *Purkinje fibers. Iron hematoxylin. Paraffin section.* × 132.

The stain utilized in preparing this section of the ventricular myocardium stains **red blood cells** (RBC) and **cardiac muscle cells** (CM) very intensely. Therefore, the thick bundle of **Purkinje fibers** (PF) is shown to advantage, due to its less dense staining quality. The **connective tissue** (CT) surrounding these fibers is highly vascularized, as evidenced by the red blood cell–filled capillaries. Purkinje fibers are composed of individual cells, each with a centrally placed single **nucleus** (N). These fibers form numerous gap junctions with each other and with cardiac muscle cells. The boxed area is presented at a higher magnification in the inset.

Inset. **Purkinje fibers. Iron hematoxylin. Paraffin section.** × 270.

Individual cells of Purkinje fibers are much larger than cardiac muscle cells. However, the presence of peripherally displaced **myofibrils** (m) displaying A and I bands (arrow) clearly demonstrates that they are modified cardiac muscle cells. The **nucleus** (N) is surrounded by a clear area, housing glycogen and mitochondria.

FIGURE 3 ■ *Heart valve. l.s. Paraffin section.* × 132.

This figure is a montage, displaying a **valve leaflet** (Le), as well as the **endocardium** (EC) of the heart. The leaflet is in the **lumen** (L) of the ventricle, as is evidenced by the numerous trapped **red blood cells** (RBC). The **endothelial** (En) lining of the endocardium is continuous with the endothelial lining of the leaflet. The three layers of the endocardium are clearly evident, as are the occasional **smooth muscle cells** (SM) and **blood vessels** (BV). The core of the leaflet is composed of dense collagenous and elastic connective tissue, housing numerous cells whose nuclei are readily observed. Since the core of these leaflets is devoid of blood vessels, the connective tissue cells receive their nutrients directly from the blood in the lumen of the heart via simple diffusion. The connective tissue core of the leaflet is continuous with the skeleton of the heart that forms a fibrous ring around the opening of the valves.

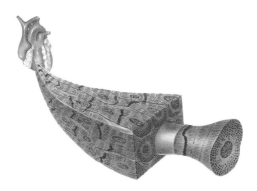

Cardiac muscle

■ **KEY**

BV	blood vessel	En	endothelium	My	myocardium
CM	cardiac muscle cell	L	lumen	N	nucleus
CT	connective tissue	Le	valve leaflet	PF	Purkinje fiber
EC	endocardium	m	myofibril	RBC	red blood cell

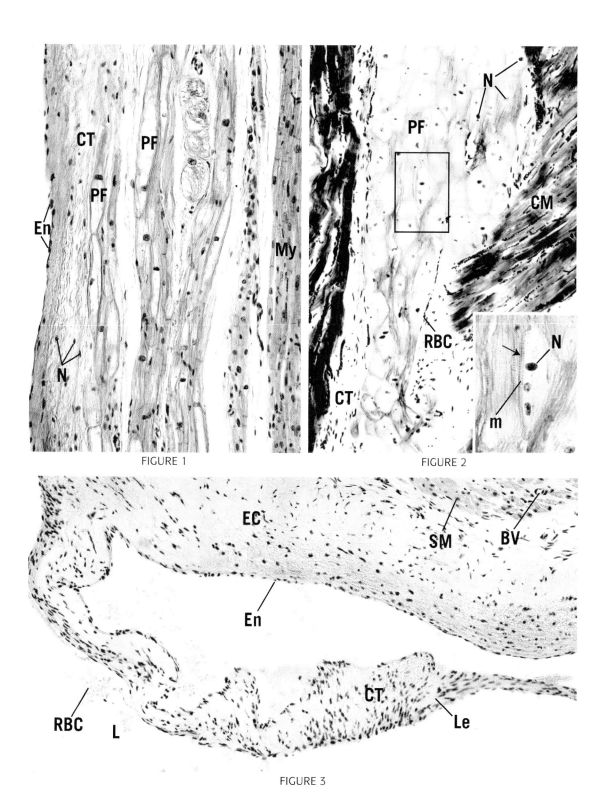

FIGURE 1

FIGURE 2

FIGURE 3

PLATE 8-5 ■ *Capillary, Electron Microscopy*

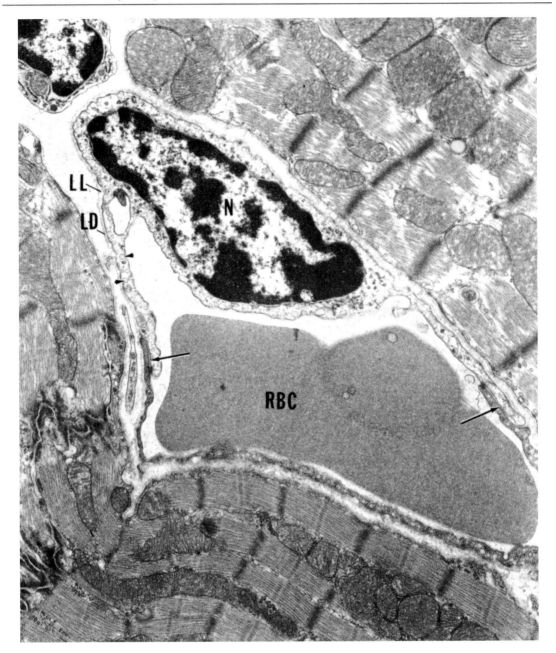

FIGURE 1 ■ *Continuous capillary. x.s. Cardiac muscle. Mouse. Electron microscopy.* × 29,330.

This electron micrograph of a continuous capillary in cross section was taken from mouse heart tissue. Observe that the section passes through the **nucleus** (N) of one of the endothelial cells constituting the wall of the vessel and that the lumen contains **red blood cells** (RBC). Note that the endothelial cells are highly attenuated and that they form tight junctions (arrows) with each other. Arrowheads point to pinocytotic vesicles that traverse the endothelial cell. The **lamina densa** (LD) and **lamina lucida** (LL) of the basal lamina are clearly evident.

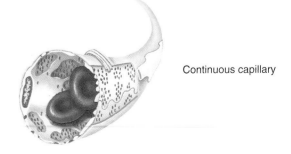

Continuous capillary

PLATE 8-6 ■ *Freeze Etch, Fenestrated Capillary, Electron Microscopy*

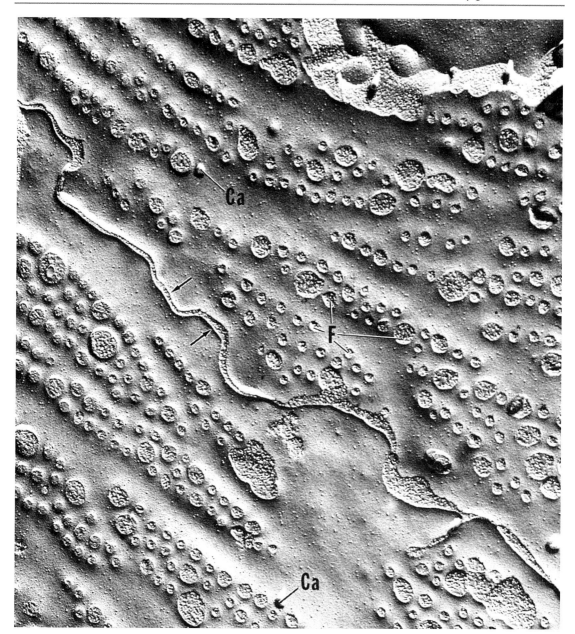

FIGURE 1 ■ *Fenestrated capillary. Hamster.*
Electron Microscopy. Freeze fracture. × 205,200.

This electron micrograph is a representative example of fenestrated capillaries from the hamster adrenal cortex, as revealed by the freeze fracture replica technique. The parallel lines (arrows) running diagonally across the field represent the line of junction between two endothelial cells, which are presented in a surface view. Note that the numerous **fenestrae** (F), whose diameters range from 57–166 nm, are arranged in tracts, with the regions between tracts nonfenestrated. Occasional **caveolae** (Ca) are also present. (From Ryan U, Ryan J, Smith D, Winkler H: *Tissue Cell* 7:181–190, 1975.)

Lymphoid Tissue

Lymphoid tissue forms the basis of the immune system of the body and is organized into diffuse and nodular lymphatic tissues (see Graphic 9-1). The lymphocyte, the principal cell of lymphoid tissue, is responsible for the proper functioning of the immune system. Although morphologically identical, small lymphocytes may be further identified according to function into three categories: null cells, **B lymphocytes**, and T lymphocytes. **Null cells** are composed of two categories of cells, namely stem cells and natural killer (NK) cells. **Stem cells** are undifferentiated cells that will give rise to the various cellular elements of blood, whereas **NK cells** are cytotoxic cells that are responsible for the destruction of certain categories of foreign cells. **B lymphocytes**, which probably mature in **bone marrow** in mammals **(bursa of Fabricius in birds)**, have the capability of transforming into **plasma cells**, and **T lymphocytes**, which are potentiated in the **thymus**. Plasma cells possess the ability to manufacture **humoral antibodies** specific against a particular antigen. Antibodies, once released, bind to and thus inactivate the antigen. Additionally, the attachment of antibodies to antigens may enhance **phagocytosis** (opsonization) or precipitate **complement activation**, resulting in **chemotaxis** of neutrophils and even **lysis** of the invader. T lymphocytes do not produce antibodies; instead, they have the capacity of functioning in the **cell-mediated immune response**. It is the T lymphocytes that participate in the graft rejection phenomenon and in the elimination of virally-transformed cells. Several subgroups of T and B lymphocytes exist, such as **memory cells**, **T helper cells** (T_H1 and T_H2 cells), **T suppressor cells**, and **T cytotoxic cells** (T killer cells); a discussion of these is found later in this chapter. Once a T lymphocyte becomes activated by the presence of an antigen, it releases **cytokines**, substances that activate macrophages, attract them to the site of antigenic invasion, and enhance their phagocytic capabilities. Frequently, T lymphocytes also assist B lymphocytes in the performance of their functions.

DIFFUSE LYMPHOID TISSUE

Diffuse lymphoid tissue occurs throughout the body, especially under wet epithelial membranes, where the loose connective tissue is infiltrated by lymphoid cells, namely lymphocytes, plasma cells, macrophages, and reticular cells. This is particularly evident in the lamina propria of the digestive tract and in the subepithelial connective tissue of the respiratory tract. It may be noted that the lymphoid cells are not arranged in any particular pattern but are scattered in a haphazard manner. Frequently, lymphoid nodules, transitory structures that are a denser aggregation of lymphoid tissue composed mainly of lymphocytes, may be observed. Lymphoid nodules present the characteristic appearance of a lighter **germinal center** and a darker, peripherally located **corona**. The germinal centers are sites of lymphocyte production, whereas the corona is composed mostly of newly formed B lymphocytes.

LYMPH NODES

Lymph nodes are ovoid- to kidney-shaped organs that filter lymph (see Graphic 9-2). They possess a convex surface, which receives afferent lymph vessels, and a hilum, where blood vessels enter and efferent lymph vessels leave and drain lymph from the organ. Each lymph node has a dense irregular collagenous connective tissue **capsule**. Connective tissue septa, derived from the capsule, subdivide the cortex into incomplete compartments. Attached to the septa and the internal aspect of the capsule is a network of reticular tissue and associated reticular cells that act as a framework for housing the numerous free cells, mostly lymphocytes, occupying the organ. The **cortex** of the lymph node houses the capsular and cortical sinuses, as well as lymphoid nodules, composed mainly of **B lymphocytes** and reticular cells. Between the cortex and the medulla is the **paracortex** populated by **T lymphocytes**. The **medulla** consists of medullary **sinusoids** and **medullary cords**. The medullary sinusoids are continuous with the capsular and cortical sinuses, whereas the **medullary cords** are composed mainly of lymphoid cells. Additional cell components of lymph nodes are **macrophages, antigen-presenting cells,** and some **granulocytes**. Aside from functioning in the maintenance and production of immunocompetent cells, lymph nodes also filter lymph. The filtering process is facilitated by the reticular cell processes that span the sinuses of the node and thus disturb and retard lymph flow, providing more time for the resident macrophages to phagocytose antigens and other debris.

TONSILS

Tonsils are aggregates of more or less **encapsulated lymphoid tissue** situated at the entrances to the oral pharynx and to the nasal pharynx. Participating in the formation of the **tonsillar ring** are the **palatine, pharyngeal,** and **lingual tonsils**. These structures produce antibodies against the numerous antigens and microorganisms that abound in their vicinity.

SPLEEN

The **spleen** is the largest lymphoid organ of the body (see Graphic 9-2). Its principal functions are to filter blood, phagocytose senescent red blood cells and invading microorganisms, supply immunocompetent **T** and **B lymphocytes,** and manufacture **antibodies**. Unlike lymph nodes, the spleen is not divided into cortical and medullary regions, nor is it supplied by afferent lymphatic vessels. Blood vessels enter and leave the spleen at its hilum and travel within the parenchyma via trabeculae derived from its connective tissue capsule. The spleen is subdivided into **red** and **white pulps;** the former consists of **pulp cords (of Billroth)** interposed between sinusoids, whereas the latter is composed of lymphoid tissue associated with arteries. This lymphoid tissue is arranged in a specific fashion, either as **periarterial lymphatic sheaths** (**PALS**) composed of T lymphocytes or as **lymphoid nodules** consisting of B lymphocytes. The region between the red and white pulps is known as the **marginal zone** and is rich in arterial vessels and avidly phagocytic macrophages. The **red pulp** is composed of a spongy network of sinusoids lined by unusual elongated endothelial cells displaying large intercellular

spaces, supported by a thick, discontinuous, hoop-like basement membrane. Reticular cells and reticular fibers associated with these sinusoids extend into the pulp cords to contribute to the cell population that consists of **macrophages, plasma cells,** and extravasated blood cells.

Understanding splenic organization depends on knowing the vascular supply of the spleen. The splenic artery entering at the hilum is distributed to the interior of the organ via trabeculae as trabecular arteries. On leaving a trabecula, the vessel enters the parenchyma to be surrounded by the periarterial lymphatic sheath and occasional lymphoid nodules and is termed the central artery. **Central arteries** enter the red pulp by losing their periarterial lymphatic sheath and subdivide into numerous straight vessels known as **penicillar arteries**. These small vessels possess three regions: **pulp arterioles, sheathed arterioles,** and **terminal arterial capillaries**. Whether these terminal arterial capillaries drain directly into the sinusoids (closed circulation) or terminate as open-ended vessels in the pulp cords (open circulation) has not been determined conclusively. Sinusoids are drained by pulp veins, which lead to trabecular veins and eventually join the splenic vein.

THYMUS

The **thymus** is a bilobed lymphoid organ located in the mediastinum, overlying the great vessels of the heart (see Graphic 9-2). Its major functions are the formation, potentiation, and destruction of T lymphocytes. Immunoincompetent T lymphocytes enter the thymus where they become immunocompetent and are released into the general circulation with the caveat that those T lymphocytes that would recognize and attack the self are not released but are destroyed in the cortex. The thin connective tissue capsule of the thymus sends septa into the organ, incompletely subdividing it into lobules. The thymus, unlike the previous lymphoid structures, is derived from endodermal primordium that becomes invaded by lymphocytes. Additionally, the thymus possesses no lymphoid nodules; instead, it is divided into an outer **cortex**, composed of **epithelial reticular cells, macrophages,** and **small T lymphocytes (thymocytes),** and an inner, lighter staining **medulla** consisting of **epithelial reticular cells, large T lymphocytes,** and **thymic (Hassall's) corpuscles**. Blood vessels gain entrance to the medulla by traveling in the connective tissue septa, which they exit at the corticomedullary junction, where they provide capillary loops to the cortex. These capillaries are the continuous type and are surrounded by epithelial reticular cells that isolate them from the cortical lymphocytes, thus establishing a **blood-thymus barrier**, providing for an antigen-free environment for the potentiation of the immunocompetent T lymphocytes. The blood vessels of the medulla are not unusual and present no blood-thymus barrier. The thymus is drained by venules in the medulla, which also receives blood from the cortical capillaries. Epithelial reticular cells form a specialized barrier between the cortex and medulla, preventing medullary material from gaining access to the cortex. The thymus attains its greatest development shortly after birth, but subsequent to puberty it involutes and becomes infiltrated by adipose tissue; however, even in the adult the thymus retains its ability to form T lymphocytes.

Histophysiology

I. THE IMMUNE RESPONSE

The immune system relies on the interactions of its primary cell components, lymphocytes and antigen-presenting cells, to effect an immune response. These responses are meticulously controlled and directed but a complete description of the mechanisms of their actions is beyond the purposes of this *Atlas*. Therefore, only the salient features of the mechanisms of the immune process will be described.

A. Cells of the Immune System

The cells of the immune system may be subdivided into three major categories, clones of T lymphocytes and B lymphocytes, NK cells, as well as antigen-presenting cells. A **clone** is a small population of identical cells each of which is capable of recognizing and responding to one specific (or very closely related) **epitope** (antigenic determinant). Resting T and B cells become activated if they come in contact with the specific epitope and certain cytokines. These activated cells proliferate and differentiate into **effector cells**. **Antigen-presenting cells**, such as macrophages, participate in the immune process by phagocytosing foreign substances, breaking them down to epitopes. They present these epitopes on their cell surface in conjunction with **major histocompatibility complex molecules** (MHC molecules) and other membrane-associated markers. It should be noted that in humans MHC molecules are also referred to as human leukocyte antigen molecules (HLA molecules).

1. T Lymphocytes

T lymphocytes (T cells) are immunoincompetent until they enter the cortex of the thymus. Here, under the influence of the cortical environment, they express their T cell receptors and **cluster of differentiation markers** (CD2, CD3, CD4, CD8, and CD28) and become immunocompetent. Once immunocompetent, the T cells are either killed if they are committed against the self or enter the medulla of the thymus. In the medulla they will lose either their CD4 or CD8 markers and thus develop into $CD8^+$ or $CD4^+$ cells, respectively. These cells enter into blood vessels of the medulla to become members of the circulating population of lymphocytes.

T cells encompass several categories of cells that are responsible not only for the **cell-mediated**

immune response, but also for facilitating the **humorally-mediated response** of B cells to **thymic dependent antigens**. In order to be able to perform their functions, T cells possess characteristic integral membrane proteins on their cell surfaces. One of these is the **T cell receptor** (TCR), which has the capability of recognizing that particular epitope for which the cell is genetically programmed; however, T cells can recognize only those epitopes that are bound to MHC molecules present on the surface of antigen presenting cells. Thus, T cells are said to be **MHC restricted**.

a. *T Helper Cells* are subdivided into two categories, T_H1 and T_H2 **cells** and they are both $CD4^+$ cells. The former coordinate the cell-mediated, whereas the latter orchestrate the humorally-mediated immune response. T_H1 cells produce and release the cytokines interleukin 2, gamma interferon, and others that modify the immune response. T_H2 cells produce and release interleukins 4, 5, and 6 that induce B cells to proliferate and differentiate into **plasma cells** that produce antibodies.

b. *T Cytotoxic Cells* (T_c cells) are $CD8^+$ cells. Upon contacting the proper MHC-epitope complex displayed by antigen-presenting cells and having been activated by interleukin 2, these cells undergo mitosis to form numerous **cytotoxic T lymphocytes** (CTLs). These newly formed cells kill foreign and virally-transformed self cells by secreting **perforins** and **fragmentins** (see Graphic 9-4).

c. *T Suppressor Cells* (T_s cells) are $CD8^+$ cells that function in repressing the activities of other cells of the immune system. In this fashion, they modulate and stop an immune response. It is believed that they may prevent the initiation of an autoimmune response. It should be understood that some investigators question the existence of T_s cells.

d. *T Memory Cells* are immunocompetent cells that are the progeny of activated T cells that undergo mitotic activity during an antigenic challenge. These cells are long lived, circulating cells that are added to and increase the number of cells of the original clone. It is this increase in the size of the clone that is responsible for the **anamnestic response** (a more rapid and more intense secondary response) against another encounter with the same antigen.

2. B Lymphocytes

B lymphocyte (B cells) are formed and become immunocompetent in the bone marrow. They enter the general circulation, establish clones whose members seed various lymphoid organs, and are responsible for the **humoral immune response**. Instead of T cell receptors, B cells have antibodies (IgD or the monomeric form of IgM) on their cell membranes. These **surface immunoglobulins** (SIGs) of a particular B cell target the same epitope. Unlike T cells, B cells have the capability of acting as antigen-presenting cells and present their MHC II-epitope complex to T_H1 cells.

Once activated, B cells manufacture and release IL-12, a cytokine that promotes the formation of T_H1 cells. B cells proliferate during a humoral immune response to form plasma cells and B memory cells (see Graphic 9-3).

a. *Plasma Cells* are differentiated cells that do not possess surface immunoglobulins but are "antibody factories" that synthesize and release an enormous number of identical copies of the same antibody that is specific against a particular epitope (although it may cross react with similar epitopes).

b. *B Memory Cells* are similar to T memory cells, in that they are long-lived, circulating cells that are added to and increase the number of cells of the original clone. Similarly, it is this increase in the size of the clone that is responsible for the **anamnestic response** against a subsequent encounter with the same antigen.

3. Natural Killer Cells

Natural killer cells (NK cells) are members of the **null cell** division of lymphocytes. NK cells do not have the cell surface determinants typical of T or B cells and they are immunocompetent as soon as they are formed in the bone marrow. These cells kill virally altered cells and tumor cells in a **nonspecific** manner and they are not MHC restricted. NK cells also recognize and become activated by the Fc portions of those antibodies that are bound to cell surface epitopes. Once activated, NK cells release perforins and fragmentins to kill these decorated cells by a procedure known as **antibody-dependent cell-mediated cytotoxicity (ADCC)**. Perforins assemble as pores within the plasmalemma of target cells, whereas fragmentins drive the target cell into apoptosis.

4. Antigen-Presenting Cells

Antigen-presenting cells (APCs), macrophages, and B lymphocytes possess class II major histocompatibility complex molecules (**MHC II molecules**), whereas all other nucleated cells possess **MHC I molecules**.

An APC phagocytoses and degrades the antigen into **epitopes**, small highly antigenic peptides 7 to 11 amino acids long. Each epitope is attached to an MHC II molecule, and this complex is placed on the external aspect of its cell membrane. The MHC II-epitope complex is recognized by the T cell receptor (**TCR**) in conjunction with the **CD4 molecule** of the T_H1 or T_H2 cells, a process known as **MHC II restriction** (see Graphic 9-5).

Antigen-presenting cells and, specifically, macrophages produce and release a variety of cytokines that modulate the immune response. These include **interleukin 1,** which stimulates T helper cells and self-activated macrophages as well as **prostaglandin E_2** that attenuates some immune responses. Cytokines, such as **interferon-γ**, released by other lymphoid cells, as well as by macrophages, enhance the phagocytic and cytolytic avidity of macrophages.

II. LYMPH NODES

The convex aspect of lymph nodes receives **afferent lymph vessels** that deliver their contents into the subcapsular sinuses. Paratrabecular (cortical) sinuses drain subcapsular sinuses and convey their lymph to the sinusoids of the medulla, which are drained by **efferent lymph vessels** at the hilum. The **cortex** is subdivided into several incomplete compartments, with each housing a lymphatic nodule rich in B cells as well as APCs and macrophages. The region of the lymph node between the cortex and medulla, the **paracortex,** houses mostly T cells, APCs, and macrophages. Cells that arise in the cortex or paracortex migrate into the medulla, where they form **medullary cords** composed of T cells, B cells, and plasma cells. T cells and B cells enter the sinusoids and leave the lymph node via efferent lymph vessels. Lymphocytes also enter lymph nodes via arterioles that penetrate the lymph node at the hilum, travel to the paracortex within connective tissue trabeculae, and form **high endothelial vessels** (postcapillary venules).

III. SPLEEN

Branches of the splenic artery, the trabecular arteries, enter the **white pulp** by leaving their trabeculae and, as they become surrounded by sheaths of T cells, the **periarterial lymphatic sheath (PALS)**, are known as central arteries. Along the path of the central arteries are occasional lymphatic nodules composed mostly of B cells but still surrounded by the PALS. As central arteries lose their lymphatic sheath, they branch repeatedly, forming straight vessels, penicillar arteries, that possess three regions: pulp arterioles, macrophage-sheathed arterioles, and terminal arterial capillaries. The terminal arterial capillaries either terminate in the splenic sinusoids (**closed circulation**) or freely in the red pulp (**open circulation**). The **red pulp** is composed of the sinusoids, the reticular fiber network, and the cells of the splenic cords. A region of smaller sinusoids forms the interface between the white and red pulps, and this interface is known as the marginal zone. Capillaries arising from the central arteries deliver their blood to sinusoids of the **marginal zone.** APCs of the marginal zone monitor this blood for the presence of antigens and foreign substances.

IV. THYMUS

The thymic cortex is completely isolated from all vascular and connective tissue elements by **reticular epithelial cells.** Additionally, within the cortex, these cells form a three-dimensional meshwork in whose interstices clusters of T cells become mature. Although there are six different types of epithelial reticular cells (three in the cortex and three in the medulla), they all present the same appearance as large, pale cells with large, ovoid nuclei. These cells are derived from the third pharyngeal pouch and migrate into the developing thymus. They manufacture the hormones **thymosin, serum thymic factor,** and **thymopoietin,** all of which facilitate the transformation of immature T cells into immunocompetent T cells. During the transformation, which occurs in the thymic **cortex,** the immature T cells (**thymocytes**) undergo **gene rearrangement,** in that they express on their cell membrane T cell receptors (**TCRs**) and cluster of differentiation (**CD**) markers (especially CD2, CD3, CD4, and CD8).

Most of the T cells die as they migrate from the cortex to the medulla; their remnants are phagocytosed by macrophages. It is believed that the cells that were killed were genetically programmed to recognize self-proteins as antigens. In the thymic **medulla,** T cells lose either their CD4 or CD8 markers and develop into $CD8^+$ and $CD4^+$ cells, respectively.

Clinical Considerations ▨ ▩ ▪

Hodgkin's Disease
Hodgkin's disease is a neoplastic transformation of lymphocytes that is prevalent mostly in young males. Its clinical signs are asymptomatic initially because of the swelling of the liver, spleen, and lymph nodes and are not accompanied by pain. Other manifestations include the loss of weight, elevated temperature, diminished appetite, and generalized weakness. Histopathologic characteristics include the presence of Reed-Sternberg cells, easily recognizable cells distinguished by their large size and the presence of two large, pale, oval nuclei in each cell.

Wiskott-Aldrich Syndrome
Wiskott-Aldrich syndrome is an immunodeficiency disorder occurring only in boys and is characterized by excema, lowered platelet count, and lymphocytopenia (of both B and T cell populations). The immunosuppressed state of these children leads to recurring bacterial infections that result in severe bacterial infections, hemorrhage, and death at an early age. Most children who survive the first decade of life are stricken with leukemia or lymphoma.

Summary of Histological Organization

Lymphoid tissue consists of **diffuse** and **dense lymphoid tissue.** The principal cell of lymphoid tissue is the **lymphocyte,** of which there are two categories: **B lymphocytes** and **T lymphocytes.** Additionally, **macrophages, reticular cells, plasma cells, dendritic cells,** and **antigen-presenting cells** perform important functions in lymphatic tissue.

I. LYMPH NODE

A. Capsule

The **capsule,** usually surrounded by **adipose tissue,** is composed of dense irregular **collagenous connective tissue** containing some **elastic fibers** and **smooth muscle.** Afferent lymphatic vessels enter the convex aspect; **efferent lymphatics** and **blood vessels** pierce the **hilum.**

B. Cortex

Lymphatic nodules, composed of a dark **corona** (mostly **B lymphocytes**) and lighter staining **germinal centers,** housing activated **B lymphoblasts, macrophages,** and **dendritic reticular cells** are found in the **cortex.** Connective tissue **trabeculae** subdivide the cortex into incomplete compartments. **Subcapsular** and **cortical sinuses** display lymphocytes, reticular cells, and **macrophages.**

C. Paracortex

The **paracortex** is the region between the cortex and medulla, composed of **T lymphocytes. Postcapillary venules,** with their characteristic **cuboidal endothelium,** are present.

D. Medulla

The **medulla** displays connective tissue **trabeculae, medullary cords** (composed of macrophages, plasma cells, and lymphocytes), and **medullary sinusoids** lined by discontinuous **endothelial cells.** Sinusoids contain **lymphocytes, plasma cells,** and **macrophages.** The region of the **hilum** is evident as a result of the thickened capsule and lack of lymphatic nodules.

E. Reticular Fibers

With the use of special stains an extensive network of **reticular fibers** may be demonstrated to constitute the framework of lymph nodes.

II. TONSILS

A. Palatine Tonsils

1. Epithelium
Covered by **stratified squamous nonkeratinized epithelium** that extends into the **tonsillar crypts. Lymphocytes** may migrate through the epithelium.

2. Lymphatic Nodules
Surround **crypts** and frequently display **germinal centers.**

3. Capsule
Dense irregular collagenous connective tissue **capsule** separates the tonsil from the underlying pharyngeal wall musculature. **Septa,** derived from the capsule, extend into the tonsil.

4. Glands
Not present.

B. Pharyngeal Tonsils

1. Epithelium
For the most part, **pseudostratified ciliated columnar epithelium** (infiltrated by lymphocytes) covers the free surface, as well as the folds that resemble crypts.

2. Lymphatic Nodules
Most **lymphatic nodules** display **germinal centers.**

3. Capsule
The thin **capsule,** situated deep to the tonsil, provides **septa** for the tonsil.

4. Glands
Ducts of the **seromucous glands,** beneath the capsule, pierce the tonsil to open onto the epithelially covered surface.

C. Lingual Tonsils

1. Epithelium
Stratified squamous nonkeratinized epithelium covers the tonsil and extends into the shallow crypts.

2. Lymphatic Nodules
Most **lymphatic nodules** present germinal centers.

3. Capsule
The **capsule** is thin, not clearly defined.

4. Glands
Seromucous glands open into the base of **crypts.**

III. SPLEEN

A. Capsule

The **capsule**, composed of **dense irregular collagenous connective tissue** thickest at the **hilum**, possesses some **elastic fibers** and **smooth muscle cells**. It is covered by **mesothelium** but is not surrounded by adipose tissue. **Trabeculae,** bearing blood vessels, extend from the capsule into the substance of the spleen.

B. White Pulp

White pulp is composed of **periarterial lymphatic sheaths** and **lymphatic nodules** with germinal centers. Both periarterial lymphatic sheaths (housing **T lymphocytes**) and lymphatic nodules (housing **B lymphocytes**) surround the acentrically located **central artery**, a distinguishing characteristic of the spleen.

C. Marginal Zone

A looser accumulation of **lymphocytes, macrophages,** and **plasma cells** are located between white and red pulps. It is supplied by **capillary loops** derived from the **central artery.**

D. Red Pulp

Red pulp is composed of **pulp cords** and **sinusoids.** Pulp cords are composed of delicate reticular fibers, stellate-shaped **reticular cells, plasma cells, macrophages,** and **cells** of the **circulating blood. Sinusoids** are lined by elongated discontinuous **endothelial cells** surrounded by thickened hoop-like **basement membrane** in association with **reticular fibers.** The various regions of **penicilli** are evident in the red pulp. These are **pulp arterioles, sheathed arterioles,** and **terminal arterial capillaries.** Convincing evidence to determine whether circulation in the red pulp is open or closed is not available.

E. Reticular Fibers

With the use of special stains an extensive network of **reticular fibers** may be demonstrated to constitute the framework of the spleen.

IV. THYMUS

A. Capsule

The thin **capsule** is composed of **dense irregular collagenous connective tissue** (with some elastic fibers) that extends **interlobular trabeculae** that incompletely subdivide the thymus into **lobules.**

B. Cortex

The **cortex** has no lymphatic nodules or plasma cells. It is composed of lightly staining **epithelial reticular cells, macrophages,** and densely packed, darkly staining, small **T lymphocytes (thymocytes)** responsible for the dark appearance of the cortex. Epithelial reticular cells also surround **capillaries,** the only blood vessels present in the cortex.

C. Medulla

The **medulla,** which stains much lighter than the cortex, is continuous from lobule to lobule. It contains **plasma cells, lymphocytes, macrophages,** and **epithelial reticular cells.** Moreover, **thymic (Hassall's) corpuscles,** concentrically arranged epithelial reticular cells, are characteristic features of the thymic medulla.

D. Involution

The thymus begins to involute subsequent to puberty. The **cortex** becomes less dense because its population of lymphocytes and epithelial reticular cells is, to some extent, replaced by fat. In the medulla, **thymic corpuscles** increase in number and size.

E. Reticular Fibers and Sinusoids

The thymus possesses neither reticular fibers nor sinusoids.

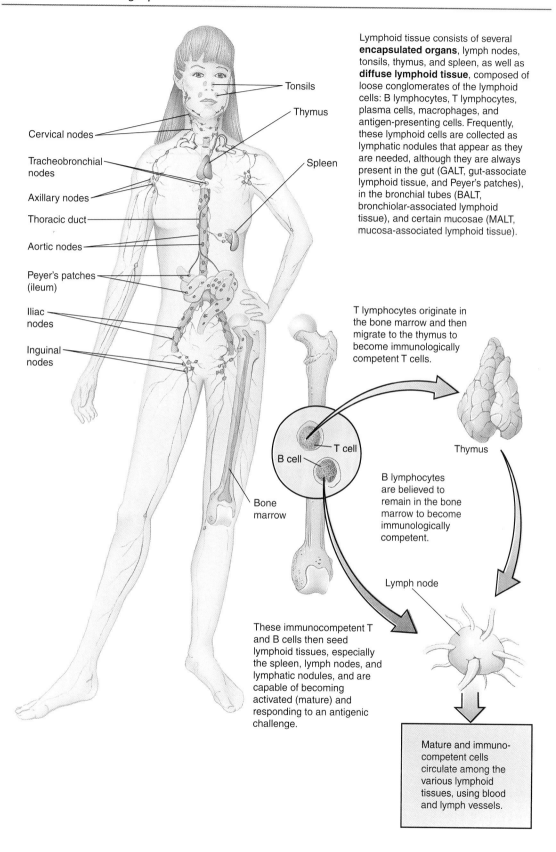

Tonsils

Thymus

Cervical nodes

Spleen

Tracheobronchial nodes

Axillary nodes

Thoracic duct

Aortic nodes

Peyer's patches (ileum)

Iliac nodes

Inguinal nodes

Lymphoid tissue consists of several **encapsulated organs**, lymph nodes, tonsils, thymus, and spleen, as well as **diffuse lymphoid tissue**, composed of loose conglomerates of the lymphoid cells: B lymphocytes, T lymphocytes, plasma cells, macrophages, and antigen-presenting cells. Frequently, these lymphoid cells are collected as lymphatic nodules that appear as they are needed, although they are always present in the gut (GALT, gut-associate lymphoid tissue, and Peyer's patches), in the bronchial tubes (BALT, bronchiolar-associated lymphoid tissue), and certain mucosae (MALT, mucosa-associated lymphoid tissue).

T lymphocytes originate in the bone marrow and then migrate to the thymus to become immunologically competent T cells.

T cell

B cell

Thymus

B lymphocytes are believed to remain in the bone marrow to become immunologically competent.

Bone marrow

Lymph node

These immunocompetent T and B cells then seed lymphoid tissues, especially the spleen, lymph nodes, and lymphatic nodules, and are capable of becoming activated (mature) and responding to an antigenic challenge.

Mature and immuno-competent cells circulate among the various lymphoid tissues, using blood and lymph vessels.

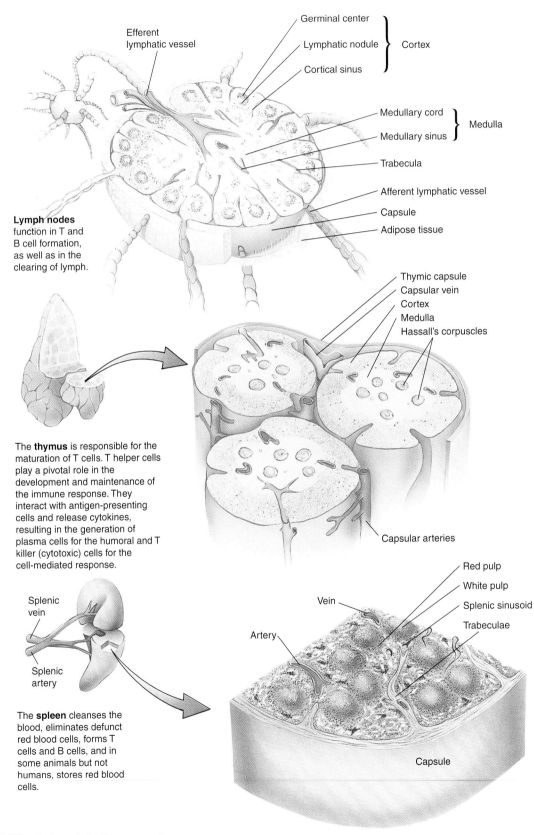

Efferent lymphatic vessel

Germinal center

Lymphatic nodule

Cortex

Cortical sinus

Medullary cord

Medulla

Medullary sinus

Trabecula

Afferent lymphatic vessel

Capsule

Adipose tissue

Lymph nodes function in T and B cell formation, as well as in the clearing of lymph.

Thymic capsule
Capsular vein
Cortex
Medulla
Hassall's corpuscles

Capsular arteries

The **thymus** is responsible for the maturation of T cells. T helper cells play a pivotal role in the development and maintenance of the immune response. They interact with antigen-presenting cells and release cytokines, resulting in the generation of plasma cells for the humoral and T killer (cytotoxic) cells for the cell-mediated response.

Splenic vein

Splenic artery

Red pulp
White pulp
Vein
Splenic sinusoid
Artery
Trabeculae

Capsule

The **spleen** cleanses the blood, eliminates defunct red blood cells, forms T cells and B cells, and in some animals but not humans, stores red blood cells.

Antigen-dependent cross linking of the surface antibodies activates the B cell which places the epitope-MHC II complex on the external aspect of its plasmalemma.

The TCR and CD4 molecules of the T_H2 cell recognize the B cell's MHC II-epitope complex. Additionally, binding of the B cell's CD40 molecule to the T_H2 cell's CD40 receptor induces the B cell to proliferate and the T_H2 cell to release of IL4, IL5, and IL6.

IL4, IL5, and IL6 induce the activation of B cells and their differentiation into B memory and plasma cells.

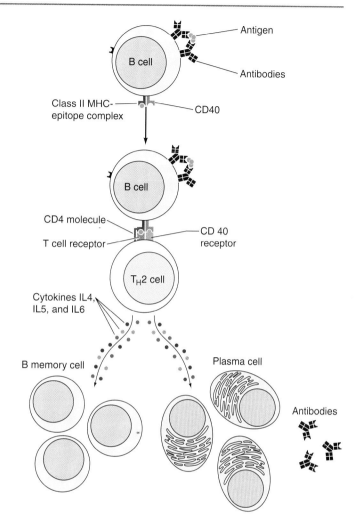

The T cell receptor (TCR) and CD4 molecule of the T_H1 cell binds to the epitope and the MHC II of the antigen-presenting cell (APC), respectively. The binding induces the APC to express B7 molecules on its plasmalemma, which then binds to the CD28 molecule of the T_H1 cell, inducing that cell to release IL2.

The same APC expresses the MHC I-epitope complex, which is recognized by the CD8 molecule and the TCR of the cytotoxic T lymphocyte (CTL). Additionally, the CD28 molecule of the CTL binds with the B7 molecule on the APC plasmalemma. These interactions induce the expression of IL2 receptors on the CTL plasma membrane. Binding of IL2 (released by the T_H1 cell) to the IL2 receptors of the CTL induces that cell to proliferate.

The plasmalemma of virally transformed cells expresses MHC I-epitope complex, which is recognized by the CD8 molecule and TCR of the newly formed cytotoxic T lymphocytes. The binding of the CTL induces these cells to secrete perforins and fragmentins. The former assemble to form pores in the plasma membrane of the transformed cell, and framentin drives the transformed cell into apoptosis.

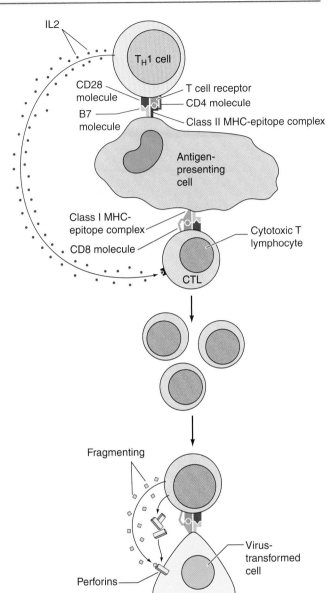

Bacteria-infected macrophages bear MHC II-epitope complexes on their plasmalemma that, if recognized by the CD4 molecule and TCR of T$_H$1 cells, activates these T cells, causing them to release IL2 and to express IL2 receptors on their plasma membrane. Binding of IL2 to the IL2 receptors induces proliferation of the T$_H$1 cell s.

The TCR and CD4 molecules of the newly formed T$_H$1 cells recognize and bind to the MHC II-epitope complexes of bacteria-infected macrophages. The binding causes activation of these T$_H$1 cells so that they release γ-interferon, a cytokine that encourages the macrophages to destroy their endocytosed bacteria.

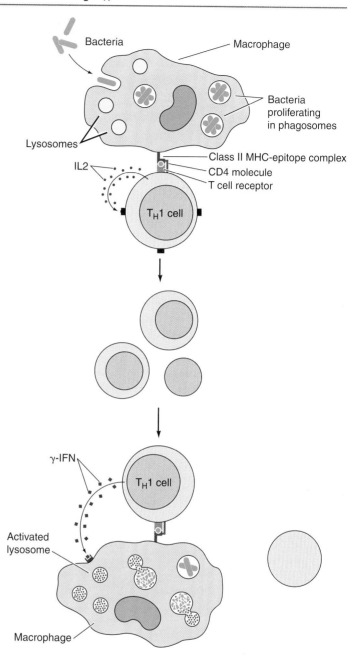

PLATE 9-1 ■ *Lymphatic Infiltration, Lymphatic Nodule*

FIGURE 1 ▨ *Lymphatic infiltration. Monkey. Plastic section.* × 540.

The **connective tissue** (CT) deep to wet epithelia is usually infiltrated by loosely aggregated **lymphocytes** (Ly) and **plasma cells** (PC), as is exemplified by this photomicrograph of monkey duodenum. Observe that the simple columnar **epithelium** (E) contains not only the **nuclei** (N) of epithelial cells, but also dark dense nuclei of lymphocytes (arrows), some of which are in the process of migrating from the lamina propria (connective tissue) into the lumen of the duodenum. Note also the presence of a **lacteal** (La), a blindly ending lymphatic channel containing lymph. These vessels may be recognized by the absence of red blood cells.

FIGURE 2 ▨ *Lymphatic nodule. Monkey. Plastic section.* × 132.

The gut-associated lymphatic nodule in this photomicrograph is part of a cluster of nodules known as **Peyer's patches** (PP) and is taken from the monkey ileum. The **lumen** (L) of the small intestine is lined by a simple columnar **epithelium** (E) with numerous **goblet cells** (GC). However, note that the epithelium is modified over the lymphoid tissue into a **follicle-associated epithelium** (FAE) whose cells are shorter, infiltrated by lymphocytes, and display no goblet cells. Observe that this particular lymphatic nodule presents no germinal center but is composed of several cell types, as recognized by nuclei of various sizes and densities. These will be described in Figures 3 and 4. Although this lymphatic nodule is unencapsulated, the **connective tissue** (CT) between the **smooth muscle** (SM) and the lymphatic nodule is free of infiltrate.

FIGURE 3 ▨ *Lymphatic nodule. Monkey. Plastic section.* × 270.

This is a higher magnification of a lymphatic nodule from Peyer's patches in the monkey ileum. Note that the lighter staining **germinal center** (Gc) is surrounded by the **corona** (Co) of darker staining cells possessing only a limited amount of cytoplasm around a dense nucleus. These cells are small **lymphocytes** (Ly). Germinal centers form in response to an antigenic challenge and are composed of lymphoblasts and plasmablasts, whose nuclei stain much lighter than those of small lymphocytes. The boxed area is presented at a higher magnification in the following figure.

FIGURE 4 ▨ *Lymphatic nodule. Monkey. Plastic section.* × 540.

This is a higher magnification of the boxed area of the previous figure. Observe the **small lymphocytes** (Ly) at the periphery of the **germinal center** (Gc). The activity of this center is evidenced by the presence of mitotic figures (arrows), as well as the **lymphoblasts** (LB) and **plasmablasts** (PB). The germinal center is the site of production of small lymphocytes that then migrate to the periphery of the lymphatic nodule to form the corona.

■ **KEY**

Co	corona	GC	goblet cell	N	nucleus
CT	connective tissue	L	lumen	PB	plasmablast
E	epithelium	La	lacteal	PC	plasma cell
FAE	follicle-associated epithelium	LB	lymphoblast	PP	Peyer's patch
Gc	germinal center	Ly	small lymphocyte	SM	smooth muscle

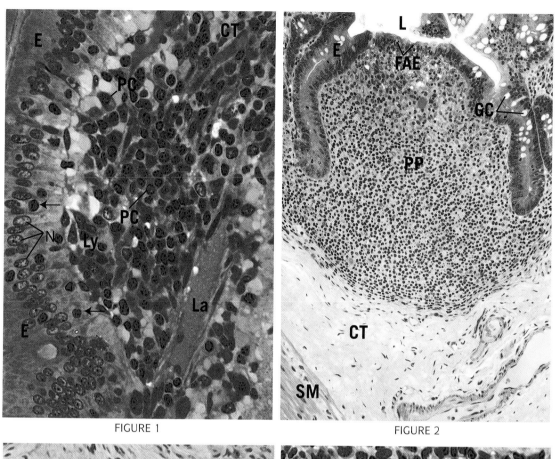

FIGURE 1

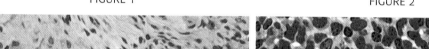

FIGURE 2

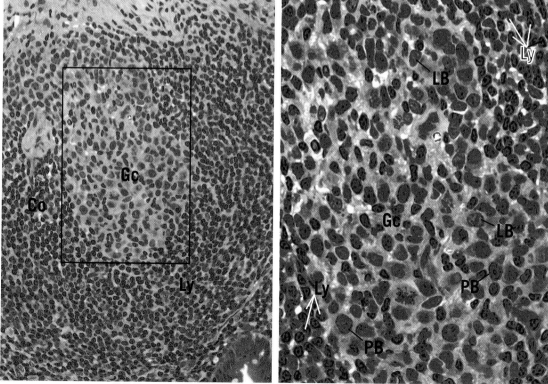

FIGURE 3

FIGURE 4

PLATE 9-2 ■ *Lymph Node*

FIGURE 1 ▨ *Lymph node. Paraffin section.* × 14.

Lymph nodes are kidney-shaped structures possessing a convex and a concave (hilus) surface. They are invested by a connective tissue **capsule** (Ca) that sends **trabeculae** (T) into the substance of the node, subdividing it into incomplete compartments. The compartmentalization is particularly evident in the **cortex** (C), the peripheral aspect of the lymph node. The lighter staining central region is the **medulla** (M), while the zone between the medulla and cortex is the **paracortex** (PC). Observe that the cortex displays numerous **lymphatic nodules** (LN), many with **germinal centers** (Gc). This is the region of B-lymphocytes, while the paracortex is particularly rich in T-lymphocytes. Note that the medulla is composed of **sinusoids** (S), **trabeculae** (T) of connective tissue conducting blood vessels, and **medullary cords** (MC). The medullary cords are composed of lymphocytes, macrophages, and plasma cells. Lymph enters the lymph node, and as it percolates through sinuses and sinusoids, foreign substances are removed from it by phagocytic activity of macrophages.

FIGURE 2 ▨ *Lymph node. Monkey. Plastic section.* × 270.

Afferent lymphatic vessels (AV) enter the lymph node at its convex surface. These vessels bear **valves** (V) that regulate the direction of flow. Lymph enters the **subcapsular sinus** (SS), which contains numerous **macrophages** (Ma), **lymphocytes** (Ly), and antigen-transporting cells. These sinuses are lined by **endothelial cells** (EC), which also cover the fine collagen fibers that frequently span the sinus to create a turbulence in lymph flow. Lymph from the subcapsular sinus enters the cortical sinus, then moves into the medullary sinusoids. It is here that lymphocytes also migrate into the sinusoids, leaving the lymph node via the efferent lymph vessels eventually to enter the general circulation.

FIGURE 3 ▨ *Lymph node. Monkey. Plastic section.* × 132.

The cortex of the lymph node is composed of numerous lymphatic nodules, one of which is presented in this photomicrograph. Observe that the lymph node is usually surrounded by **adipose tissue** (AT). The thin connective tissue **capsule** (Ca) sends **trabeculae** (T) into the substance of the lymph node. Observe that the lymphatic nodule possesses a dark staining **corona** (Co), composed mainly of **small lymphocytes** (Ly) whose heterochromatic nuclei are responsible for their staining characteristics. The **germinal center** (Gc) displays numerous cells with lightly staining nuclei, belonging to dendritic reticular cells, plasmablasts, and lymphoblasts.

FIGURE 4 ▨ *Lymph node. Human. Silver stain. Paraffin section.* × 132.

The hilus of the human lymph node displays the collagenous connective tissue **capsule** (Ca), which sends numerous **trabeculae** (T) into the substance of the lymph node. Observe that the region of the hilus is devoid of lymphatic nodules, but is particularly rich in **medullary cords** (MC). Note that the basic framework of these medullary cords, as well as of the lymph node, is composed of thin reticular fibers (arrows), which are connected to the collagen fiber bundles of the trabeculae and capsule.

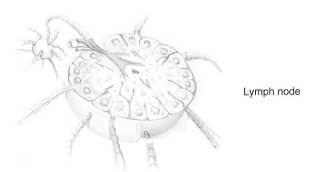

Lymph node

▨ **KEY**

AT	adipose tissue	Gc	germinal center	PC	paracortex
AV	afferent lymphatic vessel	LN	lymphatic nodule	S	sinusoid
C	cortex	Ly	small lymphocyte	SS	subcapsular sinus
Ca	capsule	M	medulla	T	trabeculae
Co	corona	Ma	macrophage	V	valve
EC	endothelial cell	MC	medullary cord		

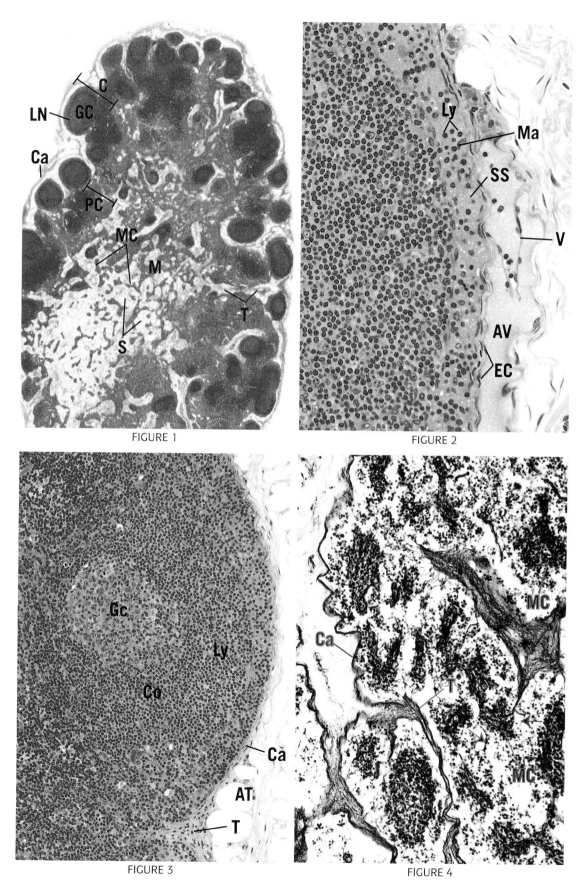

FIGURE 1

FIGURE 2

FIGURE 3

FIGURE 4

PLATE 9-3 ■ *Lymph Node, Tonsils*

FIGURE 1 ■ *Lymph node. Paraffin section.* × 132.

The medulla of the lymph node consists of numerous endothelially lined **sinusoids** (S), which receive lymph from the cortical sinuses. Surrounding the sinusoids are many **medullary cords** (MC), composed of macrophages, small lymphocytes, and plasma cells, whose nuclei (arrows) stain intensely. Both T- and B-lymphocytes are found in medullary cords, since they are in the process of migrating from the paracortex and cortex, respectively. Some of these lymphocytes will leave the lymph node using the sinusoids and efferent lymphatic vessels at the hilus. The medulla also displays connective tissue **trabeculae** (T) housing **blood vessels** (BV), which enter the lymph node at the hilus.

FIGURE 2 ■ *Lymph node. Monkey. Plastic section.* × 540.

This photomicrograph is a high magnification of a **sinusoid** (S) and surrounding **medullary cords** (MC) of a lymph node medulla. Note that the medullary cords are composed of macrophages, **plasma cells** (PC), and small **lymphocytes** (Ly). The sinusoids are lined by **endothelial cells** (EC), which do not form a continuous lining. The lumen contains lymph, small **lymphocytes** (Ly), and **macrophages** (Ma). These cells are actively phagocytosing particulate matter as is evidenced by their vacuolated appearance.

FIGURE 3 ■ *Palatine tonsil. Human. Paraffin section.* × 14.

The palatine tonsil is an aggregate of **lymphatic nodules** (LN), many of which possess **germinal centers** (Gc). The palatine tonsil is covered by a stratified squamous nonkeratinized **epithelium** (E) that lines the deep **primary crypts** (PCr) that invaginate deeply into the substance of the tonsil. Frequently **secondary crypts** (SCr) are evident, also lined by the same type of epithelium. The deep surface of the palatine tonsil is covered by a thickened connective tissue **capsule** (Ca). The crypts frequently contain debris (arrow) that consists of decomposing food particles, as well as lymphocytes that migrate from the lymphatic nodules through the epithelium to enter the crypts.

FIGURE 4 ■ *Pharyngeal tonsil. Human. Paraffin section.* × 132.

The pharyngeal tonsil, located in the nasopharynx, is an aggregate of lymphatic nodules, often displaying **germinal centers** (Gc). The **epithelial lining** (E) is pseudostratified ciliated columnar with occasional patches of stratified squamous nonkeratinized epithelium (asterisk). The lymphatic nodules are located in a loose, collagenous **connective tissue** (CT) that is infiltrated by small **lymphocytes** (Ly). Note that lymphocytes migrate through the epithelium (arrows) to gain access to the nasopharynx.

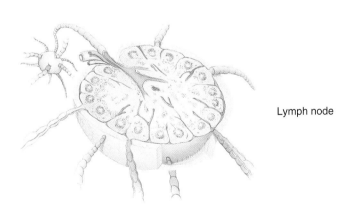

Lymph node

■ KEY

BV	blood vessel	Gc	germinal center	PC	plasma cell
Ca	capsule	LN	lymphatic nodule	PCr	primary crypt
CT	connective tissue	Ly	lymphocyte	S	sinusoid
E	epithelium	Ma	macrophage	T	trabeculae
EC	endothelial cell	MC	medullary cord	SCr	secondary crypt

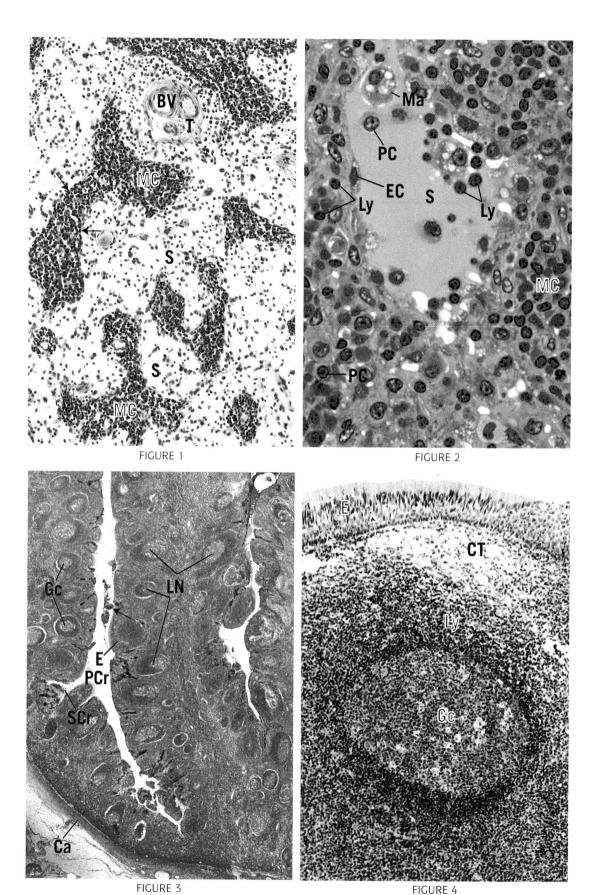

FIGURE 1

FIGURE 2

FIGURE 3

FIGURE 4

PLATE 9-4 ■ *Lymph Node, Electron Microscopy*

FIGURE 1 ■ *Lymph node. Mouse. Electron microscopy.* × 8608.

This electron micrograph of a mouse popliteal lymph node presents the **capsule** (Ca) and the subcapsular sinus. The sinus is occupied by three **lymphocytes**, one of which is labeled (L), as well as the **process** (P) of an antigen-transporting (antigen-presenting) cell, whose cell body (arrowheads) and nucleus are in the cortex, deep to the sinus. The process enters the lumen of the subcapsular sinus via a pore (arrows) in its floor (FL). It is believed that antigen-transporting cells are nonphagocytic and that they trap antigens at the site of antigenic invasion and transport them to lymphatic nodules of lymph nodes where they mature to become dendritic reticular cells. (From Szakal A, Homes K, Tew J: *J Immunol* 131:1714–1717, 1983.)

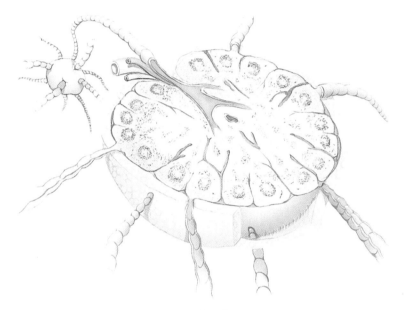

Lymph node

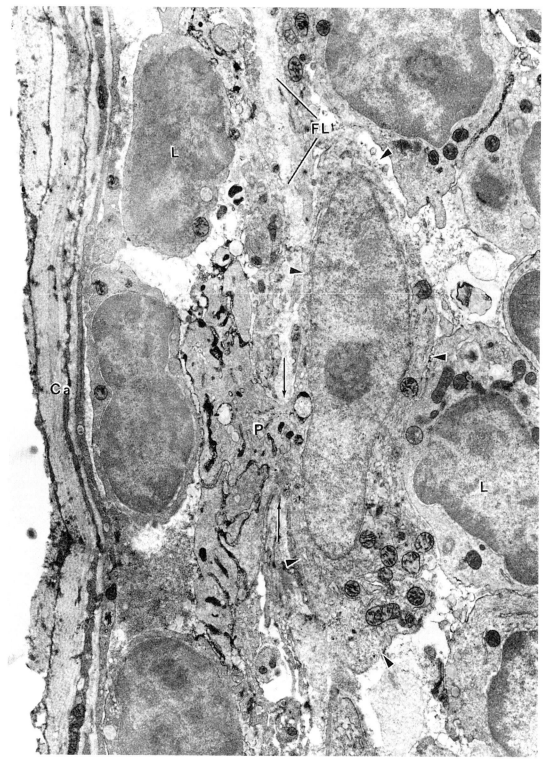

FIGURE 1

PLATE 9-5 ■ *Thymus*

FIGURE 1 ▦ *Thymus. Human infant. Paraffin section.* × 14.

The thymus of an infant is a well-developed organ that displays its many characteristics to advantage. This photomicrograph presents a part of one lobe. It is invested by a thin connective tissue **capsule** (Ca) that incompletely subdivides the thymus into **lobules** (Lo) by connective tissue **septa** (Se). Each lobule possesses a darker staining peripheral **cortex** (C) and a lighter staining **medulla** (M). The medulla of one lobule, however, is continuous with that of other lobules. The connective tissue capsule and septa convey blood vessels into the medulla of the thymus. Shortly after puberty the thymus begins to involute, and the connective tissue septa become infiltrated with adipocytes.

FIGURE 2 ▦ *Thymus. Monkey. Plastic section.* × 132.

The lobule of the thymus presented in this photomicrograph appears to be surrounded completely by connective tissue **septa** (Se); however, in a three-dimensional reconstruction, it would be seen that this lobule is continuous with surrounding **lobules** (Lo). Observe the numerous **blood vessels** (BV) in the septa, as well as the darker staining **cortex** (C) and the lighter staining **medulla** (M). The light patches of the cortex probably present epithelial reticular cells and macrophages (arrows), while the darker staining structures are nuclei of the T-lymphocyte series. The medulla contains the characteristic **thymic corpuscles** (TC), as well as blood vessels, macrophages, and epithelial reticular cells.

FIGURE 3 ▦ *Thymus. Monkey. Plastic section.* × 270.

The center of this photomicrograph is occupied by the **medulla** (M) of the thymus, presenting a large **thymic (Hassall's) corpuscle** (TC), composed of concentrically arranged **epithelial reticular cells** (ERC). The function, if any, of this structure is not known. The thymic medulla houses numerous **blood vessels** (BV), macrophages, **lymphocytes** (Ly), and occasional plasma cells.

FIGURE 4 ▦ *Thymus. Monkey. Plastic section.* × 540.

The cortex of the thymus is bounded externally by collagenous connective tissue **septa** (Se). The substance of the cortex is separated from the septa by a border of **epithelial reticular cells** (ERC), recognizable by their pale nuclei. Additional epithelial reticular cells form a cellular reticulum, in whose interstices **lymphocytes** (Ly) develop into mature T-lymphocytes. Numerous **macrophages** (Ma) are also evident in the cortex. These cells phagocytose lymphocytes destroyed in the thymus.

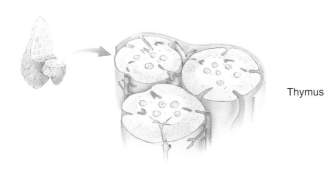

Thymus

▦ KEY

BV	blood vessel	Lo	lobule	Ma	macrophage
C	cortex	Ly	lymphocyte	Se	septum
Ca	capsule	M	medulla	TC	thymic corpuscle
ERC	epithelial reticular cell				

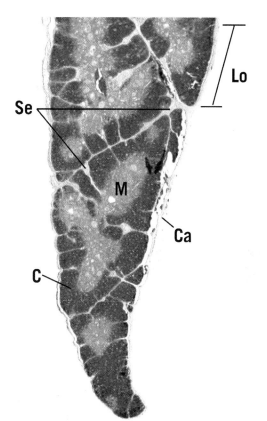

FIGURE 1

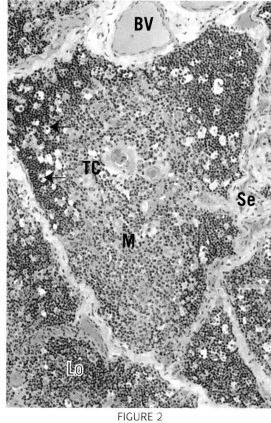

FIGURE 2

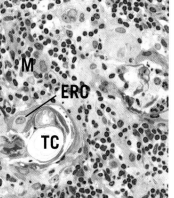

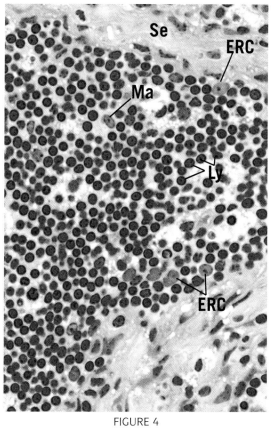

FIGURE 3

FIGURE 4

PLATE 9-6 ■ *Spleen*

FIGURE 1 ■ *Spleen. Human. Paraffin section.* × 132.

The spleen, the largest lymphoid organ, possesses a thick collagenous connective tissue **capsule** (Ca). Since it lies within the abdominal cavity, it is surrounded by a simple squamous **epithelium** (E). Connective tissue **septa** (SE), derived from the capsule, penetrate the substance of the spleen, conveying **blood vessels** (BV) into the interior of the organ. The spleen is not subdivided into cortex and medulla; instead it is composed of **white pulp** (WP) and **red pulp** (RP). White pulp is arranged as a cylindrical sheath of **lymphocytes** (Ly) surrounding a blood vessel known as the **central artery** (CA), whereas red pulp consists of **sinusoids** (S) meandering through a cellular tissue known as **pulp cords** (PC). The white pulp of the spleen is found in two different arrangements. The one represented in this photomicrograph is known as a **periarterial lymphatic sheath** (PALS) composed mostly of T lymphocytes. The zone of lymphocytes at the junction of the periarterial lymphatic sheath and the red pulp is known as the **marginal zone** (MZ).

FIGURE 3 ■ *Spleen. Monkey. Plastic section.* × 540.

The red pulp of the spleen, presented in this photomicrograph, is composed of **splenic sinusoids** (S) and **pulp cords** (PC). The splenic sinusoids are lined by a discontinuous type of epithelium, surrounded by an unusual arrangement of **basement membrane** (BM) that encircles the sinusoids in a discontinuous fashion. Sinusoids contain numerous **blood cells** (BC). **Nuclei** (N) of the sinusoidal lining cells bulge into the lumen. The regions between sinusoids are occupied by pulp cords, housing various cells of the blood, macrophages, reticular cells, and plasma cells. The vascular supply of the red pulp is derived from penicillar arteries, which give rise to **arterioles** (AR) whose **endothelial cells** (EC) and **smooth muscle** (SM) cells are evident in the center of this field.

FIGURE 2 ■ *Spleen. Monkey. Plastic section.* × 132.

Lying within the **periarterial lymphatic sheaths** (PALS) of the spleen, a second arrangement of white pulp may be noted, namely **lymphatic nodules** (LN) bearing a **germinal center** (Gc). Lymphatic nodules frequently occur at branching of the **central artery** (CA). Nodules are populated mostly by B lymphocytes (arrows), which account for the dark staining of the **corona** (CO). The germinal center is the site of active production of B lymphocytes during an antigenic challenge. The **marginal zone** (MZ), also present around lymphatic nodules, is the region where lymphocytes leave the small capillaries and first enter the connective tissue spaces of the spleen. It is from here that T lymphocytes migrate to the periarterial lymphatic sheaths, while B lymphocytes seek out lymphatic nodules. Both the marginal zone and the white pulp house numerous macrophages, as well as antigen-presenting cells (arrowheads) in addition to lymphocytes.

FIGURE 4 ■ *Spleen. Human. Silver stain. Paraffin section.* × 132.

The connective tissue framework of the spleen is demonstrated by the use of silver stain, which precipitates around reticular fibers. The **capsule** (Ca) of the spleen is pierced by **blood vessels** (BV) that enter the substance of the organ via **trabeculae** (T). The **white pulp** (WP) and **red pulp** (RP) are clearly evident. In fact, the lymphatic nodule presents a well-defined **germinal center** (Gc) as well as a **corona** (CO). The **central artery** (CA) is also evident in this preparation. **Reticular fibers** (RF), which form an extensive network throughout the substance of the spleen, are attached to the capsule and to the trabeculae.

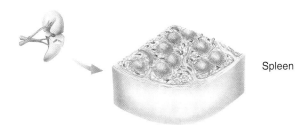

Spleen

■ KEY

AR	arteriole	EC	endothelial cell	PC	pulp cord
BC	blood cell	Gc	germinal center	RF	reticular fiber
B M	basement membrane	LN	lymphatic nodule	RP	red pulp
BV	blood vessel	Ly	lymphocyte	S	sinusoid
Ca	capsule	MZ	marginal zone	SE	septum
CA	central artery	N	nucleus	SM	smooth muscle
CO	corona	PALS	periarterial lymphatic sheath	T	trabeculae
E	epithelium			W P	white pulp

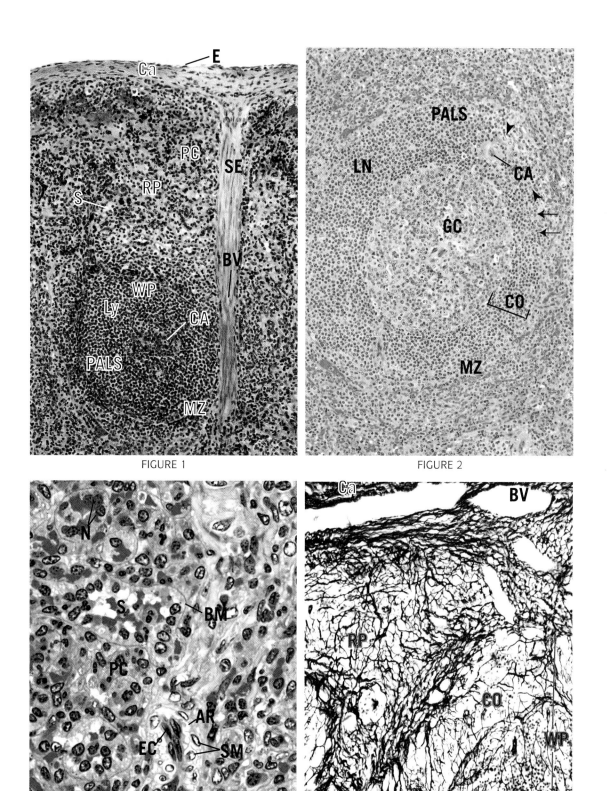

FIGURE 1

FIGURE 2

FIGURE 3

FIGURE 4

Lymphoid Tissue ■ 191

Endocrine System

The endocrine system in cooperation with the nervous system, orchestrates homeostasis by influencing, coordinating, and integrating the physiological functions of the body.

The endocrine system consists of several glands, isolated groups of cells within certain organs, and individual cells scattered among parenchymal cells of the body. This chapter considers only that part of the endocrine system that is composed of glands. Islets of Langerhans, interstitial cells of Leydig, cells responsible for ovarian hormone production, and DNES (diffuse neuroendocrine) cells are treated in more appropriate chapters.

The **endocrine glands** to be discussed here are the pituitary, thyroid, parathyroid, and suprarenal glands, and the pineal body. All of these glands produce **hormones,** low-molecular-weight molecules that are transported via the bloodstream to their target cells. Therefore, endocrine glands possess an extensive vascular supply that is particularly rich in fenestrated capillaries. Since some hormones are **proteins,** they do not cross the target cell plasmalemma, but attach to specific receptors on the plasma membrane of the target cell, thus activating its intracellular **second messenger system.** Other hormones are lipid soluble and, subsequent to entering the target cell, bind to their intracellular receptors, and thus exert their influence. Still other hormones act to modify the electrical potential difference across the plasmalemma of certain cells, such as muscle cells or neurons. Therefore, the activity of the hormone will, to a large extent, depend on the target cell receptors to which it becomes attached. The presence of most hormones also elicits a vascularly mediated negative feedback response, in that subsequent to a desired response, the further production and/or release of that particular hormone is inhibited.

PITUITARY GLAND

The **pituitary gland** (hypophysis) is composed of several regions, namely, pars anterior (pars distalis), pars tuberalis, infundibular stalk, pars intermedia, and pars nervosa (the last two are known as the pars posterior) (see Graphic 10-1). Since the pituitary gland develops from two separate embryonic origins, the epithelium of the pharyngeal roof and the floor of the diencephalon, it is frequently discussed as being subdivided into two parts: the **adenohypophysis** (**pars anterior, pars tuberalis,** and **pars intermedia**) and the **neurohypophysis** (**pars nervosa** and **infundibular stalk**). The pars nervosa is continuous with the median eminence of the hypothalamus via the thin neural stalk (infundibular stalk).

The pituitary gland receives its **blood supply** from the right and left **superior hypophyseal arteries,** serving the median eminence, pars tuberalis, and the infundibulum, and from the right and left **inferior hypophyseal arteries,** that serve the pars nervosa.

Hypophyseal Portal System: The two superior hypophyseal arteries give rise to the **primary capillary plexus** located in the region of the median eminence. **Hypophyseal portal veins** drain the primary capillary plexus and deliver the blood into the **secondary capillary plexus,** located in the pars distalis. Both capillary plexuses are composed of fenestrated capillaries.

Pars Anterior

The **pars anterior** is composed of numerous parenchymal cells arranged in thick cords, with large capillaries, known as sinusoids, richly vascularizing the intervening regions. The parenchymal cells are classified into two main categories: those whose granules readily take up stain, chromophils, and those cells that do not possess a strong affinity for stains, chromophobes. **Chromophils** are of two types, **acidophils** and **basophils.** Although considerable controversy surrounds the classification of these cells vis-à-vis their function, it is probable that at least six of the seven hormones manufactured by the pars anterior are made by separate cells. Hormones that modulate the secretory functions of the pituitary-dependent endocrine glands are **somatotropin, thyrotropin (TSH), follicle-stimulating hormone (FSH), luteinizing hormone (LH), prolactin, adrenocorticotropin (ACTH),** and **melanocyte-stimulating hormone (MSH).** It is believed that two types of acidophils produce somatotropin and prolactin, whereas various populations of basophils produce the remaining five hormones. **Chromophobes,** however, probably do not produce hormones. They are believed to be acidophils and basophils that have released their granules.

Control of Anterior Pituitary Hormone Release: Axons whose soma are located in the hypothalamus terminate at the primary capillary bed. These axons store releasing hormones (somatotropin-releasing hormone, prolactin-releasing hormone, corticotropin-releasing hormone, thyrotropin-releasing hormone, and gonadotropin-releasing hormone) and inhibitory hormones (prolacting inhibiting hormone, inhibitin, and somatostatin). The hormones are released by these axons into the primary capillary plexus and are conveyed to the secondary capillary plexus by the hypophyseal portal veins. The hormones then activate (or inhibit) chromophils of the adenohypophysis, causing them to release or prevent them from releasing their hormones.

An additional control is the mechanism of negative feedback, in that the presence of specific plasma levels of the pituitary hormones prevents the chromophils from releasing additional quantities of those hormones.

Pars Intermedia

The **pars intermedia** is not well developed. It is believed that the cell population of this region may have migrated into the pars anterior to produce **melanocyte-stimulating hormone** and **adrenocorticotropin.** It is quite probable that a single basophil can produce both of these hormones.

Pars Nervosa and Infundibular Stalk

The **pars nervosa** does not present a very organized appearance. It is composed of **pituicytes,** cells believed to be neuroglial in nature that may fulfill a supporting function for the numerous unmyelinated axons of the pars nervosa. These axons, whose cell bodies are located in the **supraoptic** and **paraventricular nuclei** of the hypothalamus, enter the pars nervosa via the **hypothalamo-hypophyseal tract.** They possess expanded axon terminals, referred to as **Herring bodies,** within the pars nervosa. Herring bodies contain **oxytocin** and **antidiuretic hormone (ADH, vasopressin),** two neurosecretory hormones that are stored in the pars nervosa but are manufactured in the cell bodies in the **hypothalamus.** The release of these neurosecretory hormones (neurosecretion) is mediated by nerve impulses.

Pars Tuberalis

The **pars tuberalis** is composed of numerous cuboidal cells whose function is not known.

THYROID GLAND

The **thyroid gland** consists of right and left lobes that are interconnected by a narrow isthmus across the thyroid cartilage and upper trachea (see Graphic 10-2). It is enveloped by a connective tissue capsule whose septa penetrate the substance of the gland, forming not only its supporting framework but also its conduit for a rich vascular supply. The parenchymal cells of the gland are arranged in numerous follicles, composed of a **simple cuboidal epithelium** lining a central **colloid-filled lumen.** The colloid, secreted and resorbed by the **follicular cells,** is composed of the thyroid hormone that is bound to a large protein and the complex is known as **thyroglobulin.** An additional secretory cell type, **parafollicular cells (clear cells),** is present in the thyroid. These cells have no contact with the colloidal material. They manufacture the hormone **calcitonin,** which is released directly into the connective tissue in the immediate vicinity of capillaries. Thyroid hormone is essential for regulating basal metabolism and for influencing growth rate and mental processes, and generally stimulates endocrine gland functioning. Calcitonin helps control calcium concentrations in the blood by inhibiting bone resorption by osteoclasts (i.e., when blood calcium levels are high, calcitonin is released).

PARATHYROID GLANDS

The **parathyroid glands,** usually four in number, are embedded in the fascial sheath of the posterior aspect of the thyroid gland. The parathyroid glands possess slender connective tissue capsules from which septa are derived to penetrate the glands and convey a vascular supply to the interior. In the adult, two types of cells are present: numerous small **chief cells** and a smaller number of large **acidophilic cells,** the **oxyphils.** Fatty infiltration of the gland is common in older individuals. Although there is no know function of oxyphils, chief cells produce **parathyroid hormone (PTH),** the most important regulator of calcium in the body. PTH helps control serum calcium levels by acting directly on osteoblasts to increase osteoclastic activity, reducing calcium loss through the kidneys, and facilitating calcium absorption in the intestines. Lack of parathyroid glands is not compatible with life.

SUPRARENAL GLANDS

The **suprarenal glands** (adrenal glands in some animals) are invested by a connective tissue capsule (see Graphics 10-2 and 10-3). The glands are derived from two different embryonic origins, namely, **mesodermal epithelium,** which gives rise to the **cortex,** and **neuroectoderm,** from which the **medulla** originates. The rich vascular supply of the gland is conveyed to the interior in connective tissue elements derived from the capsule.

Cortex

The **cortex** is subdivided into three concentric regions or zones. The outermost region, just beneath the capsule, is the **zona glomerulosa,** where the cells are arranged in arches and spherical clusters with numerous capillaries surrounding them. The second region, the **zona fasciculata,** is the most extensive. Its parenchymal cells, usually known as **spongiocytes,** are arranged in long cords, with numerous capillaries between the cords. The innermost region of the cortex, the **zona reticularis,** is arranged in anastomosing cords of cells with a rich intervening capillary network. Three types of hormones are produced by the suprarenal cortex, namely, **mineralocorticoids** (zona glomerulosa),

glucocorticoids (zona fasciculata and, to some extent, zona reticularis), and some **androgens** (zona fasciculata and zona reticularis).

Medulla

The cells of the **medulla,** disposed in irregularly arranged short cords surrounded by capillary networks, contain numerous granules that stain intensely when the freshly cut tissue is exposed to chromium salts. This is referred to as the chromaffin reaction, and the cells are called **chromaffin cells.** There are two types of chromaffin cells: one produces **epinephrine,** while the other manufactures **norepinephrine,** the two hormones of the suprarenal medulla. Since these cells are innervated by preganglionic sympathetic nerve fibers, chromaffin cells are considered to be related to postganglionic sympathetic neurons. Additionally, the medulla of the suprarenal gland also houses large, postganglionic sympathetic nerve cell bodies whose function is not known.

PINEAL BODY

The **pineal body (epiphysis)** is a projection of the roof of the diencephalon (see Graphic 10-2). The connective tissue covering of the pineal body is pia mater, which sends trabeculae and septa into the substance of the pineal body, subdividing it into incomplete lobules. Blood vessels supplying and draining the pineal body travel in these connective tissue elements. The main cellular elements of the pineal body are **pinealocytes** and **neuroglial cells.** The pinealocytes manufacture **melatonin** and **serotonin,** while neuroglial cells lend support to pinealocytes. Interestingly, serotonin is only produced during daylight, while melatonin is manufactured only at night. The intercellular spaces of the pineal body contain calcified granular material known as **brain sand (corpora arenacea),** whose significance, if any, is not known.

Histophysiology

I. MECHANISM OF HORMONAL ACTION

Hormones are substances secreted by cells of the endocrine system into the connective tissue spaces. Some hormones act in the immediate vicinity of their secretion, whereas other hormones enter the vascular system and find their target cells at a distance from their site of origin.

Some hormones (e.g., **thyroid hormone**) have a generalized effect, in that most cells are affected by them; other hormones (e.g., **aldosterone**) affect only certain cells. **Receptors** located either on the cell membrane or within the cell are specific for a particular hormone. The binding of a hormone initiates a sequence of reactions that results in a particular response. Because of the specificity of the reaction, only a minute quantity of the hormone is required. Some hormones elicit and others inhibit a particular response.

Hormones are of two types, nonsteroid and steroid based. **Nonsteroid-based hormones** may be derivatives of tyrosine (catecholamines and thyroid hormone) and small peptides (ADH and oxytocin) or small proteins (glucagon, insulin, anterior pituitary proteins, and parathormone). **Steroid-based hormones** are cholesterol derivatives (aldosterone, cortisol, estrogen, progesterone, and testosterone).

A. Nonsteroid-Based Hormones

Nonsteroid-based endocrine hormones bind to **receptors** (some are G protein linked, and some are catalytic) located on the target cell membrane, activate them, and thus initiate a sequence of intracellular reactions. These may act by altering the state of an **ion channel** (opening or closing) or by activating (or inhibiting) an **enzyme** or group of enzymes associated with the cytoplasmic aspect of the cell membrane.

Opening or closing an ion channel will permit the particular ion to traverse or inhibit the particular ion from traversing the cell membrane, thus altering the membrane potential. Neurotransmitters and **catecholamines** act on ion channels.

The binding of most hormones to their receptor will have only a single effect, which is the activation of **adenylate cyclase.** This enzyme functions in the transformation of ATP to **cAMP (cyclic adenosine monophosphate)**, the major **second messenger** of

the cell. cAMP then activates a specific sequence of enzymes that are necessary to accomplish the desired result. There are a few hormones that activate a similar compound, **cyclic guanosine monophosphate (cGMP)**, which functions in a comparable fashion.

Some hormones facilitate the opening of **calcium channels;** calcium enters the cell, and three or four calcium ions bind to the protein **calmodulin,** altering its conformation. The altered calmodulin is a **second messenger** that activates a sequence of enzymes, causing a specific response.

Thyroid hormones are unusual, in that they directly enter the nucleus, where they bind with **receptor molecules.** The hormone–receptor complexes control the activities of **operators** and/or **promoters,** resulting in mRNA transcription. The newly formed mRNAs enter the cytoplasm, where they are translated into proteins that elevate the cell's metabolic activity.

B. Steroid-Based Hormones

Steroid-based endocrine hormones diffuse into the target cell through the plasma membrane and, once inside the cell, bind to a **receptor molecule.** The receptor molecule–hormone complex enters the nucleus, seeks out a specific region of the DNA molecule, and initiates the synthesis of mRNA. The newly formed mRNA codes for the formation of specific enzymes that will accomplish the desired result.

II. THYROID HORMONE

A. Synthesis

Iodide from the bloodstream is actively transported into follicular cells at their basal aspect via **iodide pumps.** Iodide is oxidized by **thyroid peroxidase** on the apical cell membrane and is bound to **tyrosine residues** of **thyroglobulin** molecules. Within the colloid the iodinated tyrosine residues become rearranged to form **triiodothyronine** (T_3) and **thyroxine** (T_4).

B. Release

The binding of **thyroid-stimulating hormone** to receptors on the basal aspect of their plasmalemma induces follicular cells to become tall cuboidal cells. They form **pseudopods** on their apical cell membrane that engulf and endocytose colloid. The colloid-filled vesicles fuse with lysosomes, and T_3 and T_4 residues are removed from thyroglobulin, liberated into the cytosol, and are released at the basal aspect of the cell into the perifollicular capillary network.

III. PARATHYROID HORMONE AND CALCITONIN

Parathyroid hormone (PTH), produced by chief cells of the parathyroid, is responsible for maintaining proper calcium ion balance. The concentration of calcium ions is extremely important in the normal function of muscle and nerve cells and as a release mechanism for neurotransmitter substance. A drop in blood calcium concentration activates a feedback mechanism that stimulates chief cell secretion. PTH binds to receptors on osteoblasts that release osteoclast-stimulating factor followed by bone resorption and a consequent increase in blood calcium ion concentration. In the kidneys PTH prevents urinary calcium loss; thus ions are returned to the bloodstream. PTH also controls calcium uptake in the intestines indirectly by modulating kidney production of vitamin D, which is essential for calcium absorption.

Increased levels of PTH causes an elevation in plasma calcium concentration; however, it takes several hours for this level to peak. The concentration of PTH in the blood is also controlled by plasma calcium levels.

Calcitonin acts as an antagonist to PTH. Unlike PTH, calcitonin is fast acting and, since it binds directly to receptors on osteoclasts, it elicits a peak reduction in blood calcium levels within one hour. Calcitonin inhibits bone resorption thus reducing calcium ion levels in the blood. High levels of calcium ions in the blood stimulate calcitonin release.

IV. SUPRARENAL GLANDS

The suprarenal parenchyma is divided into an external cortex and an internal medulla.

A. Cortex

Parenchymal cells of the **cortex**, derived from mesoderm, are regionalized into three zones that secrete specific hormones. Control of these hormonal secretions is mostly regulated by ACTH from the pituitary gland.

Cells of the zona glomerulosa secrete **aldosterone**, a mineralocorticoid that acts on cells of the distal convoluted tubules of the kidney to modulate water and electrolyte balance.

Zona fasciculata cells secrete **cortisol** and **corticosterone**. These glucocorticoids regulate carbohydrate metabolism, facilitate the catabolism of fats and proteins, exhibit anti-inflammatory activity, and suppress the immune response.

Zona reticularis cells secrete weak **androgens** that promote masculine characteristics.

B. Medulla

Parenchymal cells of the **medulla** are derived from neural crest material. They consist of two populations of **chromaffin cells** that secrete mainly **epinephrine** (adrenaline) or **norepinephrine** (noradrenaline). Secretion of these two catecholamines is directly regulated by preganglionic fibers of the sympathetic nervous system that impinge on the postganglionic sympathetic neuron-like chromaffin cells. Catecholamine release occurs in physical and psychological stress. Moreover, scattered **sympathetic ganglion cells** in the medulla act upon smooth muscle cells of the medullary veins, thus controlling blood flow in the cortex.

V. PINEAL BODY (PINEAL GLAND; EPIPHYSIS)

Pinealocytes, parenchymal cells of the **pineal body**, synthesize serotonin during the day and melatonin during the night. However, it is unclear how the gland functions in humans. Nonetheless, melatonin is used to treat jet lag and in regulating emotional responses related to shortened daylight during winter, a condition called seasonal affective disorder (SAD).

Clinical Considerations ▨ ▨ ▪

Pituitary Gland

Galactorrhea is a condition where a male produces breast milk or a woman who is not breast feeding produces breast milk. In men it is often accompanied by impotence, headache, and loss of peripheral vision and in women by hot flashes, vaginal dryness, and an abnormal menstrual cycle. This rather uncommon condition is usually a result of prolactinoma, a tumor of prolactin-producing cells of the pituitary gland. The condition is usually treated by drug intervention or surgery, or both.

Thyroid Gland

Graves' disease is caused by binding of autoimmune IgG antibodies to TSH receptors thus stimulating increased thyroid hormone production (**hyperthyroidism**). Clinically, the thyroid gland becomes enlarged and there is evidence of exophthalmic goiter (protrusion of the eyeballs).

Parathyroid Gland

Hyperparathyroidism may be due to the presence of a benign tumor causing the excess production of parathyroid hormone. The high levels of circulating PTH cause increased bone resorption with a resultant greatly elevated blood calcium. The excess calcium may become deposited in arterial walls and in the kidneys, creating kidney stones.

Suprarenal Gland

Addison's disease is an autoimmune disease, although it may also be the aftermath of tuberculosis. It is characterized by decreased production of adrenocortical hormones due to the destruction of the suprarenal cortex and without the administration of steroid treatment it may have fatal consequences.

Summary of Histological Organization

Endocrine glands are characterized by the absence of ducts and the presence of a rich vascular network. The parenchymal cells of endocrine glands are usually arranged in short **cords, follicles,** or **clusters,** although other arrangements are also common.

I. PITUITARY GLAND

The **pituitary gland** is invested by a **connective tissue capsule.** The gland is subdivided into four component parts.

A. Pars Anterior

1. Cell Types

a. Chromophils

1. Acidophils
Stain pink with hematoxylin and eosin. They are found mostly in the center of the pars anterior.

2. Basophils
Stain darker than acidophils with hematoxylin and eosin. They are more frequently found at the periphery of the pars anterior.

b. Chromophobes
Chromophobes are smaller cells whose cytoplasm is not granular and has very little affinity for stain. They may be recognized as clusters of nuclei throughout the pars anterior.

B. Pars Intermedia

The **pars intermedia** is rudimentary in man. Small **basophils** are present, as well as **colloid**-filled **follicles.**

C. Pars Nervosa and Infundibular Stalk

These have the appearance of nervous tissue. The cells of the **pars nervosa** are **pituicytes,** resembling neuroglial cells. They probably support the **unmyelinated nerve fibers,** whose terminal portions are expanded, since they store **neurosecretions** within the pars nervosa. These expanded terminal regions are known as **Herring bodies.**

D. Pars Tuberalis

The **pars tuberalis** is composed of **cuboidal cells** arranged in cords. They may form small colloid-filled **follicles.**

II. THYROID GLAND

A. Capsule

The **capsule** of the thyroid gland consists of a thin **collagenous connective tissue** from which **septa** extend into the substance of the gland, subdividing it into lobules.

B. Parenchymal Cells

The **parenchymal cells** of the thyroid gland form **colloid**-filled **follicles** composed of

1. Follicular Cells (simple cuboidal epithelium)

2. Parafollicular Cells (clear cells) located at the periphery of the follicles

C. Connective Tissue

Slender connective tissue elements support a rich vascular supply.

III. PARATHYROID GLAND

A. Capsule

The gland is invested by a slender collagenous connective tissue **capsule** from which **septa** arise to penetrate the substance of the gland.

B. Parenchymal Cells

1. Chief Cells
Chief cells are numerous, small cells with large nuclei that form cords.

2. Oxyphils
Oxyphils are larger, acidophilic, and much fewer in number than chief cells.

C. Connective Tissue

Collagenous connective tissue **septa** as well as slender **reticular fibers** support a rich vascular supply. **Fatty infiltration** is common in older individuals.

IV. SUPRARENAL GLAND

The **suprarenal gland** is invested by a collagenous connective tissue **capsule.** The gland is subdivided into a **cortex** and a **medulla.**

A. Cortex

The **cortex** is divided into three concentric zones: **zona glomerulosa, zona fasciculata,** and **zona reticularis.**

1. Zona Glomerulosa

The **zona glomerulosa** is immediately deep to the capsule. It consists of columnar cells arranged in arches and spherical clusters.

2. Zona Fasciculata

The thickest zone of the cortex is the **zona fasciculata.** The more or less cuboidal cells (**spongiocytes**) are arranged in long, parallel cords. **Spongiocytes** appear highly vacuolated except for those of the deepest region, which are smaller and much less vacuolated.

3. Zona Reticularis

The innermost zone of the cortex is the **zona reticularis.** It is composed of small, dark cells arranged in irregularly anastomosing cords. The intervening capillaries are enlarged.

B. Medulla

The **medulla** is small in humans and is composed of large, granule-containing **chromaffin cells** arranged in short cords. Additionally, large autonomic ganglion cells are also present. A characteristic of the medulla is the presence of large veins.

V. PINEAL BODY

A. Capsule

The **capsule,** derived from **pia mater,** is thin collagenous connective tissue. **Septa** derived from the capsule divide the pineal body into incomplete lobules.

B. Parenchymal Cells

1. Pinealocytes

Pinealocytes are recognized by the large size of their nuclei.

2. Neuroglial Cells

Neuroglial cells possess smaller, denser nuclei than the pinealocytes.

C. Brain Sand

Characteristic of the pineal body are the calcified accretions in the intercellular spaces, known as **brain sand** or **corpora arenacea.**

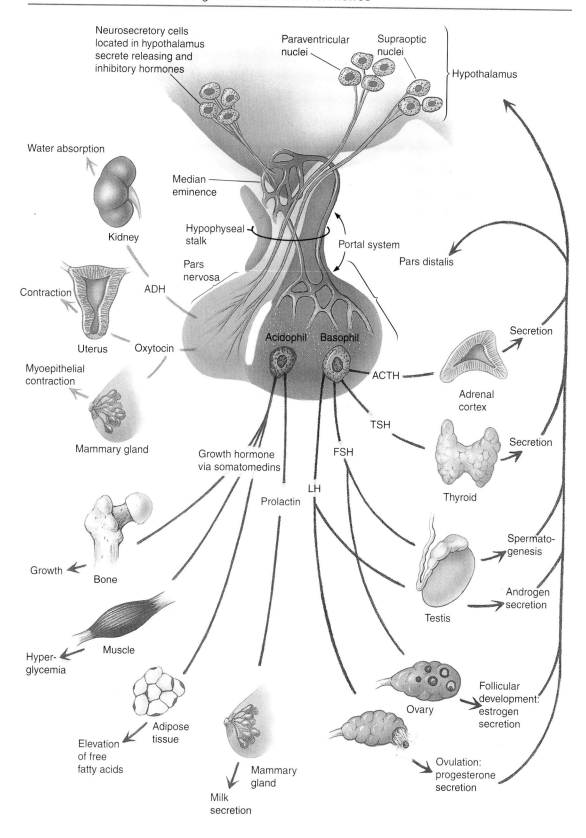

Neurosecretory cells located in hypothalamus secrete releasing and inhibitory hormones

Paraventricular nuclei

Supraoptic nuclei

Hypothalamus

Water absorption

Kidney

Median eminence

Hypophyseal stalk

Pars nervosa

Portal system

Pars distalis

ADH

Contraction

Uterus

Oxytocin

Acidophil

Basophil

ACTH

Adrenal cortex

Secretion

Myoepithelial contraction

Mammary gland

TSH

Secretion

Thyroid

Growth hormone via somatomedins

FSH

LH

Prolactin

Spermato-genesis

Androgen secretion

Testis

Growth

Bone

Hyper-glycemia

Muscle

Adipose tissue

Elevation of free fatty acids

Mammary gland

Milk secretion

Ovary

Follicular development: estrogen secretion

Ovulation: progesterone secretion

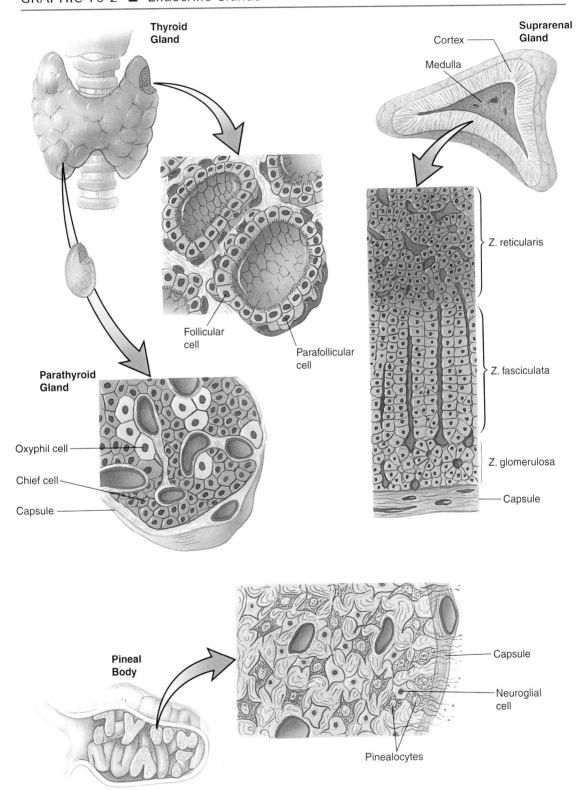

Thyroid Gland

Follicular cell

Parafollicular cell

Suprarenal Gland

Cortex

Medulla

Z. reticularis

Z. fasciculata

Z. glomerulosa

Capsule

Parathyroid Gland

Oxyphil cell

Chief cell

Capsule

Pineal Body

Capsule

Neuroglial cell

Pinealocytes

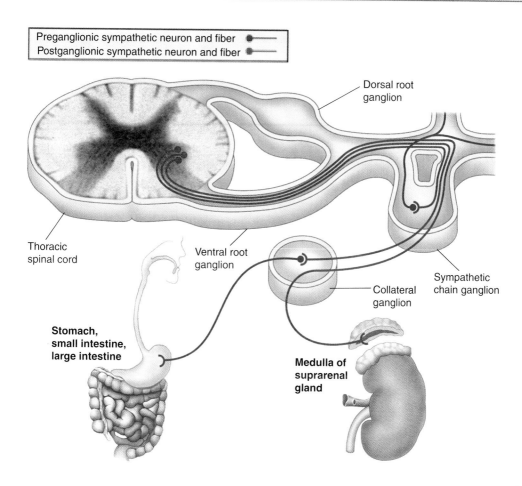

Preganglionic sympathetic neuron and fiber ●———
Postganglionic sympathetic neuron and fiber ●———

Dorsal root
ganglion

Thoracic
spinal cord

Ventral root
ganglion

Collateral
ganglion

Sympathetic
chain ganglion

Stomach,
small intestine,
large intestine

Medulla of
suprarenal
gland

PLATE 10-1 ■ *Pituitary Gland*

FIGURE 1 ■ *Pituitary gland. Paraffin section.* × 19.

This survey photomicrograph of the pituitary gland demonstrates the relationship of the gland to the **hypothalamus** (H) from which it is suspended by the infundibulum. The infundibulum is composed of a neural portion, the **infundibular stem** (IS) and the surrounding **pars tuberalis** (PT). Note that the **third ventricle** (3V) of the brain is continuous with the **infundibular recess** (IR). The largest portion of the pituitary is the **pars anterior** (PA), which is glandular and secretes numerous hormones. The neural component of the pituitary gland is the **pars nervosa** (PN) that does not manufacture its hormones, but stores and releases them. Even at this magnification, its resemblance to the brain tissue and to the substance of the infundibular stalk is readily evident. Between the pars anterior and pars nervosa is the **pars intermedia** (PI), which frequently presents an **intraglandular cleft** (IC), a remnant of Rathke's pouch.

FIGURE 2 ■ *Pituitary gland. Pars anterior. Paraffin section.* × 132.

The pars anterior is composed of large cords of cells that branch and anastomose with each other. These cords are surrounded by an extensive capillary network. However, these capillaries are wide, endothelially lined vessels known as **sinusoids** (S). The parenchymal cells of the anterior pituitary are divided into two groups: **chromophils** (Ci) and **chromophobes** (Co). With hematoxylin and eosin the distinction between chromophils and chromophobes is obvious. The former stain blue or pink, while the latter stain poorly. The boxed area is presented at a higher magnification in Figure 3.

FIGURE 3 ■ *Pituitary gland. Pars anterior. Paraffin section.* × 270.

This is a higher magnification of the boxed area of Figure 2. Note that the **chromophobes** (Co) do not take up the stain well and only their **nuclei** (N) are demonstrable. These cells are small; therefore, chromophobes are easily recognizable since their nuclei appear to be clumped together. The chromophils may be classified into two categories by their affinity to histologic dyes: blue-staining **basophils** (B) and pink-colored **acidophils** (A). The distinction between these two cell types in sections stained with hematoxylin and eosin is not as apparent as with some other stains. Note also the presence of a large **sinusoid** (S).

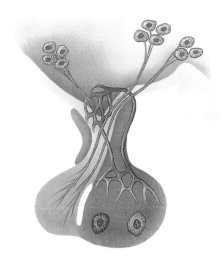

Pituitary gland

■ **KEY**

A	acidophils	IC	intraglandular cleft	PI	pars intermedia
B	basophils	IR	infundibular recess	PN	pars nervosa
Ci	chromophils	IS	infundibular stem	PT	pars tuberalis
Co	chromophobes	N	nucleus	S	sinusoids
H	hypothalamus	PA	pars anterior	3V	third ventricle

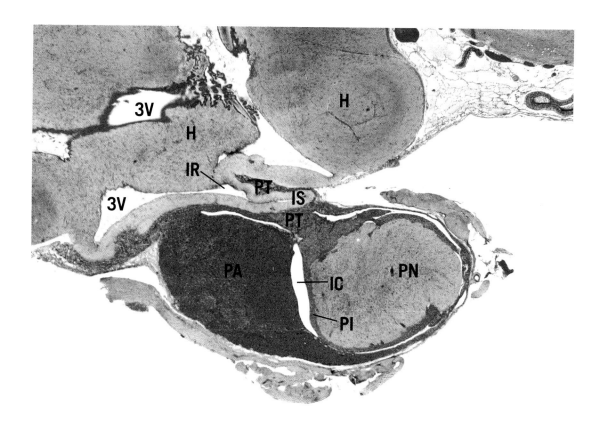

FIGURE 1

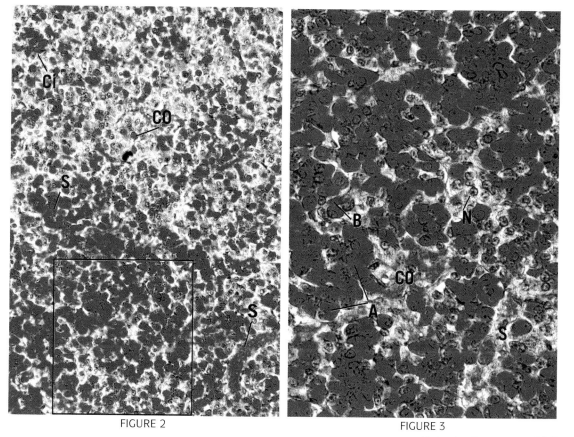

FIGURE 2

FIGURE 3

Endocrine System ■ **205**

PLATE 10-2 ■ *Pituitary Gland*

FIGURE 1 ■ *Pituitary gland. Paraffin section.* × 540.

It is somewhat difficult to discriminate between the **acidophils** (A) and **basophils** (B) of the pituitary gland stained with hematoxylin and eosin. Even at high magnification, such as in this photomicrograph, only slight differences are noted. Acidophils stain pinkish and are slightly smaller in size than the basophils, which stain pale blue. In a black and white photomicrograph, basophils appear darker than acidophils. **Chromophobes** (Co) are readily recognizable, since their cytoplasm is small and does not take up stain. Moreover, cords of chromophobes present clusters of **nuclei** (N) crowded together.

FIGURE 2 ■ *Pituitary gland. Pars intermedia. Human. Paraffin section.* × 270.

The pars intermedia of the pituitary gland is situated between the **pars anterior** (PA) and the **pars nervosa** (PN). It is characterized by **basophils** (B), which are smaller than those of the pars anterior. Additionally, the pars intermedia contains **colloid** (Cl)-filled follicles, lined by pale, small low cuboidal shaped cells (arrows). Note that some of the basophils extend into the pars nervosa. Numerous **blood vessels** (BV) and **pituicytes** (P) are evident in this area of the pars nervosa.

FIGURE 3 ■ *Pituitary gland. Pars nervosa. Paraffin section.* × 132.

The pars nervosa of the pituitary gland is composed of elongated cells with long processes known as **pituicytes** (P), which are thought to be neuroglial in nature. These cells, which possess more or less oval nuclei, appear to support numerous unmyelinated nerve fibers traveling from the hypothalamus via the hypothalamo-hypophyseal tract. These nerve fibers cannot be distinguished from the cytoplasm of pituicytes in an hematoxylin and eosin-stained preparation. Neurosecretory materials pass along these nerve fibers and are stored in expanded regions at the termination of the fibers, which are then referred to as **Herring bodies** (HB). Note that the pars nervosa resembles neural tissue. The boxed area is presented at a higher magnification in Figure 4.

FIGURE 4 ■ *Pituitary gland. Pars nervosa. Paraffin section.* × 540.

This photomicrograph is a higher magnification of the boxed area of Figure 3. Note the numerous more or less oval **nuclei** (N) of the pituicytes, some of whose processes (arrows) are clearly evident at this magnification. The unmyelinated nerve fibers and processes of pituicytes make up the cellular network of the pars nervosa. The expanded terminal regions of the nerve fibers, which house neurosecretions, are known as **Herring bodies** (HB). Also observe the presence of **blood vessels** (BV) in the pars nervosa.

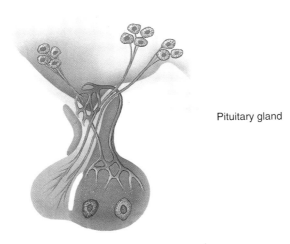

Pituitary gland

■ KEY

A	acidophils	Co	chromophobes	P	pituicytes
B	basophils	HB	Herring bodies	PA	pars anterior
BV	blood vessels	N	nucleus	PN	pars nervosa
Cl	colloid				

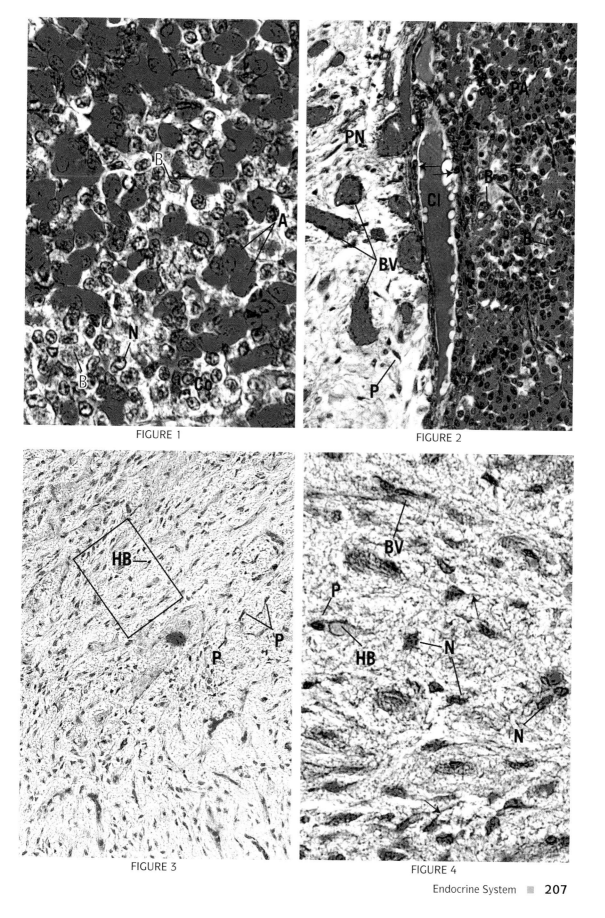

FIGURE 1

FIGURE 2

FIGURE 3

FIGURE 4

PLATE 10-3 ■ *Thyroid Gland, Parathyroid Gland*

FIGURE 1 ■ *Thyroid gland. Monkey. Plastic section.* × 132.

The capsule of the thyroid gland sends septa of connective tissue into the substance of the gland, subdividing it into incomplete lobules. This photomicrograph presents part of a lobule displaying many **follicles** (F) of varied sizes. Each follicle is surrounded by slender **connective tissue** (CT), which supports the follicles and brings **blood vessels** (BV) in close approximation. The follicles are composed of **follicular cells** (FC), whose low cuboidal morphology indicates that the cells are not producing secretory product. During the active secretory cycle, these cells become taller in morphology. In addition to the follicular cells, another parenchymal cell type is found in the thyroid gland. These cells do not border the colloid, are located on the periphery of the follicles, and are known as **parafollicular cells** (PF) or C cells. They are large and possess centrally placed round nuclei, and their cytoplasm appears paler.

FIGURE 2 ■ Thyroid gland. Monkey. Plastic section. × 540. The thyroid **follicle** (F) presented in this photomicrograph is surrounded by several other follicles and intervening **connective tissue** (CT). **Nuclei** (N) in the connective tissue may belong either to endothelial cells or to connective tissue cells. Since most capillaries are collapsed in excised thyroid tissue, it is often difficult to identify endothelial cells with any degree of certainty. The **follicular cells** (FC) are flattened, indicating that these cells are not actively secreting thyroglobulin. Note that the follicles are filled with a **colloid** (Cl) material. Observe the presence of a **parafollicular cell** (PF), which may be distinguished from the surrounding cells by its pale cytoplasm (arrow) and larger nucleus.

FIGURE 3 ■ *Thyroid and parathyroid glands. Monkey. Plastic section.* × 132.

Although the **parathyroid** (PG) and **thyroid glands** (TG) are separated by their respective **capsules** (Ca), they are extremely close to each other. The capsule of the parathyroid gland sends **trabeculae** (T) of connective tissue carrying **blood vessels** (BV) into the substance of the gland. The parenchyma of the gland consists of two types of cells, namely **chief cells** (CC), also known as principal cells, and **oxyphil cells** (OC). Chief cells are more numerous and possess darker staining cytoplasm. Oxyphil cells stain lighter and are usually larger than chief cells, and their cell membranes are evident. A region similar to the boxed area is presented at a higher magnification in Figure 4.

FIGURE 4 ■ *Parathyroid gland. Monkey. Plastic section.* × 540.

This photomicrograph is a region similar to the boxed area of Figure 3. The **chief cells** (CC) of the parathyroid gland form small cords surrounded by slender **connective tissue** (CT) elements and **blood vessels** (BV). The **nuclei** (N) of connective tissue cells may be easily recognized due to their elongated appearance. **Oxyphil cells** (OC) possess a paler cytoplasm and frequently the cell membranes are evident (arrows). The glands of older individuals may become infiltrated by adipocytes.

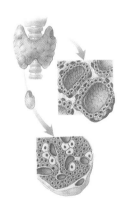

Thyroid gland and parathyroid gland

■ **KEY**

BV	blood vessels	F	follicle	PF	parafollicular cells
Ca	capsule	FC	follicular cells	PG	parathyroid gland
CC	chief cells	N	nucleus	T	trabeculae
Cl	colloid	OC	oxyphil cells	TG	thyroid gland
CT	connective tissue				

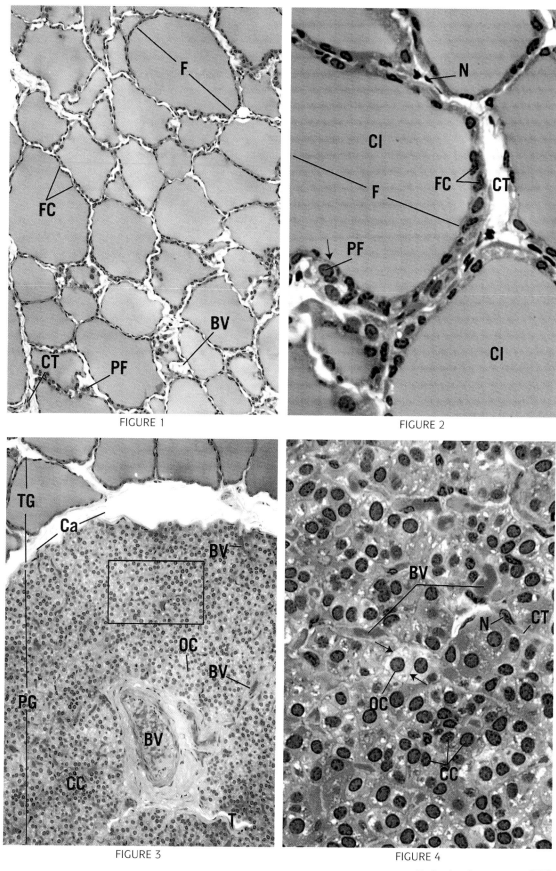

FIGURE 1

FIGURE 2

FIGURE 3

FIGURE 4

PLATE 10-4 ■ *Suprarenal Gland*

FIGURE 1 ■ *Suprarenal gland. Paraffin section.* × 14.

The suprarenal gland, usually embedded in **adipose tissue** (AT), is invested by a collagenous connective tissue **capsule** (Ca) that provides thin connective tissue elements that carry blood vessels and nerves into the substance of the gland. Since the **cortex** (Co) of the suprarenal gland completely surrounds the flattened **medulla** (M), it appears duplicated in any section that completely transects the gland. The cortex is divided into three concentric regions: the outermost **zona glomerulosa** (ZG), middle **zona fasciculata** (ZF), and the innermost **zona reticularis** (ZR). The medulla, which is always bounded by the zona reticularis, possesses several large **veins** (V), which are always accompanied by a considerable amount of connective tissue.

FIGURE 2 ■ *Suprarenal gland. Cortex. Monkey. Plastic section.* × 132.

The collagenous connective tissue **capsule** (Ca) of the suprarenal gland is surrounded by adipose tissue through which **blood vessels** (BV) and **nerves** (Ne) reach the gland. The parenchymal cells of the cortex, immediately deep to the capsule, are arranged in an irregular array, forming the more or less oval to round clusters or arch-like cords of the **zona glomerulosa** (ZG). The cells of the **zona fasciculata** (ZF) form long straight columns of cords oriented radially, each being one to two cells in width. These cells are larger than those of the zona glomerulosa. They present a vacuolated appearance due to the numerous lipid droplets that were extracted during processing and are often referred to as **spongiocytes** (Sp). The interstitium is richly vascularized by **blood vessels** (BV).

FIGURE 3 ■ *Suprarenal gland. Monkey. Plastic section.* × 132.

The columnar arrangement of the cords of the **zona fasciculata** (ZF) is readily evident by viewing the architecture of the blood vessels indicated by the arrows. The cells in the deeper region of the zona fasciculata are smaller and appear denser than the more superficially located **spongiocytes** (Sp). Cells of the **zona reticularis** (ZR) are arranged in irregular, anastomosing cords whose interstices contain wide capillaries. The cords of the zona reticularis merge almost imperceptibly with those of the zona fasciculata. This is a relatively narrow region of the cortex. The **medulla** (M) is clearly evident since its cells are much larger than those of the zona reticularis. Moreover, numerous large **veins** (V) are characteristic of the medulla.

FIGURE 4 ■ *Suprarenal gland. Monkey. Plastic section.* × 540.

The **capsule** (Ca) of the suprarenal gland displays its **collagen fibers** (Cf) and the **nuclei** (N) of the fibroblasts. The **zona glomerulosa** (ZG), which occupies the upper part of the photomicrograph, displays relatively small cells with few vacuoles (arrows). The lower part of the photomicrograph demonstrates the **zona fasciculata** (ZF), whose cells are larger and display a more vacuolated (arrowheads) appearance. Note the presence of **connective tissue** (CT) elements and **blood vessels** (BV) in the interstitium between cords of parenchymal cells.

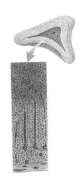

Suprarenal gland

■ **KEY**

AT	adipose tissue	CT	connective tissue	V	veins
BV	blood vessels	M	medulla	ZF	zona fasciculata
Ca	capsule	N	nuclei	ZG	zona glomerulosa
Cf	collagen fibers	Ne	nerves	ZR	zona reticularis
Co	cortex	Sp	spongiocytes		

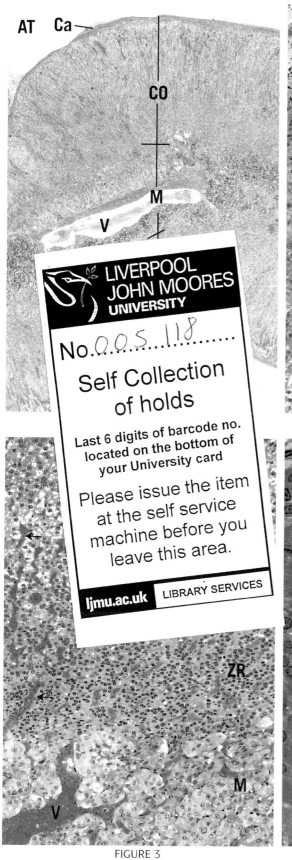

AT Ca

CO

M

V

ZR

M

V

FIGURE 3

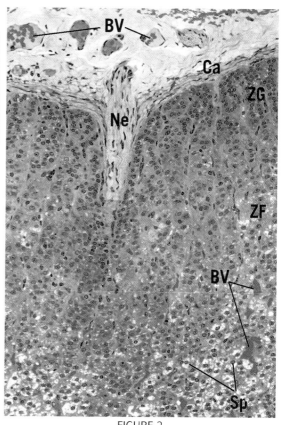

BV

Ca

ZG

Ne

ZF

BV

Sp

FIGURE 2

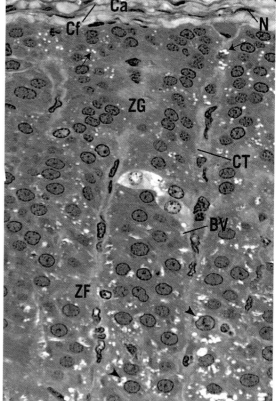

Ca

Cf

N

ZG

CT

BV

ZF

FIGURE 4

Endocrine System ■ 211

PLATE 10-5 ■ *Suprarenal Gland, Pineal Body*

FIGURE 1 ■ *Suprarenal gland. Cortex. Monkey. Plastic section.* × 540.

The upper part of this photomicrograph presents the border between the **zona fasciculata** (ZF) and the **zona reticularis** (ZR). Note that the **spongiocytes** (Sp) of the fasciculata are larger and more vacuolated than the cells of the reticularis. The parenchymal cells of the zona reticularis are arranged in haphazardly anastomosing cords. The interstitium of both regions house large capillaries containing **red blood cells** (RBC).

Inset. **Zona fasciculata. Monkey. Plastic section.** × 540.

The **spongiocytes** (Sp) of the zona fasciculata are of two different sizes. Those positioned more superficially in the cortex, as in this inset, are larger and more vacuolated (arrows) than spongiocytes close to the zona reticularis.

FIGURE 2 ■ *Suprarenal gland. Medulla. Monkey. Plastic section.* × 270.

The cells of the adrenal medulla, often referred to as **chromaffin cells** (ChC), are arranged in round to ovoid clusters or in irregularly arranged short cords. The cells are large and more or less round to polyhedral in shape with a pale **cytoplasm** (Cy) and vesicular appearing **nucleus** (N), displaying a single, large **nucleolus** (n). The interstitium presents large **veins** (V) and an extensive **capillary** (Cp) network. Large ganglion cells are occasionally noted.

FIGURE 3 ■ *Pineal body. Human. Paraffin section.* × 132.

The pineal body is covered by a capsule of connective tissue derived from the pia mater. From this capsule connective tissue **trabeculae** (T) enter the substance of the pineal body, subdividing it into numerous incomplete **lobules** (Lo). Nerves and **blood vessels** (BV) travel in the trabeculae to be distributed throughout the pineal, providing it with a rich vascular supply. In addition to endothelial and connective tissue cells, two other types of cells are present in the pineal, namely, the parenchymal cells, known as **pinealocytes** (Pi) and **neuroglial supporting cells** (Ng). A characteristic feature of the pineal body is the deposit of calcified material, known as corpora arenacea or **brain sand** (BS). The boxed area is presented at a higher magnification in Figure 4.

FIGURE 4 ■ *Pineal body. Human. Paraffin section.* × 540.

This photomicrograph is a higher magnification of the boxed area of Figure 3. With the use of hematoxylin and eosin stain, only the nuclei of the two cell types are clearly evident. The larger, paler, more numerous nuclei belong to the **pinealocytes** (Pi). The smaller, denser nuclei are those of the **neuroglial cells** (Ng). The pale background is composed of the long, intertwining processes of these two cell types. The center of the photomicrograph is occupied by **brain sand** (BS). Observe that these concretions increase in size by apposition of layers on the surface of the calcified material, as may be noted at the arrow.

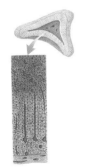

Suprarenal gland

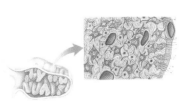

Pineal body

■ KEY

BS	brain sand	N	nucleus	Sp	spongiocytes
BV	blood vessels	n	nucleolus	T	trabeculate
ChC	chromaffin cells	Ng	neuroglial cells	V	veins
Cp	capillaries	Pi	pinealocytes	ZF	zona fasciculata
Cy	cytoplasm	RBC	red blood cells	ZR	zona reticularis
Lo	lobules				

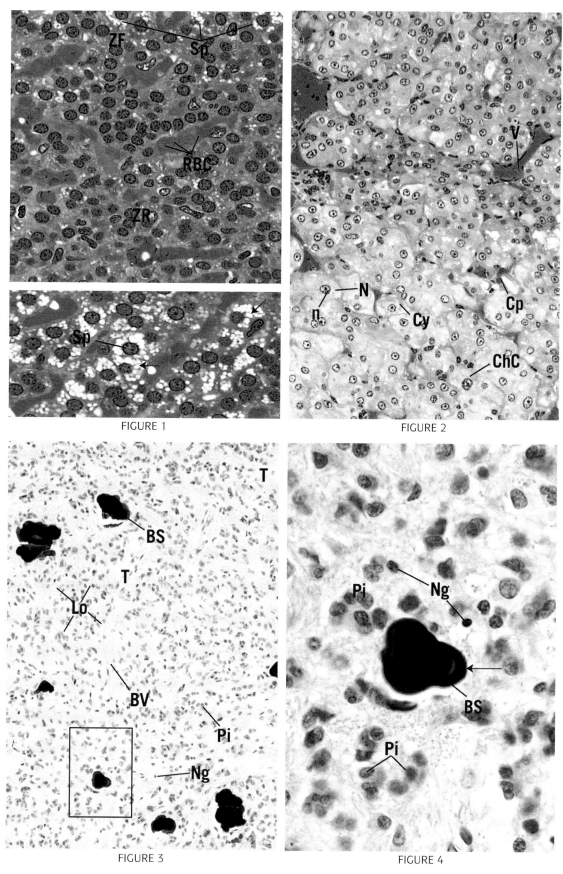

FIGURE 1

FIGURE 2

FIGURE 3

FIGURE 4

PLATE 10-6 ■ *Pituitary Gland, Electron Microscopy*

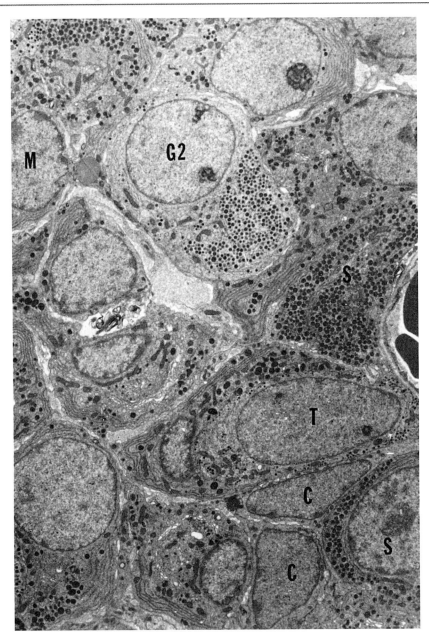

FIGURE 1 ■ *Pituitary gland. Pars anterior.*
Electron microscopy. × 4950.

Although considerable controversy surrounds the precise fine structural identification of the cells of the pars anterior, it is reasonably certain that the several cell types presented in this electron micrograph are acidophils, basophils, and chromophobes as observed by light microscopy. The acidophils are: **somatotropes** (S) and **mammotropes** (M), while only two types of basophils are included in this electron micrograph, namely, **type II gonadotropes** (G2) and **thyrotropes** (T). The **chromophobes** (C) may be recognized by the absence of secretory granules in their cytoplasm. (From Poole M: *Anat Rec* 204:45–53, 1982.)

PLATE 10-7 ■ *Pituitary Gland, Electron Microscopy*

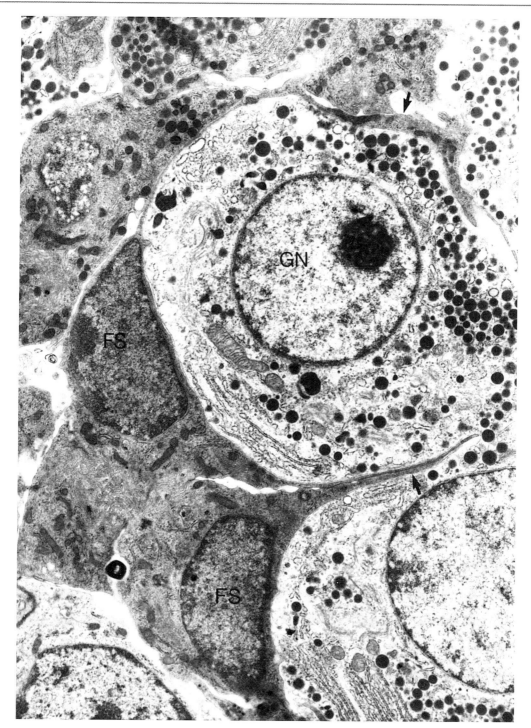

FIGURE 1 ■ *Pituitary gland. Rat. Electron microscopy.* × 8936.

The pars distalis of the rat pituitary houses various cell types, two of which are represented here. The granule-containing **gonadotrophs** (GN) are surrounded by non-granular **folliculostellate cells** (FS) whose processes are demarcated by arrows. The functions of folliculostellate cells are in question, although some believe them to be supportive, phagocytic, regenerative, or secretory in nature. (From Strokreef JC, Reifel CW, Shin SH: *Cell Tissue Res* 243:255–261, 1986.)

Integument

The integument, the largest and heaviest organ of the body, is composed of skin and its various derivatives, including sebaceous glands, sweat glands, hair, and nails. The skin covers the entire body and is continuous with the mucous membranes at the lips, at the anus, in the nose, at the leading edges of the eyelids, and at the external orifices of the urogenital system. Some of the many functions of skin include protection against physical, chemical, and biologic assaults; providing a waterproof barrier; absorbing ultraviolet radiation for both vitamin D synthesis and protection; excretion (i.e., sweat) and thermoregulation; monitoring the external milieu via its various nerve endings; and immunologic defense of the body.

SKIN

Skin is composed of a superficial **stratified squamous keratinized epithelium** known as the **epidermis** and of a deeper connective tissue layer, the **dermis** (see Graphic 11-1). The epidermis and dermis interdigitate with each other by the formation of **epidermal ridges** and **dermal ridges (dermal papillae)**, where the two are separated by a basement membrane. Evidence of this interdigitation is the ridges on the finger tips that imprint as fingerprints. Interposed between skin and deeper structures is a fascial sheath known as the hypodermis, which is not a part of skin.

Epidermis

Depending on the thickness of the keratin layer, skin is classified as thick or thin. The **epidermis** of thick skin is described first, since it is composed of all five layers, rather than just three or four present in thin skin. The deepest layer, the **stratum basale (stratum germinativum)**, is a single layer of cuboidal to columnar cells. These cells are responsible for cell renewal, via mitosis (usually at night)

and are pushed surfaceward, giving rise to the thickest layer, the **stratum spinosum.** This layer is composed of polyhedral **prickle cells** characterized by numerous processes (intercellular bridges) that form desmosomes with processes of surrounding prickle cells. Cells of the stratum spinosum also display mitotic activity (usually at night). These two layers are frequently referred to as the **stratum Malpighii** and their continued mitotic activity is responsible for the continuous migration of these cells into the next layer, known as the **stratum granulosum.** Cells of this layer accumulate **keratohyalin granules,** which eventually overfill the cells, destroying their nuclei and organelles. The fourth layer, the **stratum lucidum,** is relatively thin and not always evident. Present only in palmar and solar skin, it usually appears as a thin, translucent region, interposed between strata granulosum and corneum. The cells of the stratum lucidum have no nuclei or organelles, but contain densely packed keratin filaments and contain eleidin, a transformation product of keratohyalin. The surface-most layer is the **stratum corneum,** composed of preferentially arranged stacks of dead hulls known as **squames.** The superficial layers of the stratum corneum are desquamated at the same rate as they are being replaced by the mitotic activity of the strata basale and spinosum.

The epidermis is composed of four cell types: keratinocytes (described above), melanocytes, Langerhans cells, and Merkel cells. **Keratinocytes,** responsible for the production of **keratin,** are the most populous of epidermal cells and are derived from ectoderm. **Melanocytes,** derived from neural crest cells, are responsible for the manufacture of **melanin,** which is synthesized on specialized organelles called **melanosomes.** These melanocytes, the second most populous cell type, are interspersed among the keratinocytes of the stratum basale and are also present in hair follicles and the dermis. They possess long thin cytoplasmic processes that extend into the intercellular spaces between cells of the stratum spinosum. **Langerhans cells** (dendritic cells) derived from bone marrow and located mostly in the stratum spinosum, function as antigen-presenting cells in immune responses. **Merkel cells,** whose origin is uncertain, are interspersed among the cells of the stratum basale, and are most abundant in the fingertips. Afferent nerve terminals approximate these cells, forming complexes that are believed to function as **mechanoreceptors** (touch receptors). There is some evidence that Merkel cells may also have a neurosecretory function.

Thin skin differs from thick skin in that it has only three or four strata. Stratum lucidum is always absent in thin skin, whereas strata corneum, granulosum, and spinosum are greatly reduced in size. In fact, frequently only an incomplete layer of stratum granulosum is present.

Dermis

The **dermis** of the skin, lying directly deep to the epidermis is derived from mesoderm. It is composed of **dense irregular collagenous connective tissue** containing mostly type I collagen and numerous elastic fibers that assist in securing the skin to the underlying **hypodermis**. The dermis is subdivided into a loosely woven **papillary layer,** a superficial region that interdigitates with the epidermal ridges, and a deeper, coarser, and denser **reticular layer.** The interface between the papillary and reticular layers is indistinct. **Dermal ridges** display encapsulated nerve endings, such as **Meissner's** corpuscles, as well as capillary loops that bring nourishment to the avascular epidermis.

DERIVATIVES OF SKIN

Derivatives of skin include hair, sebaceous glands, sweat glands, and nails (see Graphic 11-2). These structures originate from epidermal downgrowths into the dermis and hypodermis, while maintaining their connection to the outside. Each **hair,** composed of a shaft of cornified cells and a root contained within a hair follicle, is associated with a **sebaceous gland** that secretes an oily **sebum** into the neck of the hair follicle. A small bundle of smooth muscle cells, the **arrector pili muscle,** attaches to the hair follicle and, cradling the sebaceous gland, inserts into the superficial aspects of the skin.

Sweat glands do not develop in association with hair follicles. These are simple coiled tubular glands whose secretory units produce sweat, which is delivered to the surface of the skin by long ducts. **Myoepithelial cells** surround the secretory portion of these glands.

Nails are cornified structures on the distal phalanx of each finger or toe. These horny plates lie on a nail bed and are bounded laterally by a nail wall. The **cuticle (eponychium)** lies over the **lunula,** an opaque, crescent-shaped area of the nail plate, while the **hyponychium** is located beneath the free edge of the nail plate.

Histophysiology

I. KERATINOCYTES AND KERATIN FORMATION

In the superficial layers of the stratum spinosum and in the stratum granulosum, the cells accumulate a histidine-rich protein, **keratohyalin granules** in which the ends of intermediate filaments are embedded. In the stratum lucidum, the cellular organelles are no longer evident, the keratohyalin granules have lost their identity, and they are now referred to as **eleidin,** a combination of filamentous material embedded in a dense matrix. Cells of the stratum corneum are filled with **keratin,** a scleroprotein composed of 10-nm-thick filaments rich in lysine residues. Additionally, the cytoplasmic aspects of the cell membranes of the keratinocytes of strata granulosum, lucidum, and corneum are reinforced by **involucrin,** a fibrous protein that forms a cross-linked mat whose individual components are 12 nm in diameter. Cells of the strata spinosum and granulosum house membrane-coating granules whose contents, a lipid-rich substance, are released into the extracellular spaces, forming a barrier that is impermeable to aqueous fluids. Moreover, lysosomal enzymes released into the cytosol of cells of the strata granulosum and lucidum digest the cell's organelles and by the time the keratinocytes reach the stratum corneum, they are non-living, keratin-filled husks. Keratin of skin is "soft" keratin, whereas keratin of nails is "hard" keratin because that of the nails has many more disulfide bonds.

Recent investigations indicate that keratinocytes produce immunogenic molecules and are probably active in the immune process. Evidence also shows that these cells are capable of producing several interleukins, colony-stimulating factors, interferons, tumor necrosis factors, as well as platelet- and fibroblast-stimulating growth factors.

II. MELANIN FORMATION

Melanin is synthesized by **melanocytes,** cells derived from neural crest cells. Although these cells are located in the stratum basale, they possess long processes that extend into the stratum spinosum. There are two types of melanin, **eumelanin,** a dark brown-to-black pigment composed of polymers of **hydroxyindole,** and **pheomelanin,** a red-to-rust-colored compound composed of **cysteinyl dopa** polymers. The former is present in individuals with dark hair, and the latter is found in individuals with red and blond hair.

Both types of melanin are derived from the amino acid **tyrosine,** which is transported into specialized **tyrosinase**-containing vesicles derived from the trans-Golgi network, known as melanosomes. Within these oval (1.0 by 0.5 μm) melanosomes, tyrosinase converts tyrosine into 3,4-dihydroxyphenylalanine, which is transformed into dopaquinone and, eventually, into melanin.

Melanosomes pass to the tips of the melanocyte processes, which are engulfed and **endocytosed** by keratinocytes of the stratum spinosum. The freed melanosomes migrate to the nucleus of the keratinocyte and form a protective umbrella, shielding the nucleus (and its chromosomes) from the ultraviolet rays of the sun. Soon thereafter, **lysosomes** attack and destroy the melanosomes.

Ultraviolet rays not only increase the rates of darkening of melanin and endocytosis of the tips of melanocytic processes but also enhance tyrosinase activity and, thus, melanin production.

Fewer melanocytes are located on the insides of the thighs and undersides of the arms and face. However, skin pigmentation is related to the location of melanin rather than to the numbers of melanocytes. Melanosomes are fewer and congregate around the keratinocyte nucleus in Caucasians, whereas in blacks they are larger and are more dispersed throughout the keratinocyte cytoplasm.

Clinical Considerations ▪ ▪ ▪

Psoriasis

Psoriasis is a condition characterized by patchy lesions on the skin, especially around joints and the scalp. This condition is produced by increased proliferation of keratinocytes and an acceleration of the cell cycle, resulting in an accumulation of cells in the stratum corneum. The condition is cyclic and is of unknown etiology.

Warts

Warts are benign epidermal growths on the skin caused by papilloma viral infection of the keratinocytes. Warts are common in young children, in young adults, and in immunosuppressed patients.

Malignancies of Skin

The three most common malignancies of skin are basal cell carcinoma, squamous cell carcinoma, and malignant melanoma.

Basal cell carcinoma, the most common human malignancy, develops in the stratum basale from damage caused by ultraviolet radiation. The most frequent site of basal cell carcinoma is on the nose, occurring as papules or nodules, which eventually craters. Surgery is usually 90% effective with no recurrence.

Squamous cell carcinoma, the second most frequent skin malignancy, is invasive and metastatic. Its probable etiology is environmental factors, such as ultraviolet radiation and x-irradiation, as well as a variety of chemical carcinogens, including arsenic. The carcinoma originates in cells of the stratum spinosum and appears clinically as a hyperkeratotic scaly plaque with deep invasion of underlying tissues, often accompanied by bleeding. Surgery is the treatment of choice.

Malignant melanoma may be a life-threatening malignancy. It develops in the melanocytes that become mitotically active and invade the dermis, eventually entering the lymphatic and circulatory system to metastasize to other organ systems. Treatment of choice is a combination of surgery and chemotherapy.

Summary of Histological Organization

I. SKIN

A. Epidermis

The **epidermis** constitutes the superficial, epithelially derived region of skin. It is composed of four cell types: **keratinocytes, melanocytes, Langerhans cells,** and **Merkel cells.** The keratinocytes are arranged in five layers, and the remaining three cell types are interspersed among them. The five layers of the epidermis are

1. Stratum Basale
A single layer of cuboidal-to-columnar cells that stand on the **basement membrane.** This is a region of cell division. It also contains **melanocytes** and **Merkel cells.**

2. Stratum Spinosum
Composed of many layers of polyhedral **prickle cells** bearing **intercellular bridges.** Mitotic activity is also present. It also contains **Langerhans cells** and processes of **melanocytes.**

3. Stratum Granulosum
Cells that are somewhat flattened and contain **keratohyalin granules.** It is absent as a distinct layer in thin skin.

4. Stratum Lucidum
A thin translucent layer whose cells contain **eleidin.** It is also absent in thin skin.

5. Stratum Corneum
Composed of **squames** packed with **keratin.** Superficial squames are desquamated.

B. Dermis

The **dermis** is a **dense irregular collagenous connective tissue** subdivided into two layers: papillary and reticular.

1. Papillary Layer
The **dermal ridges** (dermal papillae) and **secondary dermal ridges** interdigitate with the **epidermal ridges** (and **interpapillary pegs**) of the epidermis. **Collagen fibers** are slender in comparison with those of deeper layers of the dermis. Dermal ridges house **capillary loops** and **Meissner's corpuscles.**

2. Reticular Layer
The **reticular layer** of skin is composed of coarse bundles of collagen fibers. It supports a **vascular plexus** and interdigitates with the underlying **hypodermis.** Frequently, it houses **hair follicles, sebaceous glands,** and **sweat glands. Krause's end bulbs** and **pacinian corpuscles** may also be present.

II. APPENDAGES

A. Hair

Hair is an **epidermal** downgrowth embedded into dermis or hypodermis. It has a free **shaft** surrounded by several layers of cylindrical sheaths of cells. The terminal end of the hair follicle is expanded as the **hair bulb,** composed of connective tissue **papilla** and the **hair root.** The concentric layers of the follicle are

1. Connective Tissue Sheath

2. Glassy Membrane
A modified basement membrane.

3. External Root Sheath
Composed of a few layers of polyhedral cells and a single layer of columnar cells.

4. Internal Root Sheath
Composed of three layers: **Henle's layer, Huxley's layer,** and the **cuticle.** The internal root sheath stops at the neck of the follicle where sebaceous gland ducts open into the hair follicle, forming a **lumen** into which the sebum is delivered.

5. Cuticle of the Hair
Composed of highly keratinized cells that overlap each other.

6. Cortex
The bulk of the hair, composed of highly keratinized cells.

7. Medulla
A thin core of the hair whose cells contain soft keratin.

B. Sebaceous Glands

Sebaceous glands are in the forms of **saccules** associated with hair follicles. They are **branched alveolar holocrine glands** that produce an oily **sebum.** Secretions are delivered into the neck of the hair follicle via short, wide **ducts. Basal cells** are regenerative cells of sebaceous glands, located at the periphery of the **saccule.**

C. Arrector Pili Muscle

Arrector pili muscles are bundles of smooth muscle cells extending from the **hair follicle** to the **papillary layer** of the dermis. They cradle the **sebaceous gland.** Contractions of these muscle fibers elevate the hair, forming "goose bumps," release heat, and assist in the delivery of sebum from the gland into its duct.

D. Sweat Glands

1. Sweat Glands

Simple, **coiled, tubular** glands whose **secretory portion** is composed of a simple cuboidal epithelium. **Dark cells** and **light cells** are present with **intercellular canaliculi** between cells. **Myoepithelial cells** surround the secretory portion.

2. Ducts

Composed of a stratified cuboidal (two-cell-thick) epithelium. Cells of the duct are darker and smaller than those of the secretory portions. Ducts pierce the base of the epidermal ridges to deliver sweat to the outside.

E. Nail

The horny **nail plate** sits on the **nail bed.** It is bordered laterally by the **nail wall,** the base of which forms the **lateral nail groove.** The **eponychium** (cuticle) is above the nail plate, while the **hyponychium** is located below the free end of the nail plate. The posterior aspect of the nail plate is the **nail root,** which lies above the **matrix,** the area responsible for the growth of the nail.

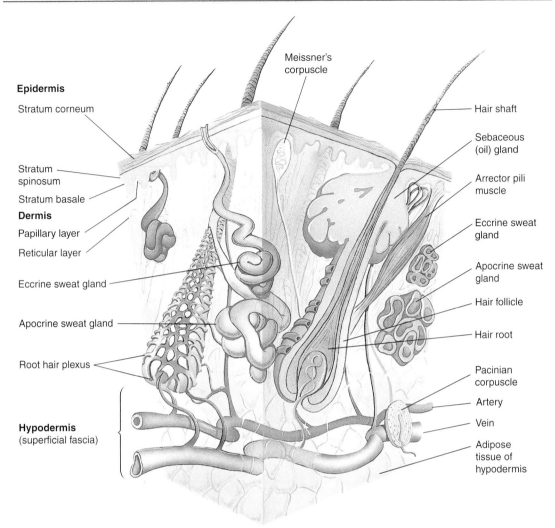

Epidermis
Stratum corneum

Stratum spinosum

Stratum basale

Dermis

Papillary layer

Reticular layer

Eccrine sweat gland

Apocrine sweat gland

Root hair plexus

Hypodermis
(superficial fascia)

Meissner's corpuscle

Hair shaft

Sebaceous (oil) gland

Arrector pili muscle

Eccrine sweat gland

Apocrine sweat gland

Hair follicle

Hair root

Pacinian corpuscle

Artery

Vein

Adipose tissue of hypodermis

Skin and its appendages, **hair**, **sweat glands** (both **eccrine** and **apocrine**), **sebaceous glands**, and **nails**, are known as the **integument**. Skin may be **thick** or **thin**, depending on the thickness of its epidermis. Thick skin epidermis is composed of five distinct layers of **keratinocytes** (strata basale, spinosum, granulosum, lucidum, and corneum) interspersed with three additional cell types, **melanocytes**, **Merkel's cells**, and **Langerhans' cells**. Thin skin epidermis lacks strata granulosum and lucidum, although individual cells that constitute the absent layers are present.

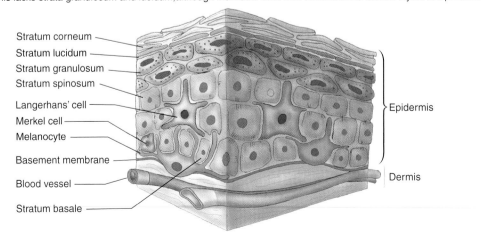

Stratum corneum

Stratum lucidum

Stratum granulosum

Stratum spinosum

Langerhans' cell

Merkel cell

Melanocyte

Basement membrane

Blood vessel

Stratum basale

Epidermis

Dermis

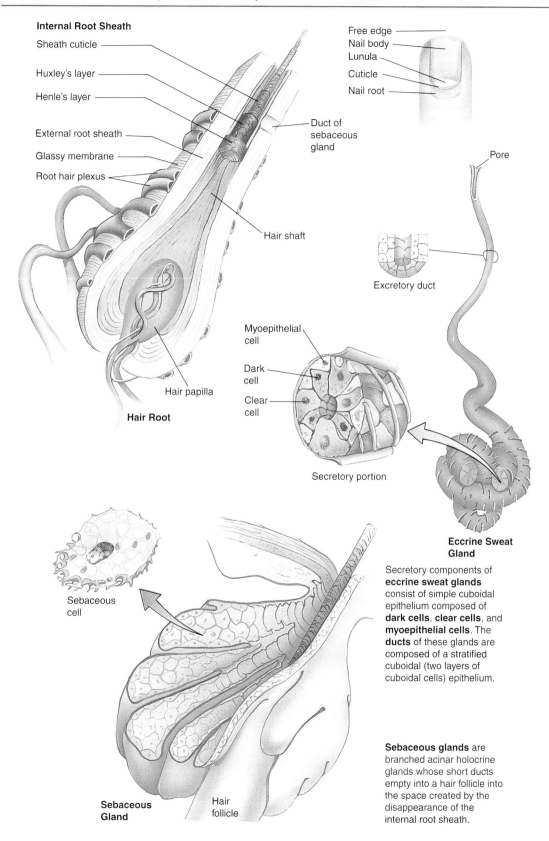

Internal Root Sheath

Sheath cuticle

Huxley's layer

Henle's layer

External root sheath

Glassy membrane

Root hair plexus

Duct of sebaceous gland

Hair shaft

Hair papilla

Hair Root

Free edge
Nail body
Lunula
Cuticle
Nail root

Pore

Excretory duct

Myoepithelial cell

Dark cell

Clear cell

Secretory portion

Eccrine Sweat Gland

Secretory components of **eccrine sweat glands** consist of simple cuboidal epithelium composed of **dark cells**, **clear cells**, and **myoepithelial cells**. The **ducts** of these glands are composed of a stratified cuboidal (two layers of cuboidal cells) epithelium.

Sebaceous cell

Sebaceous Gland

Hair follicle

Sebaceous glands are branched acinar holocrine glands whose short ducts empty into a hair follicle into the space created by the disappearance of the internal root sheath.

Integument ■ 225

PLATE 11-1 ■ *Thick Skin*

FIGURE 1 ■ *Thick skin. Paraffin section.* × 132.

Skin is composed of the superficial **epidermis** (E) and the deeper **dermis** (D). The interface of the two tissues is demarcated by **epidermal ridges** (ER) and **dermal ridges** (DR) (dermal papillae). Between successive epidermal ridges are the interpapillary pegs, which divide each dermal ridge into secondary dermal ridges. Note that in thick skin the keratinized layer, **stratum corneum** (SC), is highly developed. Observe also that the **duct** (d) of the sweat gland pierces the base of an epidermal ridge. The dermis of skin is subdivided into two regions, a **papillary layer** (PL), composed of the looser, collagenous connective tissue of the dermal ridges, and the deeper, denser, collagenous connective tissue of the **reticular layer** (RL). **Blood vessels** (BV) from the reticular layer enter the dermal ridges.

FIGURE 2 ■ *Thick skin. Monkey. Plastic section.* × 132.

This photomicrograph of thick skin presents a view similar to that in Figure 1. However, the layers of the **epidermis** (E) are much easier to delineate in this plastic section. Observe that the squames of the **stratum corneum** (SC) appear to lie directly upon the **stratum granulosum** (SG), whose cells contain keratohyalin granules. The thickest layer of lining cells in the epidermis is the **stratum spinosum** (SS), while the **stratum germinativum** (SGe) is only a single cell layer thick. The stratum lucidum is not evident, although a few transitional cells (arrows) may be identified. Note that the **secondary dermal ridges** (SDR), on either side of the **interpapillary peg** (IP), present **capillary loops** (CL). Regions similar to the boxed areas are presented in Figures 3 and 4 at higher magnification.

FIGURE 3 ■ *Thick skin. Monkey. Plastic section.* × 540.

This is a higher magnification of a region similar to the boxed area in the previous figure. The **papillary layer** (PL) of the dermis displays **nuclei** (N) of the various connective tissue cells, as well as the interface between the dermis and the **stratum germinativum** (SGe). Observe that these cells are cuboidal to columnar in shape and interspersed among them are occasional clear cells, probably inactive **melanocytes** (M), although it should be stressed that Merkel cells also appear as clear cells. Cells of the **stratum spinosum** (SS) are polyhedral in shape, possessing numerous intercellular bridges, which interdigitate with those of other cells, accounting for their spiny appearance.

FIGURE 4 ■ *Thick skin. Monkey. Plastic section.* × 540.

This is a higher magnification of a region similar to the boxed area of Figure 2. Observe that as the cells of the **stratum spinosum** (SS) are being pushed surfaceward, they become somewhat flattened. As the cells reach the **stratum granulosum** (SG) they accumulate keratohyalin granules (arrows), which increase in number as the cells progress through this layer. Occasional transitional cells (arrowheads) of the poorly defined stratum lucidum may be observed, as well as the **squames** (S) of the **stratum corneum** (SC).

Inset. **Thick skin. Paraffin section.** × 132.

This photomicrograph displays the **stratum lucidum** (SL) to advantage. Note that this layer is between the **stratum granulosum** (SG) and **stratum corneum** (SC). Observe the **duct** (d) of a sweat gland.

■ KEY

BV	blood vessel	IP	interpapillary peg	SDR	secondary dermal ridges
CL	capillary loop	M	melanocytes	SG	stratum granulosum
D	dermis	N	nucleus	SGe	stratum germinativum
d	duct	PL	papillary layer	SS	stratum spinosum
DR	dermal ridges	RL	reticular layer	S	squames
E	epidermis	SC	stratum corneum	SL	stratum lucidum
ER	epidermal ridges				

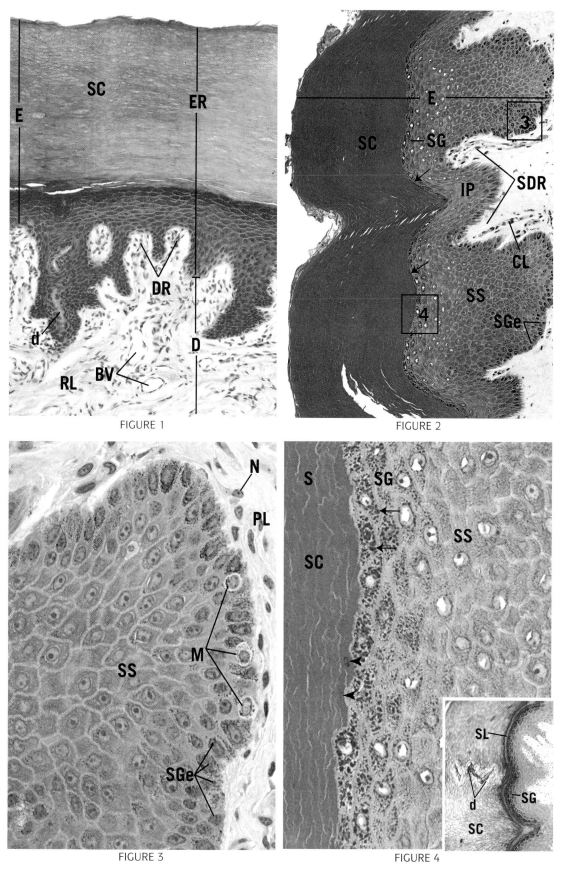

FIGURE 1

FIGURE 2

FIGURE 3

FIGURE 4

PLATE 11-2 ■ *Thin Skin*

FIGURE 1 ■ *Thin skin. Human. Paraffin section.* × 19.

Thin skin is composed of a very slender layer of **epidermis** (E) and the underlying **dermis** (D). While thick skin has no hair follicles and sebaceous glands associated with it, most thin skin is richly endowed with both. Observe the **hair** (H) and the **hair follicles** (HF), whose expanded **bulb** (B) presents the connective tissue **papilla** (P). Much of the follicle is embedded beneath the skin in the superficial fascia, the fatty connective tissue layer known as the **hypodermis** (hD), which is not a part of the integument. **Sebaceous glands** (sG) secrete their sebum into short **ducts** (d), which empty into the lumen of the hair follicle. Smooth muscle bundles, **arrector pili muscle** (AP), cradle these glands, in passing from the hair follicle to the papillary layer of the dermis. **Sweat glands** (swG) are also present in the reticular layer of the dermis. A region similar to the boxed area is presented at a higher magnification in Figure 2.

FIGURE 2 ■ *Thin skin. Human. Paraffin section.* × 132.

This is a higher magnification of a region similar to the boxed area of the previous figure. Observe that the **epidermis** (E) is much thinner than that of thick skin and that the **stratum corneum** (SC) is significantly reduced. The epidermal ridges and **interpapillary pegs** (IP) are well represented in this photomicrograph. Note that the **papillary layer** (PL) of the dermis is composed of much finer bundles of **collagen fibers** (CF) than those of the dense irregular collagenous connective tissue of the **reticular layer** (RL). The dermis is quite vascular, as evidenced by the large number of **blood vessels** (BV) whose cross-sectional profiles are readily observed. The numerous **nuclei** (N) of the various connective tissue cells attest to the cellularity of the dermis. Note also the presence of the **arrector pili muscle** (AP), whose contraction elevates the hair and is responsible for the appearance of "goose bumps." The boxed area is presented at a higher magnification in the following figure.

FIGURE 3 ■ *Thin skin. Human. Paraffin section.* × 270.

This photomicrograph is a higher magnification of the boxed area of Figure 2. Epidermis of thin skin possesses only three of four of the layers found in thick skin. The **stratum germinativum** (SGe) is present as a single layer of cuboidal to columnar cells. Most of the epidermis is composed of the prickle cells of the **stratum spinosum** (SS), while stratum granulosum and stratum lucidum are not represented as complete layers. However, individual cells of stratum granulosum (arrow) and stratum lucidum are scattered at the interface of the stratum spinosum and **stratum corneum** (SC). The papillary layer of the **dermis** (D) is richly vascularized by **capillary loops** (CL), which penetrate the **secondary dermal ridges** (sDR). Observe that the **collagen fiber** (CF) bundles of the dermis become coarser as the distance from the epidermis increases.

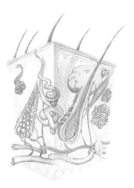

Skin

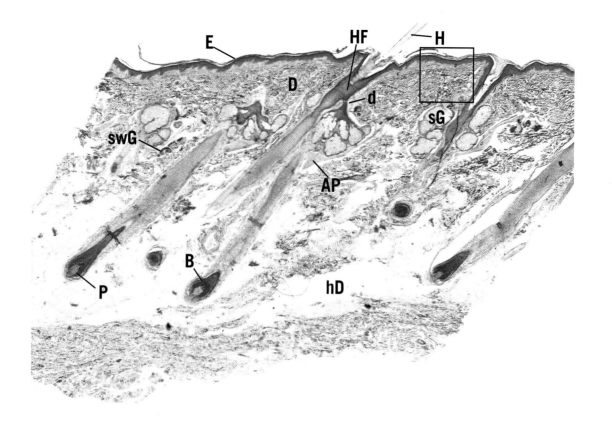

FIGURE 1

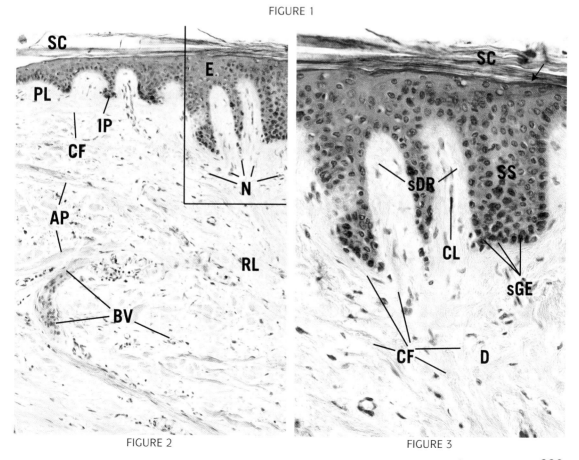

FIGURE 2

FIGURE 3

PLATE 11-3 ■ *Hair Follicles and Associated Structures, Sweat Glands*

FIGURE 1 ■ *Hair follicle. l.s. Human. Paraffin section.* × 132.

The terminal expansion of the hair follicle, known as the bulb, is composed of a connective tissue, **papilla** (P), enveloped by epithelially derived cells of the **hair root** (HR). The mitotic activity responsible for the growth of hair occurs in the matrix, from which several concentric sheaths of epithelial cells emerge to be surrounded by a **connective tissue sheath** (CTS). Color of hair is due to the intracellular pigment that accounts for the dark appearance of some cells (arrow).

FIGURE 2 ■ *Hair follicle. x.s. Human. Paraffin section.* × 132.

Many of the layers comprising the growing hair follicle may be observed in these cross-sections. The entire structure is surrounded by a **connective tissue sheath** (CTS), which is separated from the epithelially derived components by a specialized basement membrane, the **inner glassy membrane** (BM). The clear polyhedral cells compose the **external root sheath** (ERS), which surrounds the **internal root sheath** (IRS), whose cells become keratinized. At the neck of the hair follicle, where the ducts of the sebaceous glands enter, the internal root sheath disintegrates, providing a lumen into which sebum and apocrine sweat are discharged. The **cuticle** (Cu) and **cortex** (Co) constitute the highly keratinized components of the hair, while the medulla is not visible at this magnification. Note the presence of **arrector pili muscle** (AP).

FIGURE 3 ■ *Sebaceous gland. Human. Paraffin section.* × 132.

Sebaceous glands (sG) are branched, acinar holocrine glands, which produce an oily sebum. The secretion of these glands is delivered into the lumen of a **hair follicle** (HF), with which sebaceous glands are associated. **Basal cells** (BC), located at the periphery of the gland, undergo mitotic activity, to replenish the dead cells which, in holocrine glands, become the secretory product. Note that as these cells accumulate sebum in their cytoplasm, they degenerate, as evidenced by the gradual pyknosis of their **nuclei** (N). Observe the **arrector pili muscle** (AP), which cradles the sebaceous glands.

FIGURE 4 ■ *Sweat gland. Monkey. Plastic section.* × 132.

The simple coiled tubular eccrine gland is divided into two compartments, a **secretory** portion (s) and a **duct** (d). The secretory portion of the gland consists of a simple cuboidal epithelium, composed of dark and clear secretory cells (which cannot be distinguished from each other unless special procedures are utilized). Intercellular canaliculi are noted between clear cells, which are smaller than the **lumen** (L) of the gland. **Ducts** (d) may be recognized readily since they are darker staining and composed of stratified cuboidal epithelium.

Insets a and b. **Duct and secretory unit. Monkey. Plastic section.** × 540.

The duct is readily evident, since its **lumen** (L) is surrounded by two layers of cuboidal cells. **Secretory cells** (s) of the eccrine sweat gland are surrounded by darker staining **myoepithelial cells** (My).

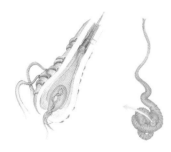
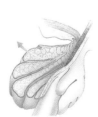

Hair root, eccrine sweat gland, and sebaceous gland

■ **KEY**

AP	arrector pili muscle	d	ducts	My	myoepithelial cells
BC	basal cells	ERS	external root sheath	N	nucleus
BM	inner glassy membrane	HF	hair follicle	P	papilla
Co	cortex	HR	hair root	s	secretory
CTS	connective tissue sheath	IRS	internal root sheath	sG	sebaceous glands
Cu	cuticle	L	lumen		

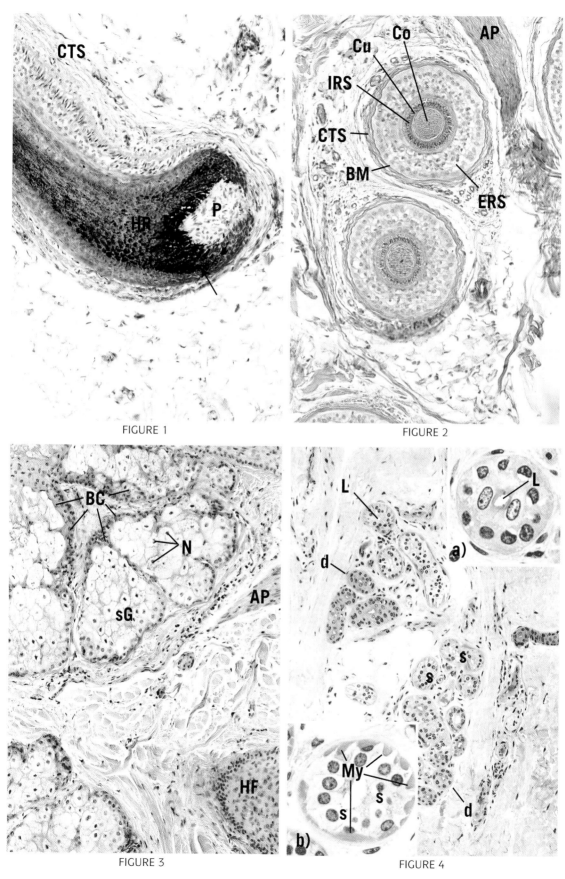

FIGURE 1

FIGURE 2

FIGURE 3

FIGURE 4

PLATE 11-4 ■ *Nail, Pacinian and Meissner's Corpuscles*

FIGURE 1 ▓ *Fingernail. l.s. Paraffin section.* × 14.

The nail is a highly keratinized structure that is located on the dorsal surface of the **distal phalanx** (Ph) of each finger and toe. The horny **nail plate** (NP) extends deep into the dermis, forming the **nail root** (NR). The epidermis of the distal phalanx forms a continuous fold, resulting in the **eponychium** (Ep), or cuticle, the **nail bed** (NB) underlying the nail plate, and the **hyponychium** (Hy). The epithelium (arrow) surrounding the nail root is responsible for the continuous elongation of the nail. The **dermis** (D) between the nail bed and the **bone** (Bo) of the distal phalanx is tightly secured to the **fibrous periosteum** (FP). Note that this is a developing finger, as evidenced by the presence of **hyaline cartilage** (HC) and endochondral osteogenesis (arrowheads).

FIGURE 2 ▓ *Fingernail. x.s. Paraffin section.* × 14.

The **nail plate** (NP) in cross-section presents a convex appearance. On either side it is bordered by a **nail wall** (NW) and the groove it occupies is referred to as the lateral **nail groove** (NG). The **nail bed** (NB) is analogous to four layers of the epidermis, while the nail plate represents the stratum corneum. The **dermis** (D), deep to the nail bed, is firmly attached to the **fibrous periosteum** (FP) of the **bone** (Bo) of the terminal phalanx. Observe that the fingertip is covered by thick skin whose **stratum corneum** (SC) is extremely well developed. The small darkly staining structures in the dermis are **sweat glands** (swG).

FIGURE 3 ▓ *Meissner's corpuscle. Paraffin section.* × 540.

Meissner's corpuscles are oval, encapsulated mechanoreceptors lying in dermal ridges just deep to the **stratum germinativum** (SGe). They are especially prominent in the genital areas, lips, fingertips, and soles of the feet. A connective tissue **capsule** (Ca) envelops the corpuscle. The **nuclei** (N) within the corpuscle belong to flattened (probably modified) Schwann cells, which are arranged horizontally in this structure. The afferent **nerve fiber** (NF) pierces the base of Meissner's corpuscle, branches, and follows a tortuous course within the corpuscle.

FIGURE 4 ▓ *Pacinian corpuscle. Paraffin section.* × 132.

Pacinian corpuscles, located in the dermis and hypodermis, are mechanoreceptors. They are composed of a **core** with an **inner** (IC) and an **outer** (OC) region, as well as a **capsule** (Ca) that surrounds the core. The inner core invests the afferent **nerve fiber** (NF), which loses its myelin sheath soon after entering the corpuscle. The core cells are modified Schwann cells, while the components of the capsule are continuous with the endoneurium of the afferent nerve fiber. Pacinian corpuscles are readily recognizable in section since they resemble the cut surface of an onion. Observe the presence of an **arrector pili muscle** (AP) and profiles of **ducts** (d) of a sweat gland in the vicinity of, but not associated with, the pacinian corpuscle.

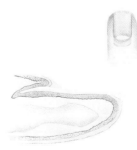

Fingernail

■ **KEY**

AP	arrector pili	Hy	hyponychium	NR	nail root
Ca	capsule	IC	inner core	NW	nail wall
Bo	bone	N	nuclei	OC	outer core
D	dermis	NB	nail bed	Ph	distal phalanx
d	duct	NF	nerve fiber	SC	stratum corneum
Ep	eponychium	NG	nail groove	SGe	stratum germinativum
FP	fibrous periosteum	NP	nail plate	swG	sweat glands
HC	hyaline cartilage				

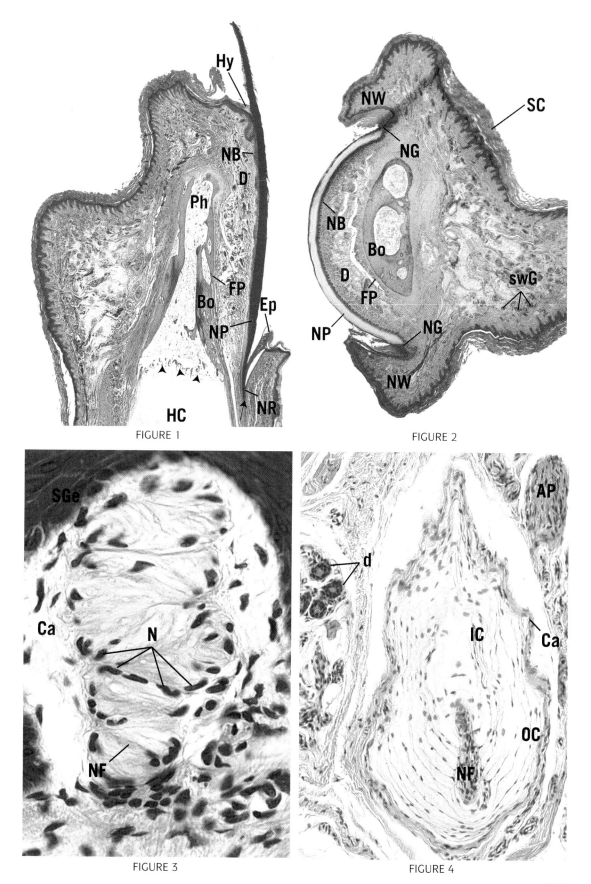

FIGURE 1

FIGURE 2

FIGURE 3

FIGURE 4

PLATE 11-5 ■ *Sweat Gland, Electron Microscopy*

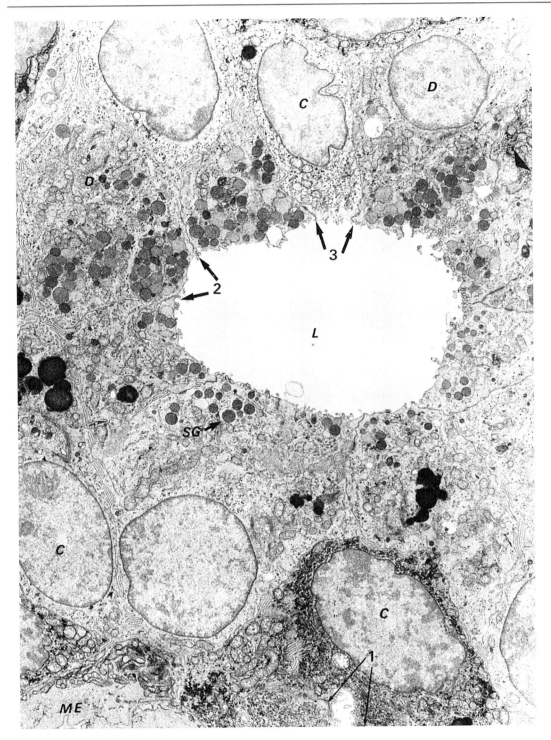

FIGURE 1 ■ *Sweat gland. x.s. Human. Electron microscopy.* × 5040.

Tight junctions (arrows) occur at three locations in the secretory coil of human sweat glands: (1) between **clear cells** (C) separating the lumen of the intercellular canaliculus (arrowhead) and the basolateral intercellular space: (2) between two **dark cells** (D) separating the main lumen and the lateral intercellular space; and (3) between a clear cell and a dark cell, separating the main lumen (L) and intercellular space. Note the presence of **secretory granules** (SG) and **myoepithelial cell** (ME). (From Briggman JV, Bank HL, Bigelow JB, Graves JS, Spicer SS: *Am J Anat* 162:357–368, 1981.)

Respiratory System

The respiratory system functions in exchanging carbon dioxide for oxygen, which will then be distributed to all of the tissues of the body. To accomplish this function, air must be brought to that portion of the respiratory system where exchange of gases can occur. The respiratory system, therefore, has a **conducting portion** and a **respiratory portion**. Some of the larger conduits of the conducting portion are extrapulmonary whereas its smaller components are intrapulmonary. The respiratory portions, however, are completely intrapulmonary. The luminal diameters of the various conduits can be modified by the presence of smooth muscle cells along their length.

CONDUCTING PORTION OF THE RESPIRATORY SYSTEM

The extrapulmonary region of the conducting portion consists of the nasal cavities, pharynx, larynx, trachea, and bronchi. The intrapulmonary region entails the intrapulmonary bronchi, bronchioles, and terminal bronchioles (see Graphic 12-1).

Extrapulmonary Region

The extrapulmonary region of the conducting portion modifies the inspired air by humidifying, cleansing, and adjusting its temperature. Cleansing and humidifying actions are accomplished by the mucosa of the respiratory tract. This **mucosa** is composed of **pseudostratified ciliated columnar epithelium** with numerous **goblet cells** and an underlying connective tissue sheath that is well endowed with **seromucous glands.** Modulation of the temperature of the inspired air is accomplished in the nasal cavity by the rich vascularity of the connective tissue just deep to its respiratory epithelium. In certain areas of this cavity the mucosa is modified to function in olfaction and is referred to

as the **olfactory mucosa.** The glands in the lamina propria of this mucosa produce a thin mucous secretion that dissolves odoriferous substances. The **olfactory cells** lying within the pseudostratified columnar olfactory epithelium perceive these sensory stimuli. In addition to the olfactory cells, two other cell types compose the olfactory epithelium, namely, supporting cells and basal cells. **Supporting cells** do not possess any sensory function. They manufacture a yellowish-brown pigment that is responsible for the coloration of the olfactory mucosa. These cells insulate and support the olfactory cells. **Basal cells** are small, dark cells that lie on the basement membrane and, probably, are regenerative in function. Axons of the olfactory cells are collected into small nerve bundles that pass through the cribriform plate of the ethmoid bone as the first cranial nerve, the olfactory nerve.

The conducting portion of the respiratory system is supported by a skeleton composed of bone and/or cartilage that assists in the maintenance of a patent lumen. The luminal diameters of these airways are controlled by smooth muscle cells located in their walls. The larynx, a region of the conducting portion, is designed to prevent foreign objects from gaining entrance into it and for phonation. It is composed of nine cartilages, three of which are paired, numerous extrinsic and intrinsic muscles, and several ligaments. The actions of these muscles on the cartilages and ligaments modulate the tension and positioning of the vocal folds, thus permitting variations in the pitch of the sound being produced. The lumen of the **larynx** is subdivided into three compartments: **vestibule, ventricle,** and **infraglottic cavity.** The last named region is continuous with the lumen of the trachea, a structure supported by 15 to 20 horseshoe-shaped segments of **hyaline cartilage.** The tracheal lumen is lined by a respiratory epithelium composed of various cell types, namely, goblet cells, basal cells, ciliated cells, brush cells, and, probably, hormone-producing DNES cells. The trachea subdivides into the two primary bronchi that lead to the right and the left lungs.

Intrapulmonary Region

The intrapulmonary region is composed of **intrapulmonary bronchi** (secondary bronchi) whose walls are supported by irregular plates of hyaline cartilage. Intrapulmonary bronchi give rise to **bronchioles,** tubes of decreasing diameters that do not possess a cartilaginous supporting skeleton. The epithelial lining of the larger bronchioles is ciliated with a few goblet cells, but those of smaller branches become simple columnar, with goblet cells being replaced by **Clara cells.** Moreover, the thickness of their walls also decreases, as does the luminal diameter. The last region of the conduction portion is composed of **terminal bronchioles** whose mucosa is further decreased in thickness and complexity. The patency of those airways whose walls do not possess a cartilaginous support is maintained by elastic fibers that radiate from their periphery and intermingle with elastic fibers emanating from nearby structures.

RESPIRATORY PORTION OF THE RESPIRATORY SYSTEM

The respiratory portion begins with branches of the terminal bronchiole, known as **respiratory bronchioles** (see Graphic 12-2). These are very similar to terminal bronchioles except that they possess outpocketings known as **alveoli,** structures whose thin walls permit gaseous exchange. Respiratory bronchioles lead to alveolar ducts that end in an expanded region, known as **alveolar sacs,** with each sac being composed of a number of alveoli. The epithelium of alveolar sacs and alveoli is composed of two types of cells: highly attenuated **type I pneumocytes,** which form much of the lining of the alveolus and alveolar sac; and **type II pneumocytes,** cells that manufacture **surfactant,** a phospholipid that reduces surface tension. Associated with the respiratory portion of the lungs is an extremely rich capillary network, supplied by the pulmonary arteries and drained by the pulmonary veins. The capillaries invest each alveolus, and their highly attenuated nonfenestrated, continuous endothelial cells closely approximate the type I pneumocytes. In fact, in many areas the basal laminae of the two fuse into a single basal lamina, providing for a minimal blood-air barrier, thus facilitating the exchange of gases. Therefore, the **blood-air barrier** is composed of the attenuated endothelial cell of the capillary, the two combined basal laminae, the attenuated type I pneumocyte, and the surfactant and fluid coating of the alveolus.

Since the lung contains a large number of alveoli, these small spaces that crowd against each other are separated from one another by walls of various thicknesses known as **interalveolar septa.** The thinnest of these portions often presents communicating **alveolar pores,** whereby air may pass between alveoli. A somewhat thicker septum may possess intervening connective tissue elements that may be as slender as a capillary with its attendant basal lamina, or it may have collagen and elastic fibers as well as smooth muscle fibers and connective tissue cells. Macrophages, known as **dust cells,** are often noted in interalveolar septa. These dust cells are derived from monocytes and enter the lungs via the bloodstream. Here they mature and become extremely efficient scavengers. It is believed that dust cells are the most numerous of all cell types, even though they are eliminated from the lungs at a rate of 50 million per day. Although it is not known whether they actively migrate to the bronchioles or reach it via fluid flow, it is known that they are transported from there within the mucus layer, via ciliary action of the respiratory epithelium, into the pharynx. Once they reach the pharynx they are either expectorated or swallowed.

Histophysiology

I. MECHANISM OF OLFACTION

The sensory cells of the olfactory epithelium are bipolar neurons whose receptor ends are modified **cilia** that extend into the overlying mucus. **Odorant-binding proteins** (integral membrane proteins) lying within the plasma membrane of the cilia are sensitive to molecules of specific odor groups, and when such a molecule binds to the receptor, one of two possibilities occurs. The receptor itself may be a **gated ion channel,** and the ion channel opens or the receptor activates **adenylate cyclase,** causing the formation of cAMP, which facilitates the opening of ion channels. In either case, opening of the ion channel results in ion flow into the cell with subsequent **depolarization** of the plasmalemma, and the olfactory cell becomes **excited.**

The odorant must satisfy at least three requirements, it must be **volatile, water soluble,** and **lipid soluble** so that it can enter the nasal cavity (volatility), penetrate the mucus (water solubility), and be able to have access to the phospholipid membrane (lipid solubility).

II. MECHANISM OF RESPIRATION

The process of inspiration requires energy, in that it depends on the contraction of the **diaphragm** and elevation of the **ribs,** increasing the size of the **thoracic cavity.** Since the **visceral pleura** adheres to the **parietal pleura,** the lungs become stretched. As the **lung volume** is increased, gas **pressure** inside the lungs becomes lower than atmospheric pressure, and air enters the lungs.

The process of expiration does not require energy, since it is dependent on **relaxation** of the muscles responsible for inspiration as well as on the stretched **elastic fibers** of the expanded lungs, which return to their **resting length.** As the muscles relax, the volume of the thoracic cage decreases, increasing the pressure inside the lung, which exceeds atmospheric pressure. The additional force of the elastic fibers returning to their resting length drives air out of the lungs.

III. MECHANISM OF GASEOUS EXCHANGE

The partial pressures of O_2 and CO_2 are responsible for the uptake or release of these gases by red blood cells. Since cells convert O_2 to CO_2 during their metabolism, the partial pressure of CO_2 is high in tissues, and this gas is preferentially taken up by red blood cells. Simultaneously they release oxygen. The converse is true in the lungs, where O_2 is taken up by red blood cells and CO_2 is released.

Oxygen uptake and release is accomplished by the **heme** moiety of the **hemoglobin** molecule without the requirement of enzymatic catalysis. Carbon dioxide, however, is ferried in three different ways: as a gas dissolved in its molecular form (7%); as **carbaminohemoglobin,** which as molecular CO_2 forms a weak bond with hemoglobin (23%); and as the bicarbonate ion, HCO_3^- (70%). Red blood cells contain the enzyme **carbonic anhydrase,** which facilitates the rapid formation of H_2CO_3, which then immediately dissociates to form bicarbonate and hydrogen ions.

Clinical Considerations ▪ ▪ ▪

Hyaline Membrane Disease
Hyaline membrane disease is frequently observed in premature infants who lack adequate amounts of pulmonary surfactant. This disease is characterized by **labored breathing**, since a high alveolar surface tension, caused by inadequate levels of surfactant, makes it difficult to expand the alveoli. The administration of glucocorticoids prior to birth can induce synthesis

of surfactant thus circumventing the appearance of the disease.

Emphysema
Emphysema is a disease that results from **destruction of alveolar walls** with the consequent formation of large cyst-like sacs, reducing

(continues)

Respiratory System ▪ 237

the surface available for gas exchange. Emphysema is marked by **decreased elasticity** of the lungs, which are unable to recoil adequately during expiration. It is associated with exposure to **cigarette smoke** and other substances that inhibit α_1-antitrypsin, a protein that normally protects the lungs from the action of elastase produced by alveolar macrophages.

Bronchial Asthma
Bronchial asthma is a condition where the bronchi become partially and reversibly obstructed by airway spasm (**bronchio-constriction**), mast cell-induced inflammatory response to allergens and/or other stimuli that would not affect a normal lung, and the formation of excess mucus. Asthma attacks vary with the individual, in some it is hardly noticed, whereas with others shortness of breath is very evident and wheezing accompanies breathing out. Most individuals who suffer from asthmatic condition use nebulizers containing bronchodilators, such as albuterol, to relieve the attack.

Summary of Histological Organization

I. CONDUCTING PORTION
A. Nasal Cavity

1. Respiratory Region
The **respiratory region** is lined by **respiratory (pseudostratified ciliated columnar) epithelium.** The subepithelial connective tissue is richly vascularized and possesses seromucous glands.

2. Olfactory Region
The epithelium of the **olfactory region** is thick **pseudostratified ciliated columnar epithelium** composed of three cell types: **basal cell, sustentacular cells,** and **olfactory cells.** The lamina propria is richly vascularized and possesses **Bowman's glands,** which produce a watery mucus.

B. Larynx

The **larynx** is lined by a **respiratory epithelium** except for certain regions that are lined by **stratified squamous nonkeratinized epithelium.** From superior to inferior, the **lumen** of the larynx presents three regions: the **vestibule, ventricle,** and **infraglottic cavity.** The **ventricular** and **vocal folds** are the superior and inferior boundaries of the ventricle, respectively. Cartilages, extrinsic and intrinsic muscles, as well as mucous and seromucous glands are present in the larynx.

C. Trachea

1. Mucosa
The **mucosa** of the trachea is composed of a **respiratory epithelium** with numerous **goblet cells,** a **lamina propria,** and a well-defined **elastic lamina.**

2. Submucosa
The **submucosa** houses **mucous** and **seromucous glands.**

3. Adventitia
The **adventitia** is the thickest portion of the tracheal wall. It houses the **C rings** of **hyaline cartilage** (or thick connective tissue between the rings). Posteriorly, the **trachealis muscle** (smooth muscle) fills in the gap between the free ends of the cartilage.

D. Extrapulmonary Bronchi

Extrapulmonary bronchi resemble the trachea in histologic structure.

E. Intrapulmonary Bronchi

These and subsequent passageways are completely surrounded by lung tissue.

1. Mucosa
Intrapulmonary bronchi are lined by **respiratory epithelium** with **goblet cells.** The subepithelial connective tissue is no longer bordered by an elastic lamina.

2. Muscle
Two ribbons of **smooth muscle** are wound helically around the mucosa.

3. Cartilage
The C rings are replaced by irregularly shaped **hyaline cartilage plates** that encircle the smooth muscle layer. **Dense collagenous connective tissue** connects the perichondria of the cartilage plates.

4. Glands
Seromucous glands occupy the connective tissue between the cartilage plates and smooth muscle. **Lymphatic nodules** and branches of the pulmonary arteries are also present.

F. Bronchioles

Bronchioles are lined by **ciliated simple columnar** to **simple cuboidal epithelium** interspersed with nonciliated **Clara cells. Goblet cells** are found only in larger bronchioles. The **lamina propria** possesses no glands and is surrounded by **smooth muscle.** The walls of bronchioles are not supported by cartilage. The largest bronchioles are about 1 mm in diameter.

G. Terminal Bronchioles

Terminal bronchioles are usually less than 0.5 mm in diameter. The lumen is lined by **simple cuboidal epithelium** (some ciliated) interspersed with **Clara cells.** The connective tissue and smooth muscle of the wall of the terminal bronchioles are greatly reduced.

II. RESPIRATORY PORTION
A. Respiratory Bronchiole

Respiratory bronchioles resemble terminal bronchioles, but they possess outpocketings of **alveoli** in their walls. This is the first region where exchange of gases occurs.

B. Alveolar Ducts

Alveolar ducts possess no walls of their own. They are long, straight tubes lined by **simple squamous epithelium** and display numerous outpocketings of alveoli. Alveolar ducts end in alveolar sacs.

C. Alveolar Sacs

Alveolar sacs are composed of groups of **alveoli** clustered around a common air space.

D. Alveolus

An **alveolus** is a small air space partially surrounded by highly attenuated epithelium. Two types of cells are present in the lining, **type I pneumocytes** (lining cells) and **type II pneumocytes** (produce surfactant). The opening of the alveolus is controlled by **elastic fibers**. Alveoli are separated from each other by richly vascularized walls known as **interalveolar septa,** some of which present **alveolar pores** (communicating spaces between alveoli). **Dust cells** (macrophages), **fibroblasts,** and other **connective tissue elements** may be noted in interalveolar septa. The **blood-air barrier** is a part of the interalveolar septum, the thinnest of which is composed of surfactant, **continuous endothelial cells, type I pneumocyte,** and their intervening **fused basal laminae.**

TABLE 12-1 ▪ *Summary Table of Respiratory System*

Division	Region	Skeleton	Glands	Epithelium	Cilia	Goblet Cells	Special Features
Nasal cavity	Vestibule	Hyaline cartilage	Sebaceous and sweat glands	Stratified squamous keratinized	No	No	Vibrissae
	Respiratory	Bone and hyaline cartilage	Seromucous	Pseudostratified ciliated columnar	Yes	Yes	Large venous plexus
	Olfactory	Nasal conchae (bone)	Bowman's glands	Pseudostratified ciliated columnar	Yes	No	Basal cells; sustentacular cells; olfactory cells; nerve fibers
Pharynx	Nasal	Muscle	Seromucous glands	Pseudostratified ciliated columnar	Yes	Yes	Pharyngeal tonsil; eustachian tube
	Oral	Muscle	Seromucous glands	Stratified squamous non-keratinized	No	No	Palatine tonsils
Larynx		Hyaline and elastic cartilage	Mucous and seromucous glands	Stratified squamous non-keratinized and pseudostratified ciliated columnar	Yes	Yes	Vocal cords; epiglottis; some taste buds
Trachea and extra-pulmonary (primary bronchi)		C-rings of hyaline cartilage	Mucous and seromucous glands	Pseudostratified ciliated columnar	Yes	Yes	Trachealis muscle; elastic lamina
Intra-pulmonary conducting	Secondary bronchi	Plates of hyaline cartilage	Seromucous glands	Pseudostratified ciliated columnar	Yes	Yes	Two helically oriented ribbons of smooth muscle
	Bronchioles	Smooth muscle	None	Simple columnar to simple cuboidal	Yes	Only in larger bronchioles	Clara cells
	Terminal bronchiole	Smooth muscle	None	Simple cuboidal	Some	None	Less than 0.5 mm in diameter; Clara cells
Respiratory	Respiratory bronchiole	Some smooth muscle	None	Simple cuboidal and simple squamous	Some	None	Outpocketings of alveoli
	Alveolar duct	None	None	Simple squamous	None	None	Outpocketings of alveoli; type I pneumocytes; type II pneumocytes; dust cells
	Alveolus	None	None	Simple squamous	None	None	Type I pneumocytes; type II pneumocytes; dust cells

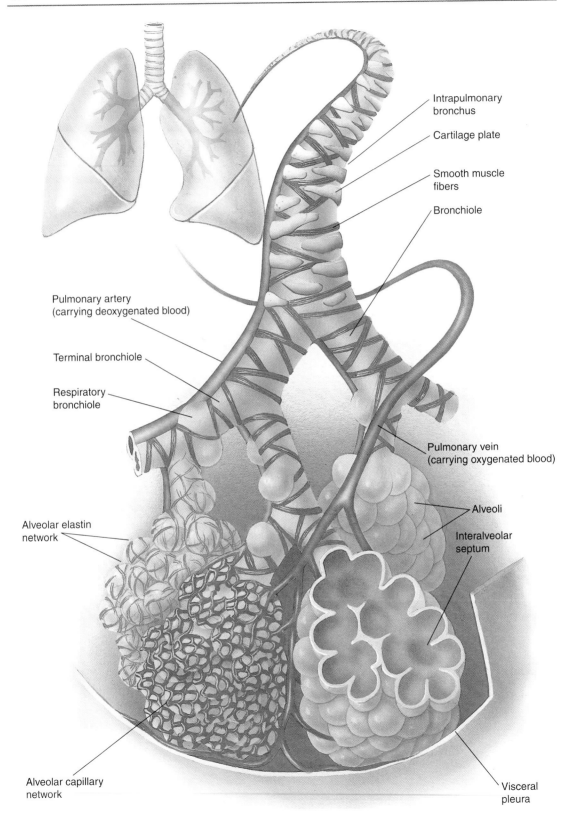

Intrapulmonary bronchus

Cartilage plate

Smooth muscle fibers

Bronchiole

Pulmonary artery (carrying deoxygenated blood)

Terminal bronchiole

Respiratory bronchiole

Pulmonary vein (carrying oxygenated blood)

Alveoli

Interalveolar septum

Alveolar elastin network

Alveolar capillary network

Visceral pleura

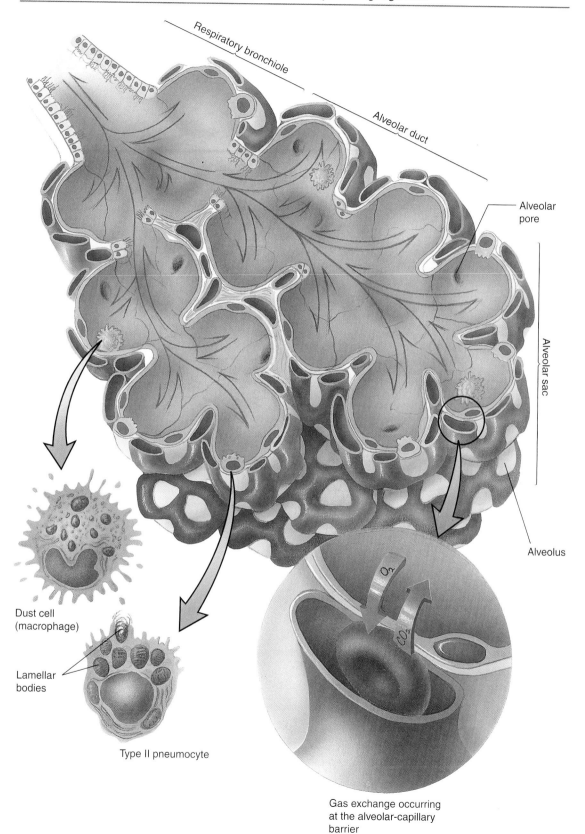

Respiratory bronchiole

Alveolar duct

Alveolar pore

Alveolar sac

Alveolus

Dust cell
(macrophage)

Lamellar
bodies

Type II pneumocyte

O_2

CO_2

Gas exchange occurring
at the alveolar-capillary
barrier

PLATE 12-1 ■ *Olfactory Mucosa, Larynx*

FIGURE 1 ■ *Olfactory area. Human. Paraffin section.* × 270.

The olfactory mucosa of the nasal cavity is composed of a thick **olfactory epithelium** (OE) and a **lamina propria** (LP) richly endowed with **blood vessels** (BV), **lymph vessels** (LV), and **nerve fibers** (NF) frequently collected into bundles. The lamina propria also contains **Bowman's glands** (BG) which produce a watery mucus that is delivered onto the ciliated surface by short ducts. The boxed area is presented at a higher magnification in Figure 2.

FIGURE 2 ■ *Olfactory epithelium. Human. Paraffin section.* × 540.

This is a higher magnification of the boxed area of the previous figure. The **epithelium** (OE) is pseudostratified ciliated columnar, whose **cilia** (C) are particularly evident. Although hematoxylin and eosin stained tissue does not permit clear identification of the various cell types, the positions of the nuclei permit tentative identification. **Basal cells** (BC) are short, and their nuclei are near the basement membrane. **Olfactory cell** (OC) nuclei are centrally located, while nuclei of **sustentacular cells** (SC) are positioned near the apex of the cell.

FIGURE 3 ■ *Intraepithelial gland. Human. Paraffin section.* × 540.

The epithelium of the nasal cavity occasionally displays small, **intraepithelial glands** (IG). Note that these structures are clearly demarcated from the surrounding epithelium. The secretory product is released into the space (asterisk) that is continuous with the **nasal cavity** (NC). The subepithelial **connective tissue** (CT) is richly supplied with **blood vessels** (BV) and **lymph vessels** (LV). Observe the **plasma cells** (PC), characteristic of the subepithelial connective tissue of the respiratory system, which also displays the presence of **glands** (GI).

FIGURE 4 ■ *Larynx. l.s. Human. Paraffin section.* × 14.

The right half of the larynx, at the level of the **ventricle** (V), is presented in this survey photomicrograph. The ventricle is bounded superiorly by the **ventricular folds** (false vocal cords) (VF) and inferiorly by the **vocal folds** (VoF). The space above the ventricular fold is the beginning of the **vestibule** (Ve) and that below the vocal fold is the beginning of the **infraglottic cavity** (IC). The **vocalis muscle** (VM) regulates the vocal ligament present in the vocal fold. Acini of mucous and seromucous **glands** (GI) are scattered throughout the subepithelial connective tissue. The **laryngeal cartilages** (LC) are also shown to advantage.

■ **KEY**

BC	basal cells	LC	laryngeal cartilages	SC	sustentacular cells
BG	Bowman's glands	LP	lamina propria	V	ventricle
BV	blood vessels	LV	lymph vessels	Ve	vestibule
C	cilia	NC	nasal cavity	VF	ventricular folds
CT	connective tissue	NF	nerve fibers	VM	vocalis muscle
GI	glands	OC	olfactory cells	VoF	vocal folds
IC	infraglottic cavity	OE	olfactory epithelium		
IG	intraepithelial glands	PC	plasma cells		

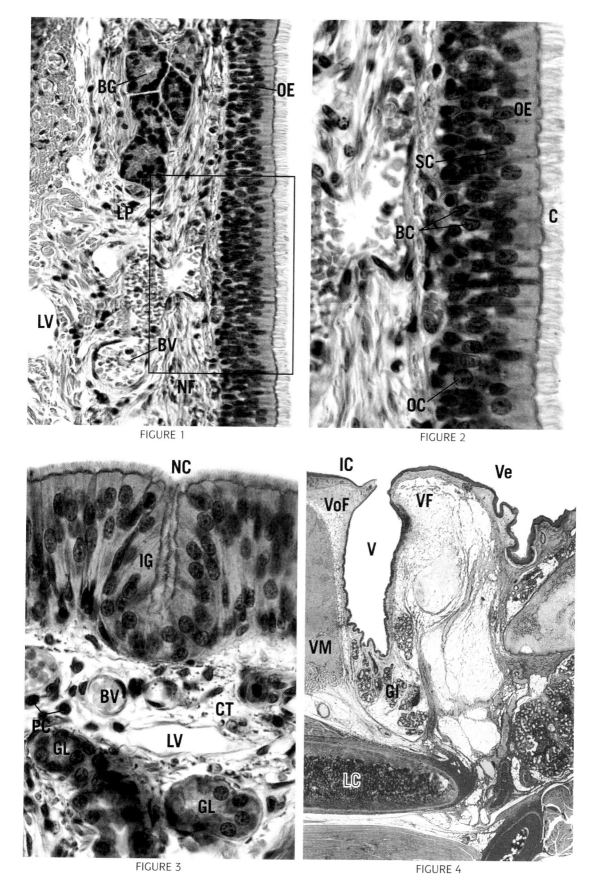

FIGURE 1

FIGURE 2

FIGURE 3

FIGURE 4

Respiratory System ■ **245**

PLATE 12-2 ■ *Trachea*

FIGURE 1 ■ *Trachea. l.s. Monkey. Paraffin section.* × 20.

This survey photomicrograph presents a longitudinal section of the **trachea** (Tr) and **esophagus** (Es). Observe that the **lumen** (LT) of the trachea is patent, due to the presence of discontinuous cartilaginous **C-rings** (CR) in its wall. The C-rings of the trachea are thicker anteriorly than posteriorly and are separated from each other by thick, fibrous connective tissue (arrows) that is continuous with the perichondrium of the C-rings. The adventitia of the trachea is adhered to the esophagus via a loose type of **connective tissue** (CT), which frequently contains adipose tissue. Note that the **lumen** (LE) of the esophagus is normally collapsed. A region similar to the boxed area is presented at a higher magnification in Figure 3.

FIGURE 2 ■ *Trachea. l.s. Monkey. Plastic section.* × 270.

The trachea is lined by a pseudostratified ciliated columnar **epithelium** (E), which houses numerous **goblet cells** (GC) that actively secrete a mucous substance. The **lamina propria** (LP) is relatively thin, while the **submucosa** (SM) is thick and contains **mucous** and **seromucous glands** (GI) whose secretory product is delivered to the epithelial surface via ducts that pierce the lamina propria. The **perichondrium** (Pc) of the hyaline cartilage C-rings (CR) merges with the submucosal connective tissue. Note a longitudinal section of a **blood vessel** (BV), indicative of the presence of a rich vascular supply.

FIGURE 3 ■ *Trachea. l.s. Monkey. Paraffin section.* × 200.

This photomicrograph is a higher magnification of a region similar to the boxed area of Figure 1. The pseudostratified ciliated columnar **epithelium** (E) lies on a basement membrane that separates it from the underlying lamina propria. The outer extent of the lamina propria is demarcated by an elastic lamina (arrows), deep to which is the **submucosa** (SM) containing a rich **vascular supply** (BV). The **C-ring** (CR), with its attendant **perichondrium** (Pc), constitutes the most substantive layer of the tracheal wall. The adventitia of the trachea, which some consider to include the C-ring, is composed of a loose type of connective tissue, housing some **adipose cells** (AC), **nerves** (N), and **blood vessels** (BV). Collagen fiber bundles of the adventitia secure the trachea to the surrounding structures.

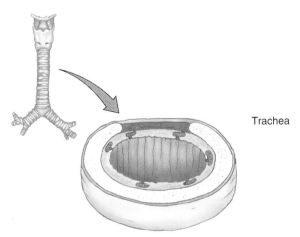

Trachea

■ **KEY**

AC	adipose cells	Es	esophagus
BV	blood vessels	GC	goblet cells
CR	C-rings	GI	mucous/seromucous glands
CT	connective tissue	LE	lumen—esophagus
E	epithelium	LP	lamina propria

LT	lumen—trachea
N	nerves
Pc	perichondrium
SM	submucosa
Tr	trachea

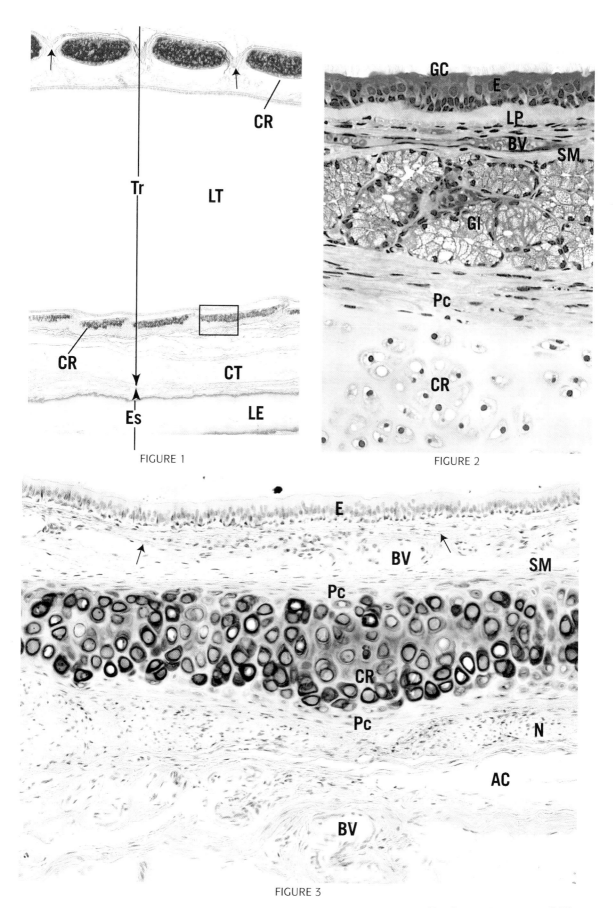

FIGURE 1

FIGURE 2

FIGURE 3

PLATE 12-3 ■ *Respiratory Epithelium and Cilia, Electron Microscopy*

FIGURE 1 ▦ *Tracheal epithelium. Hamster.*
Electron microscopy. × 7782.

The tracheal epithelium of the hamster presents mucus-producing **goblet cells** (GC) as well as **ciliated columnar cells** (CC), whose cilia (arrows) project into the lumen. Note that both cell types are well endowed with **Golgi apparatus** (GA), while goblet cells are particularly rich in **rough endoplasmic reticulum** (rER). (Courtesy of Dr. E. McDowell.)

Inset. **Bronchus. Human. Electron microscopy.** × 7782.

The apical region of a ciliated epithelial cell presents both **cilia** (C) and microvilli (arrow). (Courtesy of Dr. E. McDowell.)

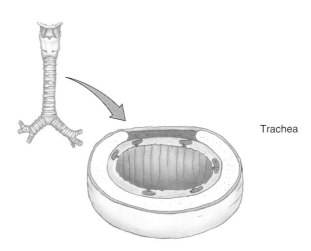

Trachea

■ **KEY**

C	cilia	GA	Golgi apparatus	rER	rough endoplasmic reticulum
CC	ciliated columnar cell	GC	goblet cell		

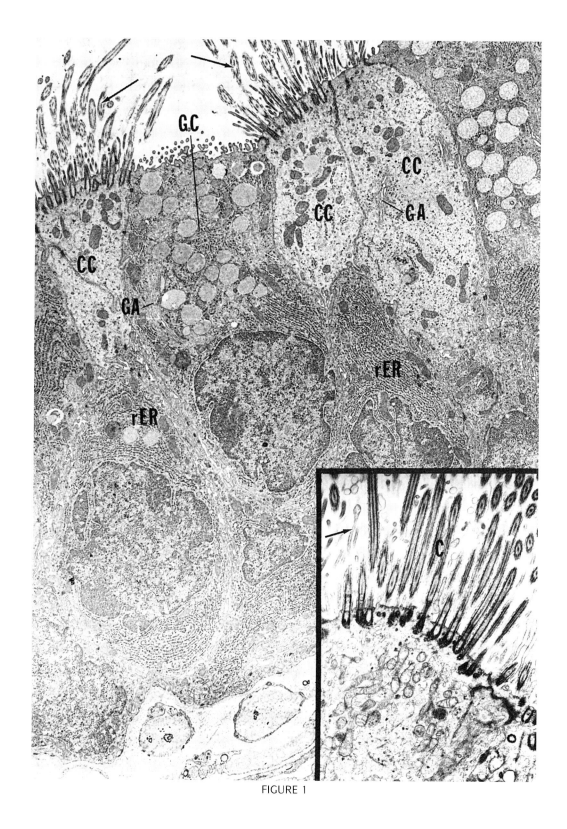

FIGURE 1

PLATE 12-4 ■ *Bronchi, Bronchioles*

FIGURE 1 ■ *Lung. Paraffin section.* × 14.

This survey photomicrograph presents a section of a lung, which permits the observation of the various conduits that conduct air and blood to and from the lung. The **intrapulmonary bronchus** (IB) is recognizable by its thick wall containing plates of **hyaline cartilage** (HC) and **smooth muscle** (Sm). Longitudinal sections of a **bronchiole** (B), **terminal bronchiole** (TB), and **respiratory bronchiole** (RB) are also evident. Smaller bronchioles (asterisks) may also be recognized, but their identification cannot be ascertained. Arrows point to structures that are probably alveolar ducts leading into alveolar sacs. Several **blood vessels** (BV), branches of the pulmonary circulatory system, may be noted. Observe that **lymphatic nodules** (LN) are also present along the bronchial tree.

FIGURE 2 ■ *Intrapulmonary bronchus. x.s. Paraffin section.* × 132.

Intrapulmonary bronchi are relatively large conduits for air, whose **lumina** (L) are lined by a typical respiratory **epithelium** (E). The **smooth muscle** (Sm) is found beneath the mucous membrane and it encircles the entire lumen. Note that gaps (arrows) appear in the muscle layer, indicating that two ribbons of smooth muscle wind around the lumen in a helical arrangement. Plates of **hyaline cartilage** (HC) act as the skeletal support, maintaining the patency of the bronchus. The entire structure is surrounded by **lung tissue** (LT).

FIGURE 3 ■ *Bronchiole. x.s. Paraffin section.* × 270.

Bronchioles maintain their patent **lumen** (L) without the requirement of a cartilaginous support, since they are attached to surrounding lung tissue by elastic fibers radiating from their circumference. The lumina of bronchioles are lined by simple columnar to simple cuboidal **epithelium** (E), interspersed with **Clara cells** (CC), depending upon the diameter of the bronchiole. The **lamina propria** (LP) is thin and is surrounded by **smooth muscle** (Sm), which encircles the lumen. Bronchioles have no glands in their walls and are surrounded by **lung tissue** (LT).

FIGURE 4 ■ *Terminal bronchioles. x.s. Paraffin section.* × 132.

The smallest conducting bronchioles are referred to as **terminal bronchioles** (TB). These possess very small diameters and their lumina are lined with a simple cuboidal **epithelium** (E) interspersed with **Clara cells** (CC). The connective tissue is much reduced and the smooth muscle layers are incomplete and difficult to recognize at this magnification. Terminal bronchioles give rise to **respiratory bronchioles** (RB) whose walls resemble those of the terminal bronchioles, except that the presence of alveoli permit the exchange of gases to occur.

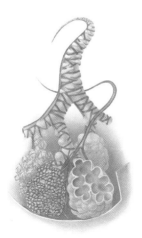

Bronchial system and lung

■ **KEY**

B	bronchiole	IB	intrapulmonary bronchus	RB	respiratory bronchiole
BV	blood vessels	L	lumen	Sm	smooth muscle
CC	Clara cells	LN	lymphatic nodule	TB	terminal bronchiole
E	epithelium	LP	lamina propria		
HC	hyaline cartilage	LT	lung tissue		

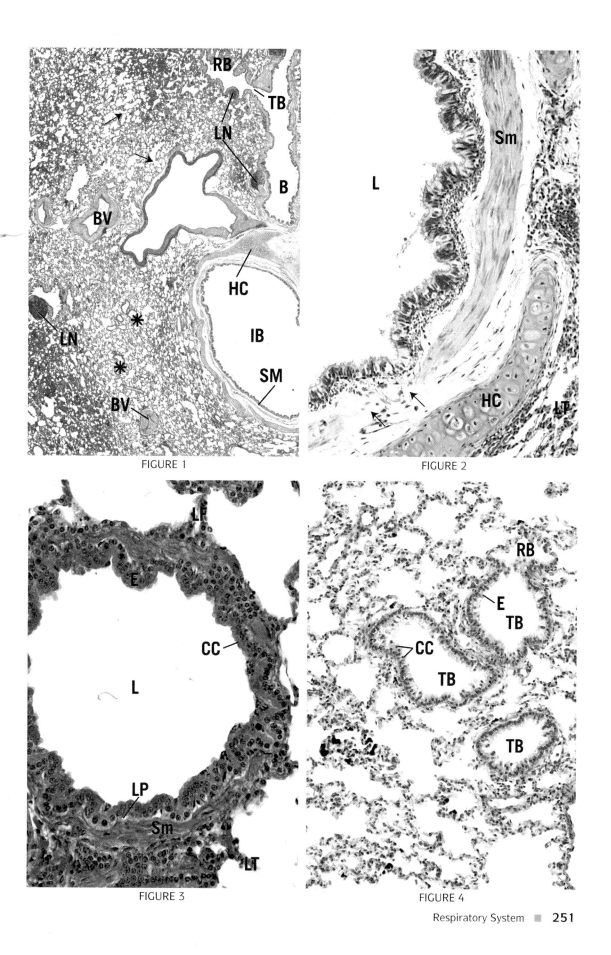

FIGURE 1

FIGURE 2

FIGURE 3

FIGURE 4

PLATE 12-5 ■ *Lung Tissue*

FIGURE 1 ■ *Respiratory bronchiole. Paraffin section.* × 270.

The respiratory bronchiole whose **lumen** (L) occupies the lower half of this photomicrograph presents an apparently thick wall with small outpocketings of **alveoli** (A). It is in these alveoli that gaseous exchanges first occur. The wall of the respiratory bronchiole is composed of a simple cuboidal epithelium, consisting of some ciliated cells and **Clara cells** (CC). The remainder of the wall presents an incomplete layer of smooth muscle cells surrounded by fibroelastic connective tissue. Careful examination of this photomicrograph reveals that the wall of the respiratory bronchiole is folded upon itself, thus giving a misleading appearance of thick walls.

FIGURE 2 ■ *Alveolar duct. l.s. Human. Paraffin section.* × 132.

Alveolar ducts (AD), unlike respiratory bronchioles, do not possess a wall of their own. These structures are lined by a simple squamous **epithelium** (E), composed of highly attenuated cells. Alveolar ducts present numerous outpocketings of **alveoli** (A), and they end in **alveolar sacs** (AS), consisting of groups of alveoli clustered around a common air space. Individual alveoli possess small smooth muscle cells that, acting like a purse string, control the opening into the alveolus. These appear as small knobs (arrow). A region similar to the boxed area is presented at a higher magnification in Figure 3.

FIGURE 3 ■ *Interalveolar septum. Monkey. Plastic section.* × 540.

This photomicrograph is a higher magnification of a region similar to the boxed area of Figure 2. Two **alveoli** (A) are presented, recognizable as empty spaces separated from each other by an **interalveolar septum** (IS). The septum is composed of a **capillary** (Ca), the nucleus (asterisk) of whose endothelial lining bulges into the lumen containing **red blood cells** (RBC). The interalveolar septum as well as the entire alveolus is lined by **type I pneumocytes** (P1), which are highly attenuated squamous epithelial cells, interspersed with **type II pneumocytes** (P2). Thicker interalveolar septa house **blood vessels** (BV) and connective tissue elements including macrophages known as **dust cells** (DC). Note the presence of **smooth muscle cells** (Sm) and connective tissue elements that appear as knobs at the entrance into the alveolus.

FIGURE 4 ■ *Lung. Dust cells. Paraffin section.* × 270.

The highly vascular nature of the lung is quite evident in this photomicrograph, since the **blood vessels** (BV) and the **capillaries** (Ca) of the interalveolar septa are filled with red blood cells. The dark blotches that appear to be scattered throughout the lung tissue represent **dust cells** (DC), macrophages that have phagocytosed particulate matter.

Inset. Lung. Dust cell. Monkey. Plastic section. × 540.

The **nucleus** (N) of a **dust cell** (DC) is surrounded by phagosomes containing particulate matter that was probably phagocytosed from an alveolus of the lung.

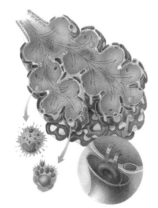

Respiratory portion of respiratory system

■ KEY

A	alveolus	CC	Clara cell	N	nucleus
AD	alveolar duct	DC	dust cell	P1	type I pneumocytes
AS	alveolar sac	E	epithelium	P2	type II pneumocytes
BV	blood vessel	IS	interalveolar septum	RBC	red blood cells
Ca	capillary	L	lumen	Sm	smooth muscle

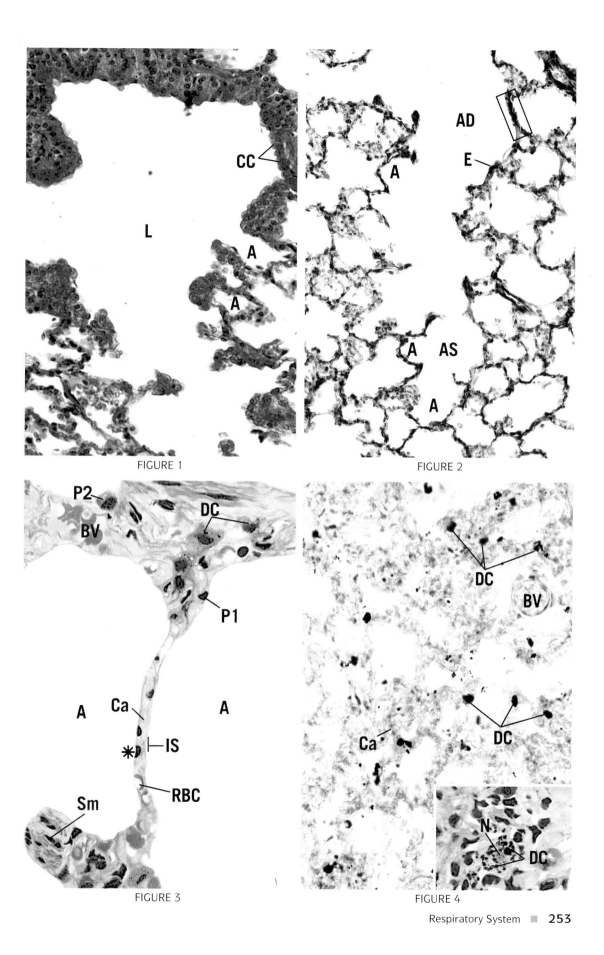

FIGURE 1

FIGURE 2

FIGURE 3

FIGURE 4

PLATE 12-6 ■ *Blood-Air Barrier, Electron Microscopy*

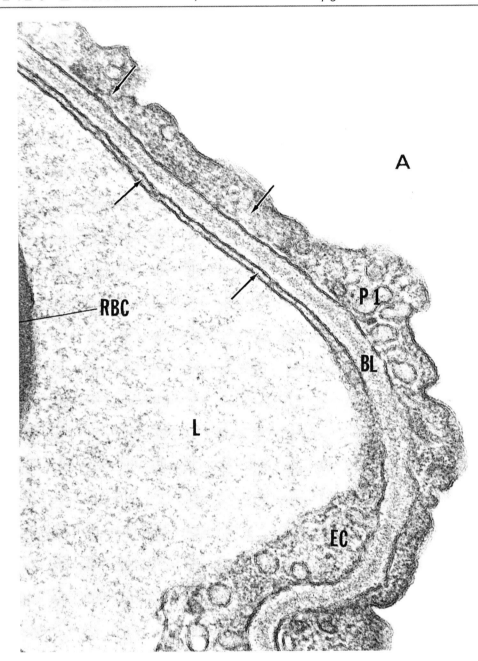

FIGURE 1 ■ *Blood-air barrier. Dog. Electron microscopy.* × 85,500.

The blood-air barrier is composed of highly attenuated **endothelial cells** (EC), **type I pneumocytes** (P1), and an intervening **basal lamina** (BL). Note that the cytoplasm (arrows) of both cell types is greatly reduced, as evidenced by the close proximity of the plasmalemma on either side of the cytoplasm. The air space of the **alveolus** (A) is empty, while the capillary **lumen** (L) presents a part of a **red blood cell** (RBC). (From DeFouw D: *Anat Rec* 209:77–84, 1984.)

Digestive System I

The digestive system functions in the ingestion, digestion, and absorption of food as well as in the elimination of unusable portions of these materials. To accomplish these functions, the digestive system is organized into three major components: 1) the oral cavity, which is responsible for reducing food in size and introducing it into the alimentary canal; 2) a muscular alimentary canal, along whose lumen the ingested foods are converted, both physically and chemically, into absorbable substances; and 3) a glandular portion, which provides fluids, enzymes, and emulsifying agents necessary for the proper functioning of the alimentary canal.

ORAL REGION: ORAL CAVITY

The **oral cavity** may be subdivided into two smaller cavities: the externally positioned vestibule and the internally placed oral cavity proper. The **vestibule** is the space bounded by the lips and cheeks anteriorly and laterally, whereas its internal boundary is formed by the dental arches. The ducts of the parotid glands deliver their secretory products into the vestibule (see Graphics 13-1 and 13-2).

The **oral cavity proper** is bounded by the teeth externally, the floor of the mouth inferiorly, and the hard and soft palates superiorly. At its posterior extent, the oral cavity proper is continuous with the oral pharynx, where the two are separated from each other by an imaginary plane. Both the oral cavity proper and the vestibule are lined by **stratified squamous epithelium,** which in regions that are subject to abrasive forces is modified into **stratified squamous keratinized** (or **parakeratinized**) **epithelium.**

Oral Mucosa

The epithelium and underlining connective tissue constitute the **oral mucosa.** If the epithelium is keratinized (or parakeratinized) the mucosa is said to be **masticatory mucosa,** and if the epithelium is not

keratinized, the mucosa is referred to as **lining mucosa.** It should be noted that most of the oral cavity possesses lining mucosa, with the exception of the gingiva, hard palate, and the dorsal surface of the tongue that are covered by masticatory mucosa. Additionally, the oral cavity has areas of specialized epithelia where intraepithelial structures, known as **taste buds,** function in taste perception. Most taste buds are located on the dorsal surface of the tongue, although the palate and pharynx also possess a few of these structures. Mucosa, whose epithelium contains taste buds is known as **specialized mucosa.** Each taste bud recognizes one or more of the four taste sensations: sour, sweet, salt, or bitter.

The contents of the oral cavity are the teeth, utilized in biting and mastication, and the tongue, a muscular structure that functions in the preparation of the bolus, tasting of the food, and beginning of deglutition (swallowing), among others.

Salivary Glands, Palate, and Tonsils

The parotid, sublingual, and submandibular glands deliver their secretions into the oral cavity proper. The hard palate assists the tongue in the preparation of the bolus, and the soft palate, a moveable structure, seals the communication between the oral and nasal pharynges, thus preventing passage of food and water from the former into the latter.

The connective tissue underlying the epithelium of the oral cavity is richly endowed with **minor salivary glands** that, secreting **saliva** in a continuous fashion, contribute to the maintenance of a moist environment. Saliva functions also in assisting in the process of deglutition by acting as a lubricant for dry foods. Moreover, enzymes present in saliva initiate digestion of carbohydrates, while secretory antibodies protect the body against antigenic substances.

The entrance to the pharynx is guarded against bacterial invasion by the **tonsillar ring,** composed of the **lingual, pharyngeal,** and **palatine tonsils.**

Histophysiology

I. TISSUE INTERACTION IN ODONTOGENESIS

Odontogenesis is induced by the ectodermally derived cells of the dental lamina that express **lymphoid enhancer factor-1** (Lef-1), a transcription factor. Lef-1 induces the epithelial cells to synthesize and release **bone morphogenic protein-4** (BMP-4), **sonic hedgehog** (Shh), and **fibroblast growth factor-8** (FGF-8). These signaling molecules act on the underlying ectomesenchymal cells to differentiate into odontogenic tissues. These neural crest-derived cells begin to express **BMP-4**, the adhesive glycoprotein **tenascin**, and the membrane-bounded proteoglycan, **syndecan**. Moreover, they also express several transcription factors, namely **Egr-1** (early growth response-1), **Msx-1** (homeobox-containing genes), and **Msx-2**. This activation of the ectomesenchyme elicits their role in the induction of the tooth morphology, so that it is the ectomesenchyme that will determine, for instance, whether the developing tooth will become a molar or an incisor. Signaling molecules from the ectomesenchyme induce the formation of the **enamel knot**, an epithelial structure that appears in the vicinity of the stratum intermedium of the enamel organ. The enamel knot synthesizes and releases its own signaling molecules, namely FGF-4, BMP-2, BMP-4, BMP-7, and sonic hedgehog. These signaling molecules promote the differentiation of the inner enamel epithelial cells into **ameloblasts** and those of the peripheralmost layer of the dental papilla into **odontoblasts**. Continued maintenance of the enamel knot is responsible for the buckling of the inner enamel epithelium resulting in the morphodifferentiation of the enamel organ into a template that is the prototype of a molar tooth, whereas if the enamel knot undergoes apoptosis morphodifferentiation is constrained and an incisor is formed.

Clinical Considerations ▨ ▨ ▪

Herpetic Stomatitis
Herpetic stomatitis, a relatively common disease caused by the herpes simplex virus (HSV) type I, is distinguished by painful **fever blisters** appearing on or in the vicinity of the lips. This is a recurring disease since the virus, in its dormant phase, inhabits the trigeminal ganglion. It travels along the axon to cause the appearance of the blisters. During the active stage the patient is highly contagious, since the virus is shed via the seeping clear exudate.

Necrotizing Ulcerative Gingivitis
Necrotizing ulcerative gingivitis is an acute ulcerative condition of the gingiva with accompanying necrosis, halitosis, erythematous appearance, and moderate to severe pain. Fever and regional lymphadenopathy may also be evident. This is usually a disease of the young adult who is experiencing stress and is not particularly attentive to dental hygiene. Frequently *Treponema vincentii* and fusiform bacillus are present in large numbers and they are also believed to be causative agents of the condition. Treatment usually consists of rinsing with dilute hydrogen peroxide several times daily and meticulous cleaning by a dental professional. Antibiotic regiment may also be recommended.

Summary of Histological Organization

I. LIPS

The **lips** control access to the **oral cavity** from the outside environment.

A. External Surface

The external surface is covered with thin **skin** and, therefore, possesses **hair follicles, sebaceous glands, and sweat glands.**

B. Transitional Zone

The **transitional zone (vermilion zone)** is the pink area of the lip. Here the connective tissue papillae extend deep into the epidermis. Hair follicles and sweat glands are absent, whereas sebaceous glands are occasionally present.

C. Mucous Membrane

The vestibular aspect of the lip is lined by a **wet epithelium** (stratified squamous nonkeratinized) with numerous **minor mixed salivary glands** in the subepithelial connective tissue.

D. Core of the Lip

The core of the lip contains **skeletal muscle.**

II. TEETH

Teeth are composed of three calcified tissues and a loose connective tissue core, the pulp.

A. Enamel

Enamel is the hardest substance in the body. It is made by **ameloblasts,** cells no longer present in the erupted tooth. Enamel is present only in the crown.

B. Dentin

Dentin is a calcified, collagen-based material that constitutes the bulk of the **crown** and **root;** it surrounds the pulp. Dentin is made by **odontoblasts,** whose long processes remain in channels, **dentinal tubules,** traversing dentin. The odontoblast cell body forms the peripheral extent of the pulp.

C. Cementum

Cementum is located on the **root** of the tooth, surrounding **dentin.** Cementum is a collagen-based calcified material manufactured by **cementoblasts,** which may become entrapped and then are referred to as **cementocytes.** Fibers of the **periodontal ligament** are embedded in cementum and bone, thus suspending the tooth in its **bony socket,** the **alveolus.**

D. Pulp

The **pulp** is a gelatinous type of mesenchymal-appearing connective tissue that occupies the **pulp chamber.** It is richly supplied by **nerves** and **blood vessels.**

III. GINGIVA

The **gingiva** (gum) is that region of the oral mucosa that is closely applied to the **neck of the tooth** and is attached to the **alveolar bone.** It is covered by a **stratified squamous partially keratinized (parakeratotic) epithelium.** The underlying connective tissue is densely populated with thick bundles of collagen fibers.

IV. TONGUE

The **tongue** is a **muscular organ** whose oral region is freely moving, while its root is attached to the floor of the pharynx. **Skeletal muscle** forms the core of the tongue, among which groups of serous and seromucous glands are interspersed.

A. Oral Region (Anterior Two-Thirds)

The mucosa of the dorsal surface of the anterior two-thirds of the tongue is modified to form four types of lingual papillae.

1. Filiform Papillae
Filiform papillae are long and slender and are the most numerous. They form a roughened surface (especially in animals such as cats) and are distributed in parallel rows along the entire surface. They are covered by a **parakeratinized stratified squamous epithelium** (but bear no taste buds) over a **connective tissue core.**

2. Fungiform Papillae

Fungiform papillae are mushroom shaped, are scattered among the filiform papillae, and may be recognized by their appearance as red dots. They contain **taste buds** along their dorsal aspect.

3. Foliate Papillae

Foliate papillae appear as longitudinal furrows along the side of the tongue near the posterior aspect of the anterior two-thirds. Their **taste buds** degenerate at an early age in humans. Serous **glands of von Ebner** are associated with these papillae.

4. Circumvallate Papillae

Circumvallate papillae are very large and form a V-shaped row at the border of the oral and pharyngeal portions of the tongue. Circumvallate papillae are each surrounded by a moat or groove, the walls of which contain **taste buds** in their **stratified squamous nonkeratinized epithelium**. Serous **glands of von Ebner** open into the base of the furrow. The connective tissue core of the circumvallate papilla possesses a rich nerve and vascular supply.

B. Pharyngeal Region (Posterior One-Third)

The **mucosa** of the posterior one-third of the tongue presents numerous **lymphatic nodules** that constitute the **lingual tonsils**.

V. PALATE

The **palate**, composed of hard and soft regions, separates the **oral** and **nasal cavities** from each other. Therefore, the palate possesses a **nasal** and an **oral aspect**. The **oral** aspect is covered by **stratified squamous epithelium (partially keratinized** on the hard palate), while the **nasal** aspect is covered by a **respiratory epithelium**. The subepithelial **connective tissue** presents dense collagen fibers interspersed with **adipose tissue** and **mucous glands**. The **core** of the hard palate houses a **bony shelf**, while that of the soft palate is composed of **skeletal muscle**.

VI. TOOTH DEVELOPMENT

Tooth development (odontogenesis) may be divided into several stages (see Graphic 13-1). These are named according to the morphology and/or the functional state of the developing tooth. **Dental lamina**, the first sign of odontogenesis, is followed by **bud, cap,** and **bell stages**. Dentin formation initiates the **appo-sition stage**, followed by **root formation** and **erup-tion**. These stages occur in both **primary** (deci-duous teeth) and **secondary** (permanent teeth) **dentition**.

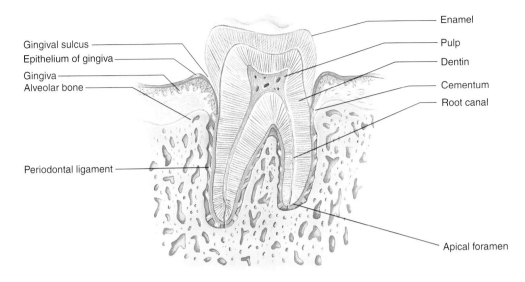

Tooth

The tooth, composed of a crown and root, is suspended in its bony socket, the alveolus, by a dense, collagenous connective tissue, the **periodontal ligament**. The crown of the tooth consists of two calcified tissues, **dentin** and **enamel**, whereas the root is composed of dentin and **cementum**. The pulp chamber of the crown and the root canal of the root are continuous with one another. They are occupied by a gelatinous connective tissue, the **pulp**, which houses blood and lymph vessels, nerve fibers, connective tissue elements, as well as **odontoblasts**, the cells responsible for the maintenance and repair of dentin. Vessels and nerves serving the pulp enter the root canal via the **apical foramen**, a small opening at the apex of the root.

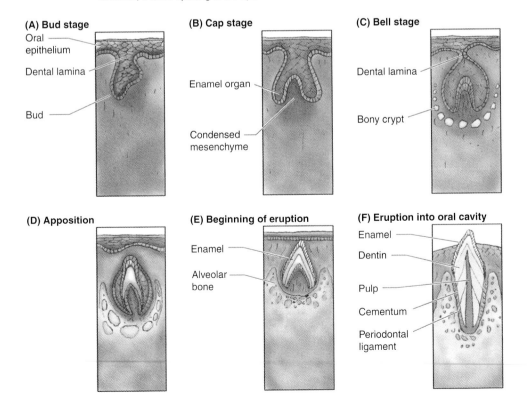

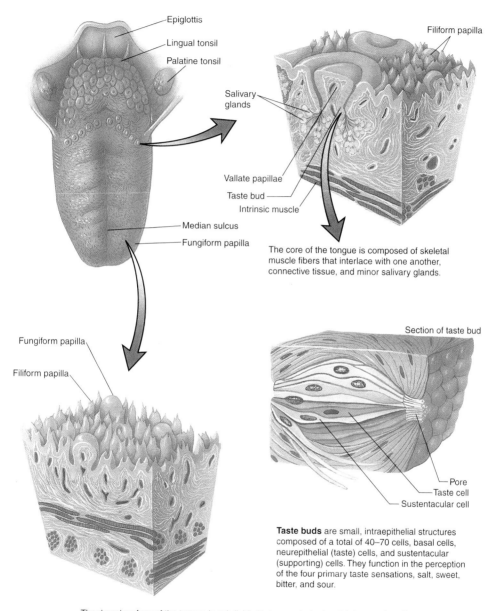

Epiglottis

Lingual tonsil

Palatine tonsil

Filiform papilla

Salivary glands

Vallate papillae

Taste bud

Intrinsic muscle

Median sulcus

Fungiform papilla

The core of the tongue is composed of skeletal muscle fibers that interlace with one another, connective tissue, and minor salivary glands.

Fungiform papilla

Filiform papilla

Section of taste bud

Pore

Taste cell

Sustentacular cell

Taste buds are small, intraepithelial structures composed of a total of 40–70 cells, basal cells, neurepithelial (taste) cells, and sustentacular (supporting) cells. They function in the perception of the four primary taste sensations, salt, sweet, bitter, and sour.

The dorsal surface of the tongue is subdivided into an anterior two-thirds, populated by the four types of lingual papillae, and a posterior one-third housing the lingual tonsils. The two regions are separated from one another by a "V-shaped" depression, the sulcus terminalis. **Filiform papillae** are short, conical, and highly keratinized. **Fungiform papillae** are mushroom-shaped, and the dorsal aspect of their epithelia houses three to five taste buds. **Circumvallate papillae**, the largest of the lingual papillae, are six to twelve in number. Each circumvallate papilla is depressed into the surface of the tongue and is surrounded by a moat-like trough. The lateral aspect of the papilla as well as the lining of the trough houses numerous taste buds. **Foliate papillae** are located on the lateral aspect of the tongue.

PLATE 13-1 ■ *Lip*

FIGURE 1 ■ *Lip. Human. Paraffin section.* × 14.

The human lip presents three surfaces and a core (C). The external surface is covered by skin, composed of **epidermis** (E) and **dermis** (D). Associated hair follicles (arrow) and glands are clearly evident. The **vermillion (red) zone** (VZ) is only found in humans. The high dermal papillae (arrowheads) carry blood vessels close to the surface, accounting for the pinkish coloration of this region. The internal aspect is lined by a wet, stratified, squamous nonkeratinized **epithelium** (Ep) and the underlying connective tissue houses minor salivary glands. The core of the lip is composed of skeletal muscle interspersed with fibroelastic connective tissue.

FIGURE 2 ■ *Lip. Human. Internal aspect. Paraffin section.* × 270.

The internal aspect of the lip is lined by a mucous membrane that is continuously kept moist by saliva secreted by the three major and numerous minor salivary glands. The thick **epithelium** (Ep) is a stratified squamous nonkeratinized type, which presents deep **rete ridges** (RR) that interdigitate with the **connective tissue papillae** (CP). The connective tissue is fibroelastic in nature, displaying a rich **vascular supply** (BV).

FIGURE 3 ■ *Lip. Human. External aspect. Paraffin section.* × 132.

The external aspect of the lip is covered by thin skin. Neither the **epidermis** (E) nor the **dermis** (D) present any unusual features. Numerous **hair follicles** (HF) populate this aspect of the lip, and **sebaceous glands** (Sg) as well as sweat glands are noted in abundance.

FIGURE 4 ■ *Lip. Human. Vermilion zone. Paraffin section.* × 132.

The vermilion zone of the lip is covered by a modified skin, composed of stratified squamous keratinized **epithelium** (Ep) that forms extensive interdigitations with the underlying **dermis** (D). Neither hair follicles nor sweat glands populate this area (though occasional sebaceous glands may be present). Note the cross-sectional profiles of **skeletal muscle fibers** (SM) and the rich **vascular supply** (BV) of the lip.

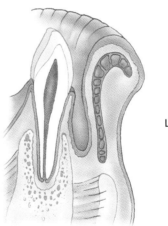

Lip

■ KEY

BV	vascular supply	D	dermis	RR	rete ridges
C	core	E	epidermis	Sg	sebaceous glands
CP	connective tissue papillae	Ep	epithelium	SM	skeletal muscle
		HF	hair follicles	VZ	vermillion (red) zone

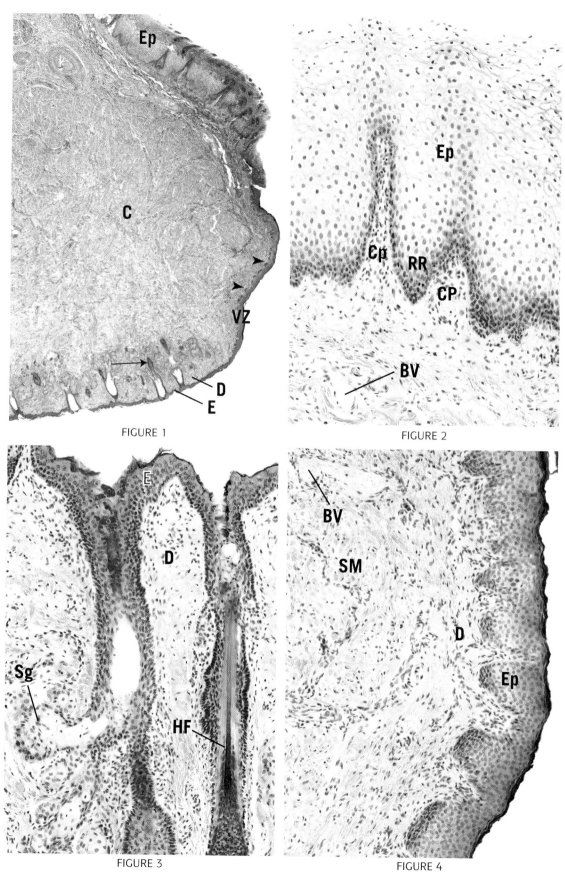

FIGURE 1

FIGURE 2

FIGURE 3

FIGURE 4

PLATE 13-2 ■ *Tooth and Pulp*

FIGURE 1 ■ *Tooth. Human. Ground section.* × 14.

The tooth consists of a crown, neck, and root, composed of calcified tissue surrounding a chamber housing a soft, gelatinous pulp. In ground section only the hard tissues remain. The crown is composed of **enamel** (e) and **dentin** (d), whose interface is known as the **dentinoenamel junction** (DEJ). At the neck of the tooth, enamel meets **cementum** (c), forming the **cementoenamel junction** (CEJ). The **pulp chamber** (PC) is reduced in size as the individual ages. The gap in the enamel (arrows) is due to the presence of a carious lesion (cavity). A region similar to the boxed area is presented at a higher magnification in Figure 2.

FIGURE 2 ■ *Tooth. Human. Ground section.* × 132.

This photomicrograph is a higher magnification of a region similar to the boxed area of the previous figure. The **enamel** (e) is composed of enamel rods (arrows) each surrounded by a rod sheath. Hypomineralized regions of enamel present the appearance of tufts of grass, **enamel tufts** (ET), which extend from the **dentinoenamel junction** (DEJ) partway into the enamel. **Dentin** (d), not as highly calcified as enamel, presents long narrow canals, **dentinal tubules** (DT), which in the living tooth house processes of odontoblasts, cells responsible for the formation of dentin.

FIGURE 3 ■ *Pulp. Human. Paraffin section.* × 132.

The pulp is surrounded by **dentin** (d) from which it is separated by a noncalcified **dentin matrix** (DM). The pulp is said to possess four regions: the **odontoblastic layer** (OL), the **cell-free zone** (CZ), the **cell-rich zone** (CR), and the **core** (C). The core of the pulp is composed of **fibroblasts** (F), delicate collagen fibers, numerous **nerve bundles** (NB), and **blood vessels** (BV). Branches of these neurovascular structures reach the periphery of the pulp, where they supply the cell-rich zone and the odontoblasts with capillaries and fine nerve fibers.

FIGURE 4 ■ *Pulp. Human. Paraffin section.* × 270.

This is a higher magnification of the lower right corner of the previous figure. Note the presence of **blood vessels** (BV) and **nerve fibers** (NF), as well as the numerous **fibroblasts** (F) of this gelatinous connective tissue.

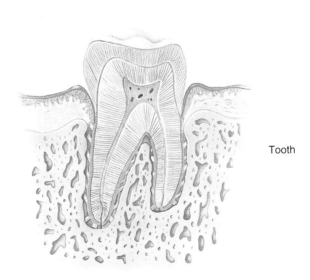

Tooth

■ **KEY**

BV	blood vessel	d	dentin	F	fibroblasts
C	core	DEJ	dentinoenamel junction	NB	nerve bundles
c	cementum	DM	dentin matrix	OL	odontoblastic layer
CEJ	cementoenamel junction	DT	dentinal tubule	PC	pulp chamber
CR	cell-rich zone	e	enamel		
CZ	cell-free zone	ET	enamel tufts		

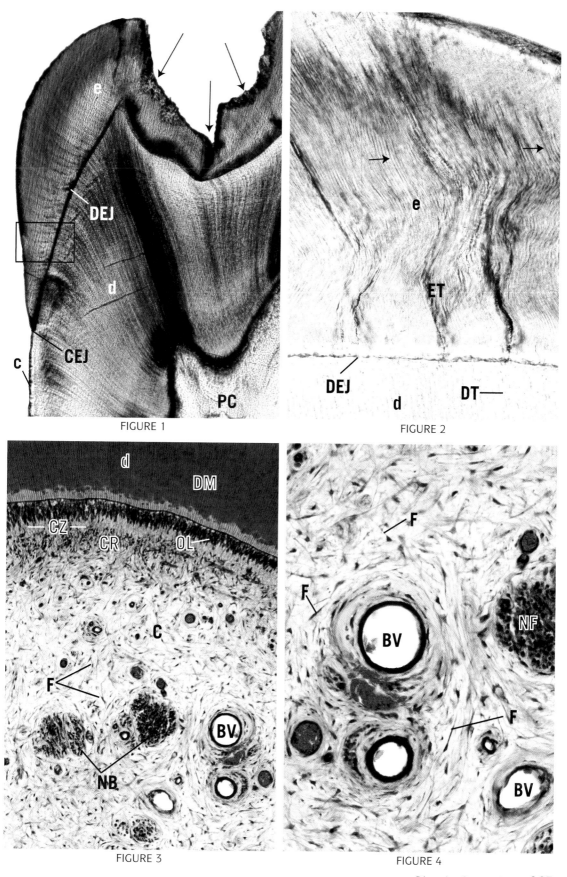

FIGURE 1

FIGURE 2

FIGURE 3

FIGURE 4

Digestive System I ■ **265**

PLATE 13-3 ■ *Periodontal Ligament and Gingiva*

FIGURE 1 ▓ *Periodontal ligament. Human. Paraffin section.* × 132.

The root of the tooth, composed of **dentin** (d) and **cementum** (c), is suspended in its **alveolus** (A) by a collagenous tissue, the **periodontal ligament** (PL). The strong bands of **collagen fibers** (CF) are embedded in the bone via **Sharpey's fibers** (SF). **Blood vessels** (BV) from the bone enter and supply the periodontal ligament. The dentinocemental junction (arrows) is clearly evident. Near the apex of the root, the cementum becomes thicker and houses cementocytes.

FIGURE 2 ■ *Periodontal ligament. Human. Paraffin section.* × 270.

The root of the tooth, composed of **dentin** (d) and **cementum** (c), is suspended in its bony **alveolus** (A) by fibers of the **periodontal ligament** (PL). Note that this photomicrograph is taken in the region of the **crest** (cr) of the alveolus above which the periodontal ligament is continuous with the connective tissue of the **gingiva** (G). Note that both the gingiva and the periodontal ligament are highly vascular, as evident from the abundance of **blood vessels** (BV).

FIGURE 3 ▓ *Gingiva. Human. Paraffin section.* × 14.

This is a decalcified longitudinal section of an incisor tooth, thus all of the calcium hydroxyapatite crystals have been extracted from the tooth and from its bony **alveolus** (A). Since enamel is composed almost completely of calcium hydroxyapatite crystals, only the space where enamel used to be, the **enamel space** (ES), is represented in this photomicrograph. The **crest** (cr) of the alveolus is evident, as are the **periodontal ligament** (PL) and the **gingiva** (G). The **gingival margin** (GM), **free gingiva** (FG), **attached gingiva** (AG), **sulcular epithelium** (SE), **junctional epithelium** (JE), and **alveolar mucosa** (AM) are also identified.

FIGURE 4 ▓ *Gingiva. Human. Paraffin section.* × 132.

This photomicrograph is a higher magnification of the gingival margin region of the previous figure. Note that the **enamel space** (ES) is located between the **dentin** (d) of the incisor tooth's crown and the **junctional epithelium** (JE). The **sulcular epithelium** (SE) of the free gingiva (FG) borders a space known as the **gingival sulcus** (GS), which would be clearly evident if the enamel were still present in this photomicrograph. Observe the well-developed interdigitations of the epithelium and connective tissue, known as the rete apparatus (arrows) of the **free gingiva** (FG) and **attached gingiva**, indicative of the presence of abrasive forces that act upon these regions of the oral cavity.

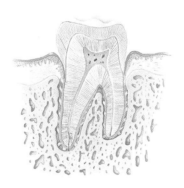

Tooth

■ **KEY**

A	alveolus	CF	collagen fibers	G	gingiva
AM	alveolar mucosa	d	dentin	GM	gingival margin
AT	attached gingiva	DEJ	dentinoenamel junction	GS	gingival sulcus
BV	blood vessel	DT	dentinal tubule	JE	junctional epithelium
c	cementum	ES	enamel space	PC	pulp chamber
cr	crest of alveolus	ET	enamel tufts	PL	periodontal ligament
CEJ	cementoenamel junction	FG	free gingiva	SE	sulcular epithelium

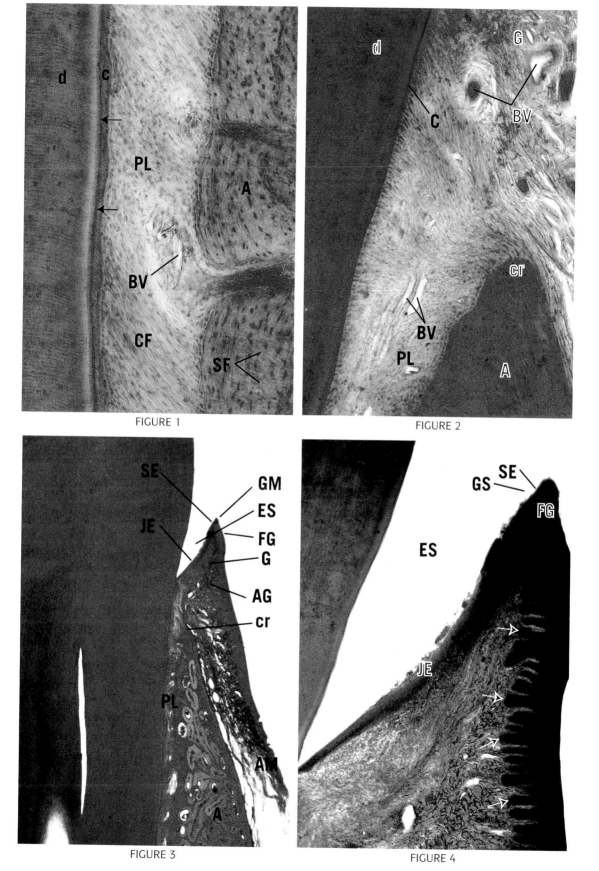

FIGURE 1

FIGURE 2

FIGURE 3

FIGURE 4

PLATE 13-4 ■ *Tooth Development*

FIGURE 1A ■ *Tooth development. Dental lamina. Frontal section. Pig. Paraffin section.* × 132.

The **dental lamina** (DL) is a horseshoe-shaped band of epithelial tissue that arises from the **oral epithelium** (OE) and is surrounded by **mesenchymal cells** (MC). A frontal section of the dental lamina is characterized by the club-shaped appearance in this photomicrograph. The mesenchymal cells in discrete regions at the distal aspect of the dental lamina become rounded and congregate to form the precursor of the dental papilla responsible for the formation of the pulp and dentin of the tooth.

FIGURE 1B ■ *Tooth development. Bud stage. Frontal section. Pig. Paraffin section.* × 132.

At various discrete locations along the **dental lamina** (DL), an epithelial thickening, the **bud** (B), makes its appearance. Each bud will provide the cells necessary for enamel formation for a single tooth. The **dental papilla** (DP) forms a crescent-shaped area at the distal aspect of the bud.

FIGURE 3 ■ *Tooth development. Bell stage. Frontal section. Pig. Paraffin section.* × 132.

As the enamel organ expands in size, it resembles a bell, hence the bell stage of tooth development. This stage is characterized by four cellular layers: **outer enamel epithelium** (OEE), **stellate reticulum** (SR), **inner enamel epithelium** (IEE), and **stratum intermedium** (SI). Observe that the enamel organ is still connected to the **dental lamina** (DL). The **dental papilla** (DP) is composed of rounded mesenchymal cells, whose peripheral-most layer (arrows) will differentiate to form odontoblasts. Note the wide basement membrane (arrowheads) between the future odontoblasts and inner enamel epithelium (the future ameloblasts). Observe also the spindle-shaped cells of the **dental sac** (DS).

FIGURE 2 ■ *Tooth development. Cap stage. Frontal section. Pig. Paraffin section.* × 132.

Increased mitotic activity transforms the bud into a cap-shaped structure. Observe that three epithelial layers of the enamel organ may be recognized: the **outer enamel epithelium** (OEE), the **inner enamel epithelium** (IEE), and the intervening **stellate reticulum** (SR). The inner enamel epithelium has begun to enclose the **dental papilla** (DP). Note that mesenchymal cells become elongated, forming the **dental sac** (DS), which will envelop the enamel organ and dental papilla. Moreover, a **bony crypt** (BC) will enclose the dental sac.

FIGURE 4 ■ *Tooth development. Apposition. Frontal section. Pig. Paraffin section.* × 132.

The elaboration of **dentin** (d) and **enamel** (e) is indicative of apposition. Dentin is manufactured by **odontoblasts** (O), the peripheralmost cell layer of the **dental papilla** (DP). The odontoblastic processes (arrows) are visible in this photomicrograph as they traverse the **dentin matrix** (DM). **Ameloblasts** (A) are highly elongated columnar cells that manufacture enamel. The long epithelial structure located to the left is the **succedaneous lamina** (SL) that is responsible for the development of the permanent tooth.

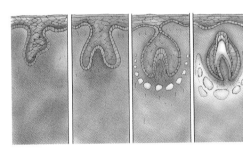

Bud stage, Cap stage, Bell stage, Apposition

■ **KEY**

A	ameloblast	DP	dental papilla	OE	oral epithelium
B	bud	DS	dental sac	OEE	outer enamel epithelium
BC	bony crypt	e	enamel	SI	stratum intermedium
d	dentin	IEE	inner enamel epithelium	SL	succedaneous lamina
DL	dental lamina	MC	mesenchymal cell	SR	stellate reticulum
DM	dentin matrix	O	odontoblast		

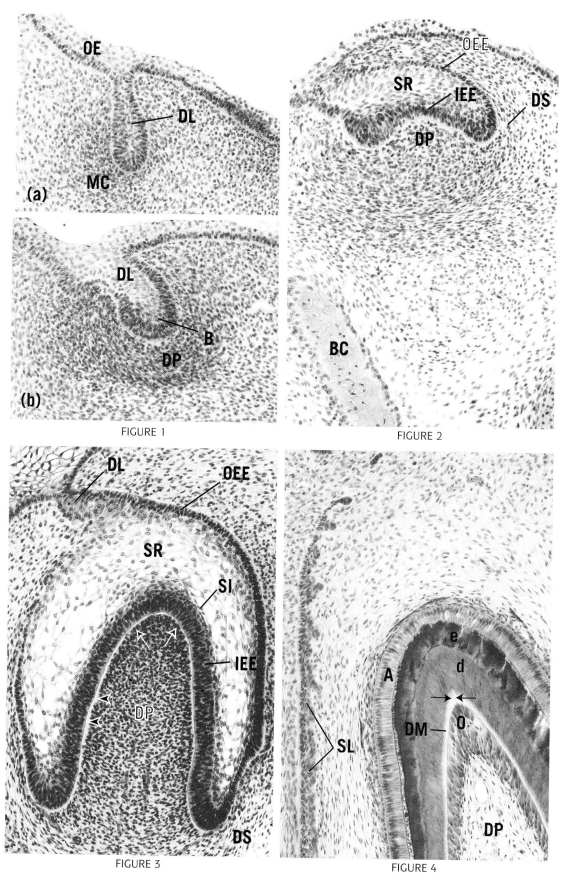

FIGURE 1

FIGURE 2

FIGURE 3

FIGURE 4

PLATE 13-5 ■ *Tongue*

FIGURE 1 ■ *Tongue. Human. l.s. Paraffin section.* × 20.

Part of the anterior two-thirds of the tongue is presented in this photomicrograph. This muscular organ bears numerous **filiform papillae** (FP) on its dorsal surface, whose stratified squamous epithelium is keratinized (arrow). The ventral surface of the tongue is lined by stratified squamous nonkeratinized **epithelium** (Ep). The intrinsic muscles of the tongue are arranged in four layers: **superior longitudinal** (SL), **vertical** (V), **inferior longitudinal** (IL), and **horizontal** (not shown here). The mucosa of the tongue is tightly adhering to the perimysium of the intrinsic tongue muscles by the subepithelial **connective tissue** (CT).

FIGURE 2 ■ *Tongue. Human. l.s. Paraffin section.* × 14.

The posterior aspect of the anterior two-thirds of the tongue presents **circumvallate papillae** (Cp). These papillae are surrounded by a deep groove (arrow), the base of which accepts a serous secretion via the **ducts** (Du) of the **glands of von Ebner** (GE). The **epithelium** (Ep) of the papilla houses taste buds along its lateral aspects, but not on its superior surface. The core of the tongue contains **skeletal muscle** (SM) fibers of the extrinsic and intrinsic lingual muscles, as well as glands and **adipose tissue** (AT). A region similar to the boxed area is presented at a higher magnification in Figure 3.

FIGURE 3 ■ *Circumvallate papilla. Monkey.* *x.s. Plastic section.* × 132.

This photomicrograph is a higher magnification of a region similar to the boxed area of the previous figure rotated 90°. Note the presence of the **groove** (G) separating the **circumvallate papilla** (Cp) from the wall of the groove. **Glands of von Ebner** (GE) deliver a serous secretion into this groove, whose contents are monitored by numerous intraepithelial **taste buds** (TB). Observe that taste buds are not found on the superior surface of the circumvallate papilla, only on its lateral aspect. The connective tissue core of the papilla is richly endowed by **blood vessels** (BV) and **nerves** (N).

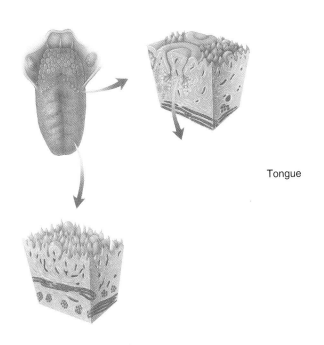

Tongue

■ **KEY**

AT	adipose tissue	FP	filiform papillae	SL	superior longitudinal muscle
BV	blood vessels	G	groove		
Cp	circumvallate papillae	GE	glands of von Ebner	SM	skeletal muscle
CT	connective tissue	IL	inferior longitudinal muscle	TB	taste buds
Du	ducts	N	nerves	V	vertical muscle
Ep	epithelium				

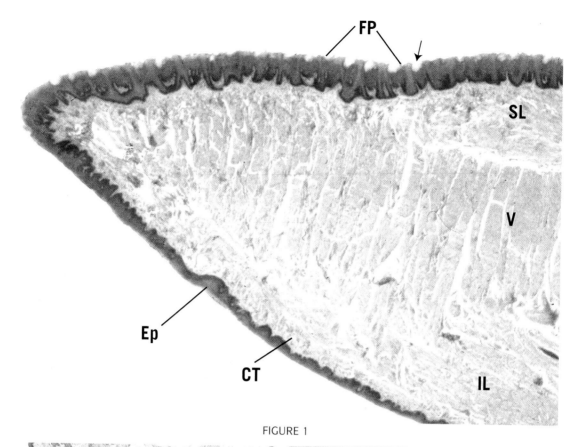

FP

SL

V

Ep

CT

IL

FIGURE 1

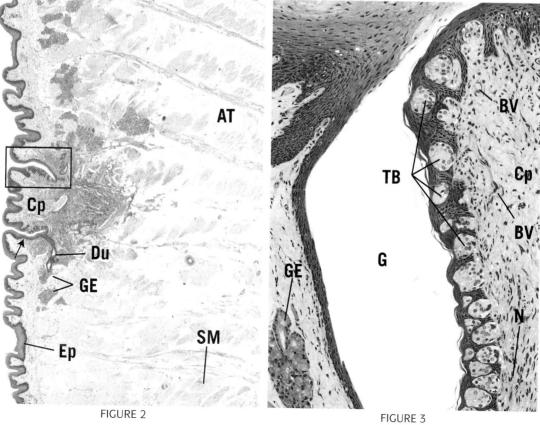

AT

Cp

Du

GE

Ep

SM

FIGURE 2

BV

Cp

TB

BV

GE

G

N

FIGURE 3

PLATE 13-6 ■ *Tongue and Palate*

FIGURE 1 ▦ *Circumvallate papilla. Monkey. Paraffin section.* × 132.

The base of the **circumvallate papilla** (Cp), the surrounding **groove** (G), and the wall of the groove are evident in this photomicrograph. The **glands of von Ebner** (GE) deliver their serous secretions via short **ducts** (Du) into the base of the groove. Observe the rich **vascular** (BV) and **nerve** (N) supply to this region. Numerous **taste buds** (TB) populate the epithelium of the lateral aspect of the circumvallate papilla. Each taste bud possesses a taste pore (arrows) through which taste hairs (microvilli) protrude into the groove. A region similar to the boxed area is presented at a higher magnification in Figure 2.

FIGURE 2 ■ *Taste bud. Monkey. x.s. Plastic section.* × 540.

This is a higher magnification of a region similar to the boxed area of Figure 1. Note that the stratified squamous parakeratinized **epithelium** (Ep) displays squames in the process of desquamation (arrowheads). The **taste buds** (TB) are composed of at least three cell types. **Basal (lateral) cells** (BC) are believed to be regenerative in nature, whereas **light** (LC) and **dark** (DC) cells are probably gustatory and sustentacular, respectively. Observe the presence of **blood vessels** (BV) in the subepithelial **connective tissue** (CT).

FIGURE 3 ▦ *Hard palate. Human. Paraffin section.* × 132.

The hard palate possesses a nasal and an oral surface. The stratified squamous parakeratinized **epithelium** (Ep) of the oral surface forms deep invaginations, **rete ridges** (RR), which interdigitate with the subepithelial **connective tissue** (CT). The thick **collagen fiber bundles** (CF) firmly bind the palatal mucosa to the periosteum of the underlying bone. The hard palate also houses large deposits of adipose tissue and mucous glands.

FIGURE 4 ▦ *Soft palate. Human. Paraffin section.* × 132.

The oral surface of the soft palate is lined by a stratified squamous nonkeratinized **epithelium** (Ep), which interdigitates with the **lamina propria** (LP) by the formation of shallow **rete ridges** (RR). The soft palate is a moveable structure as attested by the presence of **skeletal muscle fibers** (SM). The core of the soft palate also houses numerous **mucous glands** (MG) that deliver their secretory products into the oral cavity via short, straight ducts.

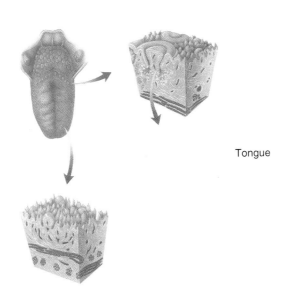

Tongue

KEY

BC	basal cells	Du	ducts	MG	mucous glands
BV	blood vessels	Ep	epithelium	N	nerve
CF	collagen fiber bundles	G	groove	RR	rete ridges
Cp	circumvallate papilla	GE	glands of von Ebner	SM	skeletal muscle
CT	connective tissue	LC	light cells	TB	taste buds
DC	dark cells	LP	lamina propria		

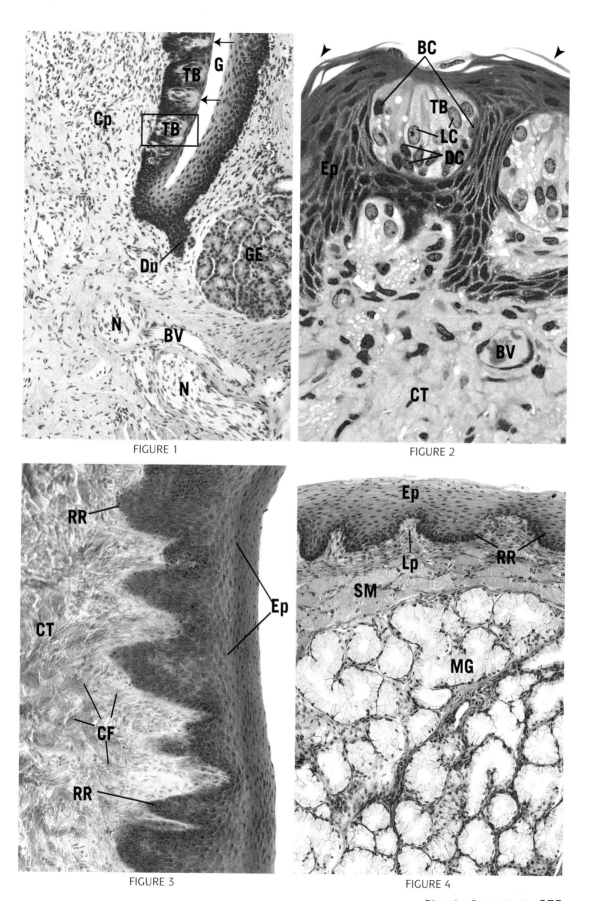

FIGURE 1

FIGURE 2

FIGURE 3

FIGURE 4

PLATE 13-7 ■ *Teeth and Nasal Aspect of the Hard Palate*

FIGURE 1 ■ *Human central incisor roots. Paraffin section.* × 132.

The roots of two human central incisors and their supporting tissues are noted in this composite photomicrograph. Note that the root of one incisor, **Root 1**, is at the top of the figure and progressing down the page the **hyaline layer of Hopewell-Smith** (HL) separates the **dentin** (d) of the root from the **cementum** (c). The **periodontal ligament** (PL1), with its attendant **blood vessels** (BV), of this tooth suspends tooth 1 in its alveolus. The interdental septum (IS), positioned between the two incisors and composed of woven bone, is formed by the fusion of the **alveolar bones proper** (ABP 1 and 2) of each root. Note the presence of **osteons** (Os) in the woven bone and the center of these osteons approximates the line of fusion between the two alveolar bones proper. The **periodontal ligament** of the other incisor (PL 2) is located between the alveolar bone proper (ABP 2) and the **cementum** of this tooth. Its **dentin** (d) and **hyaline layer of Hopewell-Smith** (HL) of root 2 are clearly evident.

FIGURE 2 ■ *Hard palate. Human. Paraffin section.* × 132.

The hard palate possesses a nasal and an oral surface. Note that the pseudostratified ciliated columnar **epithelium** (Ep) displays cilia and an **intraepithelial gland** (IeGL). Observe the presence **glands** (Gl) and **blood vessels** (BV) in the subepithelial **connective tissue** (CT). The epithelium and the subepithelial connective tissue are collectively referred to as the **mucoperiosteum** (MP) which is firmly attached to the **bony shelf** (B) of the palate. A higher magnification of the boxed area is presented in Figure 3.

FIGURE 3 ■ *Hard palate. Human. Paraffin section.* × 132.

This is a higher magnification of a region similar to the boxed area of Figure 2. Note the presence of **glands** (GL), **blood vessels** (BV), and **lymph vessels** (LV) within the subepithelial **connective tissue** (CT). The thick **collagen fiber bundles** (CF) firmly bind the palatal mucosa to the periosteum of the underlying bone. Observe the clearly visible **cilia** (c) of the pseudostratified ciliated columnar **epithelium** (Ep) covering the nasal surface of the hard palate.

■ **KEY**

ABP	alveolar bone proper	d	dentin	IeGL	intraepithelial gland
B	bony shelf	Ep	epithelium	IS	interdental septum
BV	blood vessel	Gl	gland	MP	palatal mucosa
C	cementum	HL	hyaline layer of Hopewell-Smith	Os	osteon
CT	connective tissue			PL	periodontal ligament

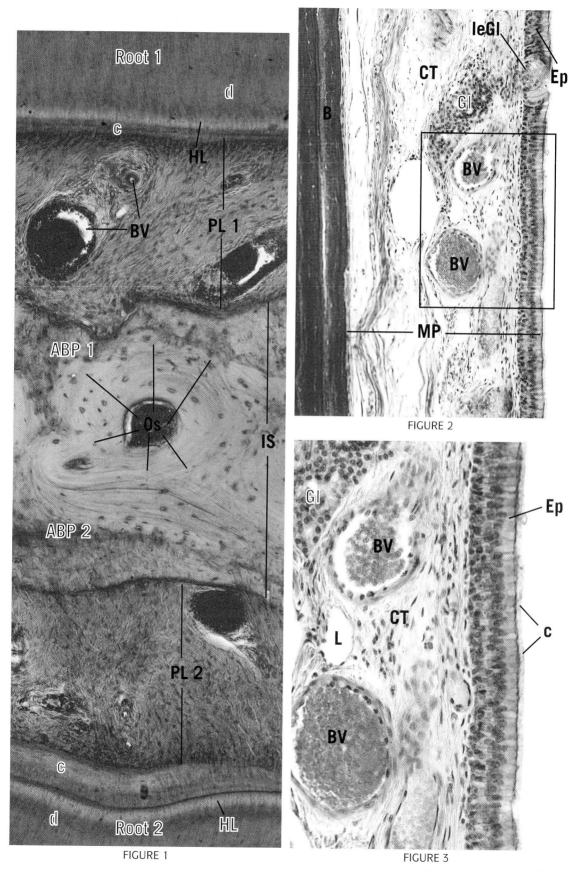

Root 1

d

c

HL

BV

PL 1

ABP 1

Os

IS

ABP 2

PL 2

c

d

Root 2

HL

FIGURE 1

leGl

CT

Ep

Gl

BV

B

BV

MP

FIGURE 2

Gl

BV

Ep

CT

L

c

BV

FIGURE 3

14

Digestive System II

The **alimentary canal** is a long, hollow, tubular structure that extends from the oral cavity to the anus and is modified along its length to perform the various facets of digestion. The oral cavity receives food and, via mastication and bolus formation, delivers it into the oral pharynx, from where it enters the esophagus and eventually the stomach. The gastric contents are reduced to an **acidic chyme,** which is dispensed in small spurts to the small intestine, where most digestion and absorption occur. The liquefied food residue passes into the large intestine, where the digestion is completed and water is resorbed. The solidified feces are then passed to the anus for elimination.

A common architectural plan is evident for the alimentary tract from the esophagus to the anus, in that four distinct concentric layers may be recognized to constitute the wall of this long tubular structure. These layers are described from the lumen outward.

LAYERS OF THE WALL OF THE ALIMENTARY CANAL

Mucosa

The innermost layer directly surrounding the lumen is known as the **mucosa,** which is composed of three concentric layers: a **wet epithelial lining** with secretory and absorptive functions; a connective tissue **lamina propria** containing glands and components of the circulatory system; and a **muscularis mucosae,** usually consisting of two thin smooth muscle layers, responsible for the mobility of the mucosa.

Submucosa

The **submucosa** is a coarser connective tissue component that physically supports the mucosa and provides nerve, vascular, and lymphatic supply to the mucosa. Moreover, in some regions of the alimentary canal the submucosa houses glands.

Muscularis Externa

The **muscularis externa** usually consists of an **inner circular** and an **outer longitudinal smooth muscle layer,** which is modified in certain regions of the alimentary canal. Although these layers are described as circularly or longitudinally arranged, they are actually wrapped around the alimentary canal in tight and loose helices, respectively. Vascular and neural plexuses reside between the muscle layers. The muscularis externa functions in churning and propelling the luminal contents along the digestive tract via peristaltic action.

Serosa or Adventitia

The outermost layer of the alimentary canal is either a serosa or an adventitia. The intraperitoneal regions of the alimentary canal, i.e., those that are suspended by peritoneum, possess a **serosa.** This structure consists of connective tissue covered by a **mesothelium** (simple squamous epithelium), which reduces frictional forces during digestive movement. Other regions of the alimentary tract are firmly attached to surrounding structures by connective tissue fibers. These regions possess an **adventitia.**

REGIONS OF THE ALIMENTARY CANAL

Esophagus

The **esophagus** is a short muscular tube whose mucosa is composed of a **stratified squamous nonkeratinized epithelium,** a loose type of connective tissue housing mucus-producing esophageal **cardiac glands** in the lamina propria, and longitudinally oriented smooth muscle fibers of the muscularis mucosae. The submucosa of this organ is composed of dense irregular collagenous connective tissue interspersed with elastic fibers. This is one of the two regions of the alimentary canal (the other is the duodenum) that houses glands in its submucosa. These glands are the mucus-producing **esophageal glands proper**. The **muscularis externa** of the esophagus is composed of **inner circular** and **outer longitudinal layers**. Those in the upper one-third are **skeletal**, those in the middle one-third are **skeletal** and **smooth**, whereas those in the lower one-third are **smooth**. The esophagus functions in conveying a bolus of food from the pharynx into the stomach.

Stomach

Based on the glands of its lamina propria, histologically, the stomach is subdivided into three regions: **cardia, fundus,** and **pylorus** (see Graphic 14-1). The mucosa of the empty stomach is thrown into longitudinal folds, the **rugae**. The luminal surface, lined by a simple columnar epithelium (**surface lining cells**), displays **foveolae (gastric pits)**, whose base is perforated by several gastric glands of the lamina propria. All **gastric glands** are composed of **parietal (oxyntic) cells, mucous neck cells, surface lining cells, diffuse neuroendocrine system (DNES, also APUD) cells,** and **regenerative cells**. Fundic glands, in addition, also house **chief (zymogenic) cells**.

Oxyntic cells produce HCl and **gastric intrinsic factor,** a factor that assists the ileum in absorbing vitamin B_{12}. These cells possess intracellular canaliculi and a complex tubulovesicular system. **Mucous neck cells,** along with **surface lining cells,** are responsible for the formation of mucus that presumably protects the stomach lining from autodigestion. The various types of **DNES** cells produce hormones such as **gastrin, somatostatin, secretin,** and **cholecystokinin**. Regenerative cells, located mainly in the neck and isthmus, replace the epithelial lining of the stomach and the cells of the glands. Chief cells, located in the base of the fundic glands, produce precursors of enzymes (**pepsin, rennin,** and **lipase**).

Small Intestine

The **small intestine** is composed of the **duodenum, jejunum,** and **ileum**. The mucosa of all three regions displays **villi,** extensions of the lamina propria, covered by a simple columnar type of epithelium. The epithelium is composed of goblet, surface absorptive, and DNES cells. **Goblet cells** produce a **mucus**. **DNES cells** release various hormones (e.g., **secretin, cholecystokinin, gastric inhibitory peptide,** and **gastrin**). The tall, columnar **surface absorptive cells** possess numerous **microvilli** covered by a thick glycocalyx composed of several enzymes. These cells function in absorption of lipids, amino acids, and carbohydrates. Long chained lipids, in the form of **chylomicrons,** are delivered to the **lacteals,** blindly ending lymphatic channels of the villus.

Simple tubular glands of the mucosa, **the crypts of Lieberkühn,** open into the intervillar spaces. These crypts are composed of simple columnar cells (similar to surface absorptive cells), goblet (and oligomucous) cells, DNES, and regenerative cells, as well as **Paneth cells**. The last are located in the base of the crypts and house large secretory granules believed to contain the antibacterial enzyme **lysozyme**. The lamina propria of the ileum houses large accumulations of lymphatic nodules, **Peyer's patches**. The surface epithelium interposed between Peyer's patches and the lumen of the ileum displays the presence of **M cells**.

The submucosa of the duodenum contains numerous glands, **duodenal (Brunner's) glands,** that produce an alkaline, mucin-containing fluid that protects the intestinal lining. They also manufacture **urogastrone,** a polypeptide that inhibits HCl production and enhances epithelial cell division.

Large Intestine

The **large intestine** is subdivided into the **cecum,** the **ascending, transverse, descending,** and **sigmoid colons,** the **rectum,** the **anal canal,** and the **appendix** (see Graphic 14-2). The large intestine possesses no villi but does house **crypts of Lieberkühn** in its lamina propria. The epithelial lining of the lumen and of the crypts is composed of **goblet (and oligomucous) cells, surface absorptive cells, regenerative cells,** and occasional **DNES cells**. There are no Paneth cells in the large intestine, with the possible exception of the appendix. The large intestine functions in the absorption of the remaining amino acids, lipids, and carbohydrates, as well as fluids, electrolytes, and certain vitamins and in the compaction of feces.

Histophysiology

I. STOMACH

The **stomach** functions in acidifying and converting the semisolid **bolus** into the viscous fluid, **chyme,** which undergoes initial digestion and is delivered into the **duodenum** in small quantities.

The gastric mucosa is lined by a simple columnar epithelium whose **surface lining cells** (not goblet cells) produce a mucous substance that coats and protects the stomach lining from the low pH environment and from autodigestion.

The lamina propria of the stomach houses **gastric glands;** depending on the region of the stomach, these are cardiac, fundic, or pyloric. **Fundic glands** are composed of five cell types: parietal (oxyntic), mucous neck, chief (zymogenic), DNES, and regenerative cells. Neither **cardiac** nor **pyloric glands** possess chief cells.

Parietal cells secrete hydrochloric acid (HCl) into **intracellular canaliculi.** These cells alter their morphology during HCl secretion, in that they increase their number of **microvilli** that project into the intracellular canaliculi. It is believed that these microvilli are stored as the **tubulovesicular system,** flanking the intracellular canaliculi when the cell is not secreting HCl. Additionally, parietal cells also secrete **gastric intrinsic factor,** a glycoprotein required for the absorption of vitamin B_{12} in the ileum.

Mucous neck cells are located in the neck of the gastric glands. They secrete a **mucus** that is distinct from that secreted by surface lining cells.

Chief cells are located in the deep aspect of fundic glands. They secrete precursors of enzymes **pepsin, rennin,** and **lipase,** which initiate digestion in the stomach.

Enteroendocrine cells (DNES cells) belong to cells of the diffuse neuroendocrine system and are known by several synonyms. Although as a group these cells produce a number of different hormones, it is believed that each cell is capable of producing only a single hormone. The hormones that these cells produce may enter vascular or lymphatic channels, but the target cells for most of these hormones are in the vicinity of their release, therefore, these hormones are referred to as **paracrine hormones.** (See Table 14-1 for hormones produced by the alimentary canal.)

II. SMALL INTESTINE

The luminal aspect of the small intestine is modified to increase its surface area. These modifications range from the macroscopic, **plicae circulares** (increase 3X), through the microscopic, **villi** (increase 10X), to the submicroscopic, **microvilli** (increase 20X).

A. Villi

Villi are lined by a simple columnar epithelium composed of surface absorptive cells, goblet cells, and DNES cells.

Surface absorptive cells possess dense accumulations of microvilli, forming the **striated border.** Their tips have a thick coat of **glycocalyx,** rich in **disaccharidases** and **dipeptidases.** These cells function in absorption of sugars, amino acids, fatty acids, monoglycerides, electrolytes, water, and many other beneficial substances. These epithelial cells also participate in the immune defense of the body by manufacturing **protein J (secretory protein),** which binds to and protects **immunoglobulin A (IgA)** as it traverses the epithelial cell and enters the intestinal lumen.

Goblet cells produce **mucinogen,** which, when released into the intestinal lumen, becomes hydrated, forming **mucin,** a slippery substance that, when mixed with material in its vicinity, becomes the substance known as **mucus.** It is the mucus that protects the intestinal lining.

B. Crypts of Lieberkühn

The simple tubular glands of the lamina propria are known as the **crypts of Lieberkühn.** They open into the intervillar spaces and are lined by a simple columnar epithelium composed of columnar cells (surface absorptive cells), goblet cells, DNES cells, regenerative cells, and Paneth cells.

Regenerative cells are located in the basal half of the crypts of Lieberkühn and function as a population of stem cells that replace the entire intestinal epithelium every 4–6 days.

Paneth cells are located in the base of the crypts of Lieberkühn and are easily recognized by their large apical granules. These cells manufacture the enzyme **lysozyme,** an antibacterial agent.

TABLE 14-1 ■ *Hormones Produced by Cells of the Alimentary Canal*

Hormone	Location	Action
Cholecystokinin (CCK)	Small intestine	Contraction of gallbladder; release of pancreatic enzymes
Gastric inhibitory peptide	Small intestine	Inhibits secretion of HCl
Gastrin	Stomach and duodenum	Stimulates secretion of HCl and gastric enzymes
Glicentin	Stomach, small and large intestines	Stimulates glycogenolysis by hepatocytes
Glucagon	Stomach and duodenum	Stimulates glycogenolysis by hepatocytes
Motilin	Small intestine	Increases intestinal peristalsis
Neurotensin	Small intestine	Decreases peristalsis in intestines; stimulates blood supply to ileum
Secretin	Small intestine	Stimulates bicarbonate secretion by pancreas
Serotonin	Stomach, small and large intestines	Increases intestinal peristalsis
Somatostatin	Stomach and duodenum	Inhibits DNES cells in its vicinity of release
Substance P	Stomach, small and large intestines	Increases intestinal peristalsis
Urogastrone	Duodenal glands (Brunner's)	Inhibits secretion of HCl; increases epithelial cell mitosis
Vasoactive intestinal peptide	Stomach, small and large intestines	Increases intestinal peristalsis; stimulates secretion of ions and water by the alimentary canal

C. Duodenal Glands (Brunner's Glands)

Brunner's glands are located in the **submucosa** of the duodenum. These glands produce an alkaline-rich mucin-containing fluid that buffers the acidic chyme entering the duodenum from the stomach. Additionally, Brunner's glands manufacture and release **urogastrone**.

III. GUT-ASSOCIATED LYMPHOID TISSUE

Since the lumen of the digestive tract is rich in antigenic substances, bacteria, and toxins and since only a thin simple columnar epithelium separates the richly vascularized connective tissue from this threatening milieu, the lamina propria of the intestines is well endowed with lymphoid elements. These include scattered cells (B cells, T cells, plasma cells, mast cells, macrophages, etc.), individual lymphatic nodules, and, in the ileum, **Peyer's patches**, clusters of lymphatic nodules. Regions where lymphatic nodules come in contact with the epithelial lining of the intestines display flattened cells that form the interface between the lumen and the lymphatic nodule. These cells are **M cells** (**microfold cells**) that phagocytose antigens and transport them, via clathrin-coated vesicles, to the basal aspect of the cell. The antigens are released into the lamina propria for uptake by antigen-presenting cells and dendritic cells.

IV. DIGESTION AND ABSORPTION

A. Carbohydrates

Amylases, present in the saliva and in the pancreatic secretion, hydrolyze carbohydrates to disaccharides. **Disaccharidases,** present in the glycocalyx of surface absorptive cells, break down disaccharides into monosaccharides that enter the lamina propria by a transepithelial route, requiring active transport.

B. Proteins

Proteins, denatured by HCl in the lumen of the stomach, are hydrolyzed (by the enzyme **pepsin**) into **polypeptides.** These are further broken down into **dipeptides** by proteases of the pancreatic secretions. **Dipeptidases** of the glycocalyx hydrolyze dipeptides into individual amino acids, which enter the lamina propria by a transepithelial route involving active transport.

C. Lipids

Pancreatic lipase breaks lipids down into **fatty acids, monoglycerides,** and **glycerol** within the lumen of the duodenum and proximal jejunum. Bile salts, delivered from the gallbladder, emulsify the fatty acids and monoglycerides, forming **micelles,** which, along with glycerol, diffuse into the surface absorptive cells. Within these cells they enter the **smooth endoplasmic reticulum,** are reesterified to **triglycerides,** and are covered by a coat of protein within the Golgi apparatus, forming lipoprotein droplets known as **chylomicrons.** Chylomicrons exit these cells at their basolateral membranes and enter the **lacteals** of the villi, contributing to the formation of **chyle.** Fatty acids that are shorter than 12 carbon chains in length pass through the surface absorptive cells without being reesterified and gain entrance to the blood capillaries of the villi.

D. Water and Ions

Water and ions are absorbed through the surface absorptive cells of the small and the large intestine.

Clinical Considerations ▪ ▪ ▪

Crohn's Disease

Crohn's disease is a subcategory of **inflammatory bowel disease**, a condition of unknown etiology. It usually involves the small intestine or the colon, but may affect any region of the alimentary canal, from the esophagus to the anus, as well as extra-alimentary canal structures, such as the skin, kidney, and the larynx. It is characterized by patchy ulcers and deep fistulas in the intestinal wall. Clinical manifestations include abdominal pain, diarrhea, and fever, and these recur after various periods of ever shortening remission.

Hiatal Hernia

Hiatal hernia is a condition where a region of the stomach herniates through the **esophageal hiatus** of the diaphragm. It may be of two types, sliding and paraesophageal hiatal hernia. In the former condition the cardioesophageal junction and the cardiac region of the stomach slides in and out of the thorax, whereas in the latter case the cardioesophageal junction remains in its normal place, below the diaphragm, but a part (or occasionally all) of the stomach pushes into the thorax and is positioned next to the esophagus. Usually, hiatal hernia is asymptomatic although acid reflux disease is quite common in patients afflicted with this condition. Patients are advised to eat smaller meals more frequently and the acid reflux disease is treated. Infrequently, paraesophageal hiatal hernias may result in strangulation of the protruded region with a possible loss of blood supply. In these cases surgical intervention may be indicated.

Summary of Histological Organization

I. ESOPHAGUS

The **esophagus** is a long muscular tube that delivers the **bolus** of food from the **pharynx** to the **stomach.** The esophagus, as well as the remainder of the alimentary tract, is composed of four concentric layers: **mucosa, submucosa, muscularis externa,** and **adventitia.** The **lumen** of the esophagus is normally collapsed.

A. Mucosa

The **mucosa** has three regions: **epithelium, lamina propria,** and **muscularis mucosae.** It is thrown into longitudinal folds.

1. Epithelium
The **epithelium** is **stratified squamous nonkeratinized.**

2. Lamina Propria
The **lamina propria** is a loose connective tissue that contains mucus-producing **esophageal cardiac glands** in some regions of the esophagus.

3. Muscularis Mucosae
The **muscularis mucosae** is composed of a single layer of **longitudinally** oriented **smooth muscle.**

B. Submucosa

The **submucosa,** composed of fibroelastic connective tissue, is thrown into longitudinal folds. The **esophageal glands proper** of this layer produce a mucous secretion. **Meissner's submucosal plexus** houses postganglionic parasympathetic nerve cells.

C. Muscularis Externa

The **muscularis externa** is composed of **inner circular** (tight helix) and **outer longitudinal** (loose helix) **muscle layers.** In the upper one-third of the esophagus these consist of **skeletal muscle,** in the middle one-third they consist of **skeletal** and **smooth muscle,** and in the lower one-third they consist of **smooth muscle. Auerbach's myenteric plexus** is located between the two layers of muscle.

D. Adventitia

The **adventitia** of the esophagus is composed of fibrous connective tissue. Inferior to the diaphragm the esophagus is covered by a **serosa.**

II. STOMACH

The **stomach** is a sac-like structure that receives food from the **esophagus** and delivers its contents, known as chyme, into the **duodenum.** The stomach has three histologically recognizable regions: **cardiac, fundic,** and **pyloric.** The **mucosa** and **submucosa** of the empty stomach are thrown into folds, known as **rugae,** that disappear in the distended stomach.

A. Mucosa

The **mucosa** presents **gastric pits,** the bases of which accept the openings of **gastric glands.**

1. Epithelium
The **simple columnar epithelium** has no goblet cells. The cells composing this epithelium are known as **surface lining cells** and extend into the gastric pits.

2. Lamina Propria
The **lamina propria** houses numerous **gastric glands,** slender blood vessels, and various connective tissue and **lymphoid cells.**

a. Cells of Gastric Glands
Gastric glands are composed of the following cell types: **parietal (oxyntic) cells, chief (zymogenic) cells, mucous neck cells, DNES (enteroendocrine) cells,** and **stem cells.** Glands of the **cardiac region** have no **chief** and only a few **parietal cells.** Glands of the **pyloric region** are short and possess no chief cells and only a few parietal cells. Most of the cells are mucus-secreting cells resembling **mucous neck cells.** Glands of the **fundic region** possess all five cell types.

3. Muscularis Mucosae
The **muscularis mucosae** is composed of an **inner circular** and an **outer longitudinal smooth muscle** layer. A third layer may be present in certain regions.

B. Submucosa

The **submucosa** contains no glands. It houses a vascular plexus, as well as **Meissner's submucosal plexus.**

C. Muscularis Externa

The **muscularis externa** is composed of three smooth muscle layers: the **inner oblique, middle circular,** and **outer longitudinal.** The middle circular forms the **pyloric sphincter. Auerbach's myenteric plexus** is located between the circular and longitudinal layers.

D. Serosa

The stomach is covered by a connective tissue coat enveloped in visceral peritoneum, the **serosa**.

III. SMALL INTESTINE

The **small intestine** is composed of three regions: **duodenum, jejunum,** and **ileum.** The **mucosa** of the small intestine presents folds, known as **villi,** that change their morphology and decrease in height from the duodenum to the ileum. The submucosa displays spiral folds, **plicae circulares** (valves of Kerckring).

A. Mucosa

The **mucosa** presents **villi,** evaginations of the epithelially covered **lamina propria.**

1. Epithelium
The **simple columnar epithelium** consists of **goblet, surface absorptive,** and **DNES cells.** The number of goblet cells increases from the duodenum to the ileum.

2. Lamina Propria
The **lamina propria,** composed of **loose connective tissue,** houses glands, known as the **crypts of Lieberkühn,** that extend to the muscularis mucosae. The cells composing these glands are **goblet cells, columnar cells,** and, especially at the base, **Paneth cells, DNES cells, and stem cells.** An occasional **caveolated cell** may also be noted. A central **lacteal,** a blindly ending lymphatic vessel, **smooth muscle cells, blood vessels,** solitary **lymphatic nodules,** and **lymphoid cells** are also present. Lymphatic nodules, with **M cell** epithelial caps, are especially abundant as **Peyer's patches** in the ileum.

3. Muscularis Mucosae
The **muscularis mucosae** consists of an **inner circular** and an **outer longitudinal** layer of **smooth muscle.**

B. Submucosa

The **submucosa** is not unusual except in the **duodenum,** where it contains **Brunner's glands.**

C. Muscularis Externa

The **muscularis externa** is composed of the usual **inner circular** and **outer longitudinal** layers of smooth muscle, with **Auerbach's myenteric plexus** intervening.

D. Serosa

The duodenum is covered by **serosa** and **adventitia,** while the jejunum and ileum are covered by a serosa.

IV. LARGE INTESTINE

The **large intestine** is composed of the **appendix, cecum, ascending, transverse,** and **descending colons, rectum,** and **anal canal.** The appendix and anal canal are described separately, although the remainder of the large intestine presents identical histologic features.

A. Colon

1. Mucosa
The **mucosa** presents no specialized folds. It is thicker than that of the small intestine.

a. Epithelium
The **simple columnar epithelium** has goblet cells and columnar cells.

b. Lamina Propria
The **crypts of Lieberkühn** of the **lamina propria** are longer than those of the small intestine. They are composed of numerous **goblet cells,** a few **DNES cells,** and **stem cells.** Lymphatic nodules are frequently present.

c. Muscularis Mucosae
The **muscularis mucosae** consists of **inner circular** and **outer longitudinal smooth muscle** layers.

2. Submucosa
The **submucosa** resembles that of the jejunum or ileum.

3. Muscularis Externa
The **muscularis externa** is composed of **inner circular** and **outer longitudinal smooth muscle** layers. The outer longitudinal muscle is modified into **teniae coli,** three flat ribbons of longitudinally arranged smooth muscles. These are responsible for the formation of **haustra coli** (sacculations). **Auerbach's plexus** occupies its position between the two layers.

4. Serosa
The colon possesses both **serosa** and **adventitia.** The serosa presents small, fat-filled pouches, the **appendices epiploicae.**

B. Appendix

The **lumen** of the **appendix** is usually stellate shaped, and it may be obliterated. The **simple columnar epithelium** covers a **lamina propria** rich in **lymphatic nodules** and some **crypts of Lieberkühn.** The **muscularis mucosae, submucosa,** and **muscularis externa** conform to the general plan of the digestive tract. It is covered by a **serosa.**

C. Anal Canal

The **anal canal** presents longitudinal folds, **anal columns,** which become joined at the orifice of the anus to form **anal valves,** and intervening **anal sinuses.** The epithelium changes from the **simple columnar** of the rectum, to **simple cuboidal** at the anal valves, to **stratified squamous** distal to the anal valves, to **epidermis** at the orifice of the anus.

Circumanal glands, hair follicles, and **sebaceous glands** are present here. The **submucosa** is rich in vascular supply, while the **muscularis externa** forms the internal anal sphincter muscle. An **adventitia** connects the anus to the surrounding structures.

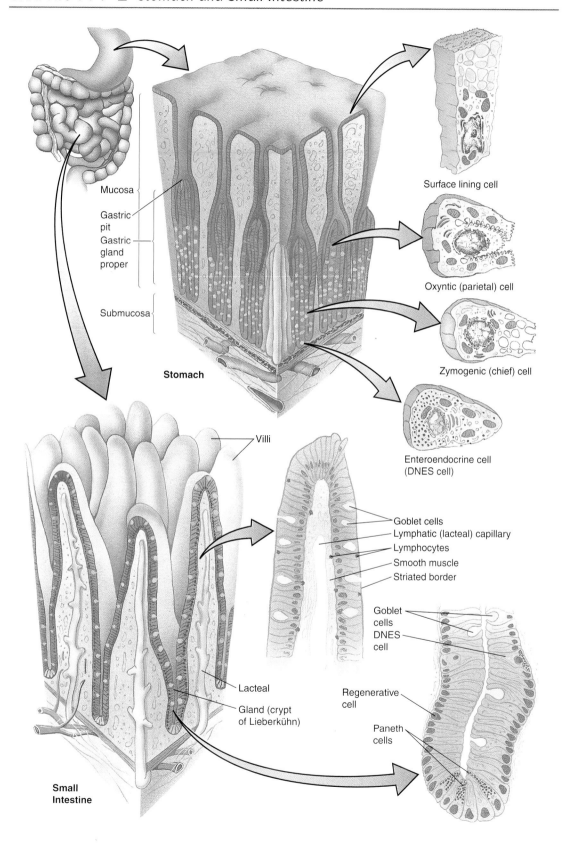

Surface lining cell

Oxyntic (parietal) cell

Zymogenic (chief) cell

Enteroendocrine cell
(DNES cell)

Mucosa

Gastric
pit

Gastric
gland
proper

Submucosa

Stomach

Villi

Goblet cells
Lymphatic (lacteal) capillary
Lymphocytes
Smooth muscle
Striated border

Goblet
cells
DNES
cell

Regenerative
cell

Paneth
cells

Lacteal

Gland (crypt
of Lieberkühn)

**Small
Intestine**

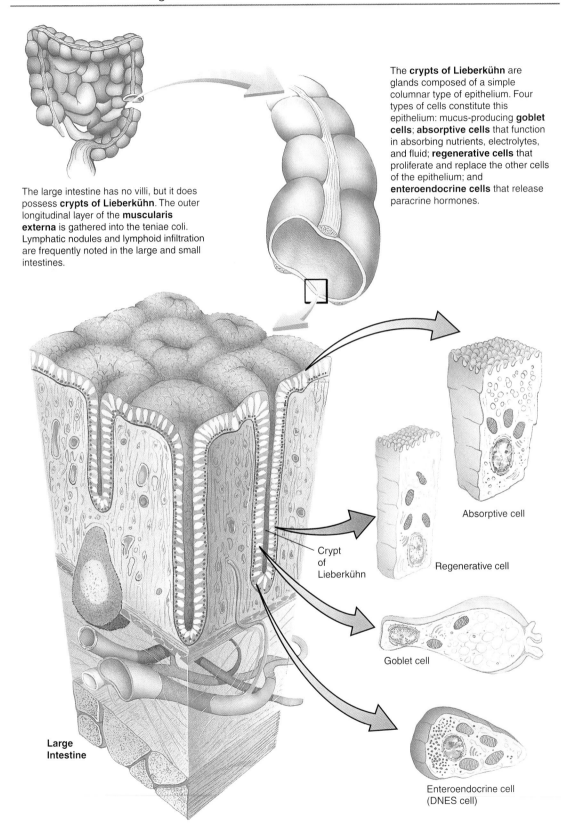

The **crypts of Lieberkühn** are glands composed of a simple columnar type of epithelium. Four types of cells constitute this epithelium: mucus-producing **goblet cells**; **absorptive cells** that function in absorbing nutrients, electrolytes, and fluid; **regenerative cells** that proliferate and replace the other cells of the epithelium; and **enteroendocrine cells** that release paracrine hormones.

The large intestine has no villi, but it does possess **crypts of Lieberkühn**. The outer longitudinal layer of the **muscularis externa** is gathered into the teniae coli. Lymphatic nodules and lymphoid infiltration are frequently noted in the large and small intestines.

Absorptive cell

Regenerative cell

Crypt of Lieberkühn

Goblet cell

Large Intestine

Enteroendocrine cell (DNES cell)

PLATE 14-1 ■ *Esophagus*

FIGURE 1 ■ *Esophagus. x.s. Paraffin section.* × 14.

This photomicrograph of a cross-section of the lower one-third of the esophagus clearly displays the general structure of the digestive tract. The **lumen** (L) is lined by a stratified squamous nonkeratinized **epithelium** (Ep) lying upon a thin **lamina propria** (LP) that is surrounded by the **muscularis mucosae** (MM). The **submucosa** (Sm) contains glands and is surrounded by the **muscularis externa** (ME), composed of an **inner circular** (IC) and an **outer longitudinal** (OL) layer. The outermost tunic of the esophagus is the fibroelastic **adventitia** (Ad). A region similar to the boxed area is presented at a higher magnification in Figure 2.

FIGURE 2 ■ *Esophagus. Human. x.s. Paraffin section.* × 132.

This photomicrograph is a higher magnification of a region similar to the boxed area of the previous figure. The **mucosa** (M) of the esophagus consists of a stratified squamous nonkeratinized **epithelium** (Ep), a loose collagenous connective tissue layer, the **lamina propria** (LP), and a longitudinally oriented smooth muscle layer, the **muscularis mucosae** (MM). The **submucosa** (Sm) is composed of a coarser collagenous **connective tissue** (CT), housing **blood vessels** (BV) and various connective tissue cells whose **nuclei** (N) are readily evident.

FIGURE 3 ■ *Esophagus. Human. x.s. Paraffin section.* × 132.

The **lamina propria** (LP) and **submucosa** (Sm) of the esophagus are separated from each other by the longitudinally oriented smooth muscle bundles, the **muscularis mucosae** (MM). Observe that the lamina propria is a very vascular connective tissue, housing numerous **blood vessels** (BV) and **lymph vessels** (LV), whose valves (arrow) indicate the direction of lymph flow. The submucosa also displays numerous **blood vessels** (BV), as well as the presence of the **esophageal glands proper** (EG) that produce a mucous secretion to lubricate the lining of the esophagus.

FIGURE 4 ■ *Esophagogastric junction. l.s. Dog. Paraffin section.* × 14.

The junction of the **esophagus** (Es) and **cardiac stomach** (CS) is very abrupt as evidenced by the sudden change of the **stratified squamous epithelium** (SE) to the **simple columnar epithelium** (CE) of the stomach. Note that the **esophageal glands proper** (EG) continue for a short distance into the **submucosa** (Sm) of the stomach. Observe also the presence of gastric pits (arrows) and the increased thickness of the **muscularis externa** (ME) of the stomach compared to that of the esophagus. The outermost tunic of the esophagus inferior to the diaphragm is a **serosa** (Se) rather than an adventitia. The boxed area is presented at a higher magnification in Figure 1 of the next plate.

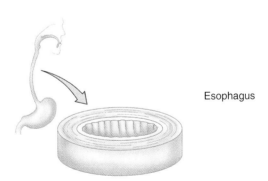

Esophagus

■ **KEY**

Ad	adventitia	Es	esophagus	N	nucleus
BV	blood vessels	IC	inner circular muscle	OL	outer longitudinal muscle
CE	simple columnar epithelium	L	lumen	SE	stratified squamous epithelium
CS	cardiac stomach	LP	lamina propria	Se	serosa
CT	connective tissue	LV	lymph vessels	Sm	submucosa
EG	esophageal glands proper	M	mucosa		
EP	epithelium	ME	muscularis externa		
		MM	muscularis mucosae		

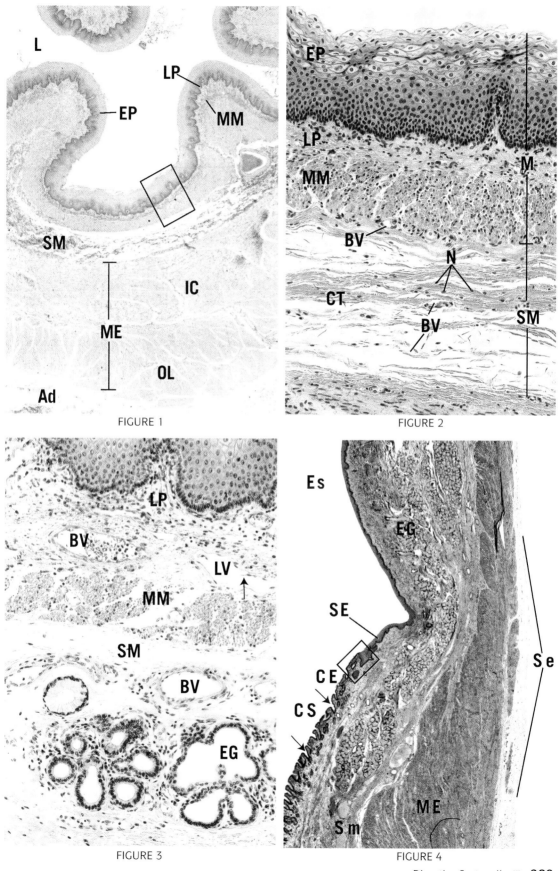

L

LP

EP

MM

EP

SM

IC

ME

OL

Ad

FIGURE 1

EP

LP

MM

M

BV

N

CT

BV

SM

FIGURE 2

LP

BV

LV

MM

SM

BV

EG

FIGURE 3

Es

EG

SE

CE

CS

Se

ME

Sm

FIGURE 4

PLATE 14-2 ■ *Stomach*

FIGURE 1 ■ *Esophagogastric junction. l.s. Dog. Paraffin section.* × 132.

This photomicrograph is a higher magnification of the boxed region of Figure 4, Plate 14-1. The **stratified squamous epithelium** (SE) of the esophagus is replaced by the **simple columnar epithelium** (CE) of the stomach in a very abrupt fashion (arrow). The **lamina propria** (LP) displays **gastric pits** (GP), lined by the typical mucus-secreting **surface lining cells** (SC), characteristic of the stomach. The structure labeled with an asterisk is not a lymphatic nodule, but a more or less tangential section through the esophageal epithelium. Note the presence of the **muscularis mucosae** (MM).

FIGURE 2 ■ *Fundic stomach. l.s. Paraffin section.* × 14.

The fundic region presents all of the characteristics of the stomach, as demonstrated by this low-power photomicrograph. The **lumen** (L) is lined by a simple columnar epithelium, deep to which is the **lamina propria** (LP) housing numerous **gastric glands** (GG). Each gland opens into the base of a **gastric pit** (GP). The **muscularis mucosae** (MM) separates the lamina propria from the **submucosa** (Sm), a richly **vascularized** (BV) connective tissue, thrown into folds (rugae) in the empty stomach. The **muscularis externa** (ME) is composed of three poorly defined layers of smooth muscle: **innermost oblique** (IO), **middle circular** (MC), and **outer longitudinal** (OL). Serosa (arrow) forms the outermost tunic of the stomach. A region similar to the boxed area is presented at a higher magnification in Figure 3.

FIGURE 3 ■ *Fundic stomach. x.s. Dog. Paraffin section.* × 132.

This photomicrograph presents a higher magnification of a region similar to the boxed area of Figure 2. The mucosa of the fundic stomach displays numerous **gastric pits** (GP) that are lined by a simple columnar epithelium, consisting mostly of mucus-producing **surface lining (surface mucous) cells** (SC). The base of each pit accepts the isthmus of two to four **fundic glands** (FG). Although fundic glands are composed of several cell types, only two, **parietal cells** (PC) and **chief cells** (CC), are readily distinguishable in this preparation. The **lamina propria** (LP) is richly **vascularized** (BV). Note the **muscularis mucosae** (MM) beneath the lamina propria. A region similar to the boxed area is presented at a higher magnification (positioned at a 90° angle) in Figure 4.

FIGURE 4 ■ *Fundic glands. x.s. Paraffin section.* × 540.

This photomicrograph presents a higher magnification (positioned at a 90° angle) of a region similar to the boxed area of Figure 3. The **lumina** (L) of several glands can be recognized. Note that **chief cells** (CC) are granular in appearance and are much smaller than the round, plate-like **parietal cells** (PC). Parietal cells, as their name implies, are located at the periphery of the gland. Slender **connective tissue elements** (CT), housing blood vessels, occupy the narrow spaces between the closely packed glands.

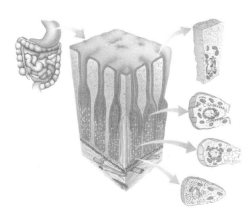

Stomach and cells

■ **KEY**

BV	blood vessels	GP	gastric pits	MM	muscularis mucosae
CC	chief cells	IO	innermost oblique muscle	OL	outer longitudinal muscle
CE	columnar epithelium	L	lumen	PC	parietal cells
CT	connective tissue	LP	lamina propria	SC	surface lining cells
FG	fundic glands	ME	muscularis externa	SE	squamous epithelium
GG	gastric glands	MC	middle circular muscle	Sm	submucosa

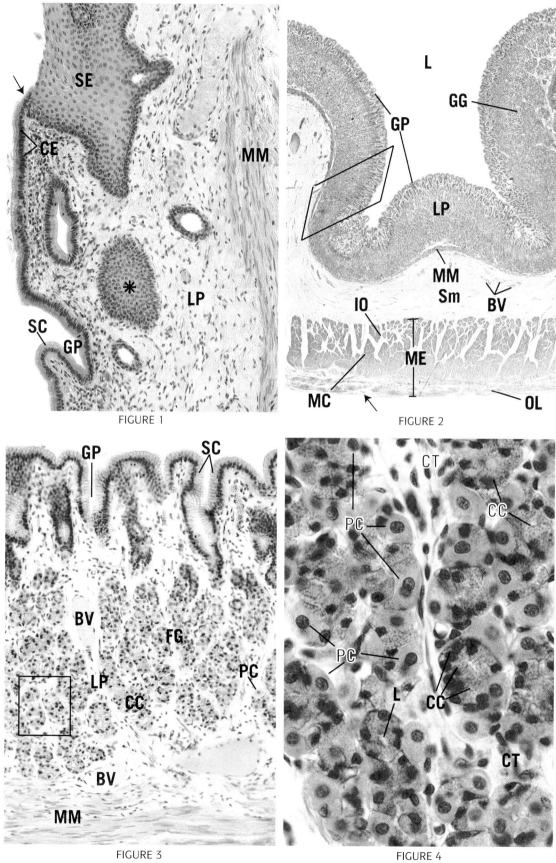

FIGURE 1

FIGURE 2

FIGURE 3

FIGURE 4

PLATE 14-3 ■ *Stomach*

FIGURE 1 ■ *Fundic stomach. x.s. Monkey. Plastic section.* × 270.

The **gastric pits** (GP) of the fundic stomach are lined mostly by mucus-producing **surface lining cells** (SC). Each gastric pit receives two to four fundic glands, simple tubular structures that are subdivided into three regions: isthmus, neck, and base. The isthmus opens directly into the gastric pit and is composed of **immature cells** (Ic), which are responsible for the renewal of the lining of the gastric mucosa, **surface lining cells** (SC), and **parietal cells** (PC). The neck and base of these glands are presented in Figure 2.

FIGURE 2 ■ *Fundic gland. Stomach. x.s. Monkey. Plastic section.* × 270.

The **neck** (n) and **base** (b) of the fundic gland both contain the large, plate-shaped **parietal cells** (PC). The neck also possesses a few immature cells, as well as **mucous neck cells** (Mn), which manufacture a mucous substance. The base of the fundic glands contains numerous acid-manufacturing **parietal cells** (PC) and **chief cells** (CC), which produce digestive enzymes. Note that the lamina propria is tightly packed with glands and that the intervening **connective tissue** (CT) is flimsy in character. The bases of these glands extend to the **muscularis mucosae** (MM).

FIGURE 3 ■ *Pyloric gland. Stomach. x.s. Monkey. Plastic section.* × 132.

The mucosa of the pyloric region of the stomach presents **gastric pits** (GP) that are deeper than those of the cardiac or fundic regions. The deep aspects of these pits are coiled (arrows). As in the other regions of the stomach, the **epithelium** (Ep) is simple columnar, consisting mainly of **surface lining cells** (SC). Note that the **lamina propria** (LP) is loosely packed with **pyloric glands** (PG) and that considerable **connective tissue** (CT) is present. The pyloric glands are composed mainly of **mucous cells** (mc). Observe the two muscle layers of the **muscularis mucosae** (MM). A region similar to the boxed area is presented in Figure 4.

FIGURE 4 ■ *Pyloric gland. Stomach. x.s. Human. Paraffin section.* × 270.

This is a photomicrograph of a region similar to the boxed area of Figure 3. The simple columnar **epithelium** (Ep) of the **gastric pit** is composed mostly of surface lining cells. These pits are not only much deeper than those of the fundic or cardiac regions, but are also somewhat coiled (arrow) as are the **pyloric glands** (PG), which empty into the base of the pits. These glands are populated by **mucus-secreting cells** (mc) similar to mucous neck cells whose **nuclei** (N) are flattened against the basal cell membrane. Note that the glands are not closely packed and that the **lamina propria** (LP) is very cellular and possesses a rich **vascular supply** (BV).

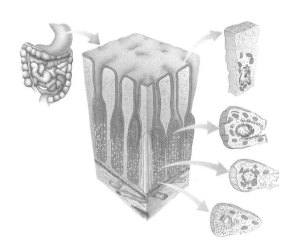

Stomach and cells

■ KEY

b	base	Ic	immature cells	n	neck
BV	blood vessels	LP	lamina propria	PC	parietal cells
CC	chief cells	mc	mucous cells	PG	pyloric glands
CT	connective tissue	MM	muscularis mucosae	SC	surface lining cells
EP	epithelium	Mn	mucous neck cell		
GP	gastric pits	N	nucleus		

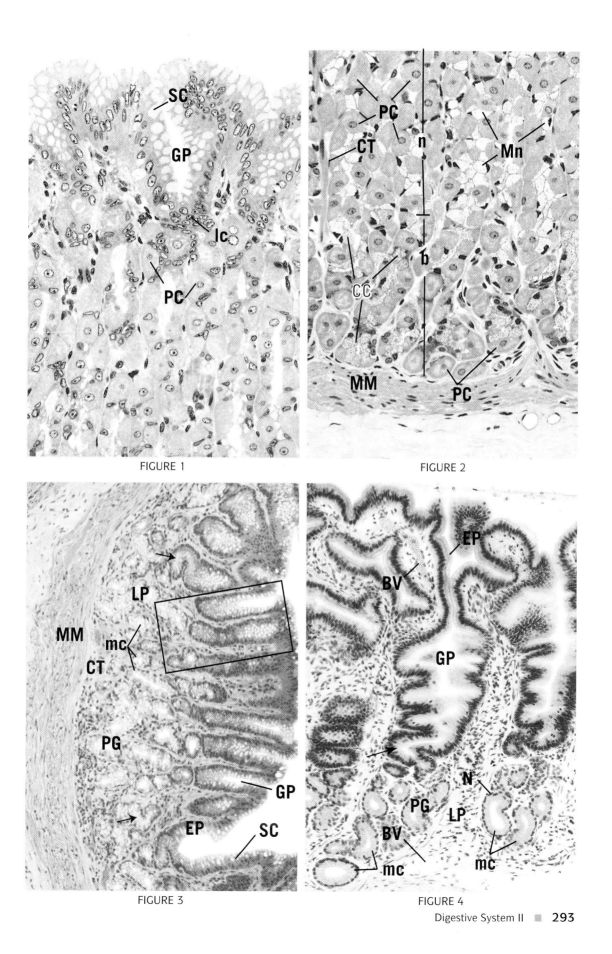

FIGURE 1

FIGURE 2

FIGURE 3

FIGURE 4

Digestive System II ■ 293

PLATE 14-4 ■ *Duodenum*

FIGURE 1A ▨ *Duodenum. l.s. Monkey. Plastic section. Montage.* × 132.

The lamina propria of the duodenum possesses finger-like evaginations, known as **villi** (V), which project into the **lumen** (L). The villi are covered by **surface absorptive cells** (SA), a simple columnar type of epithelium with a brush border. Interspersed among these surface absorptive cells are **goblet cells** (GC), as well as occasional APUD cells. The **connective tissue** (CT) core (lamina propria) of the villus is composed of lymphoid and other cellular elements whose nuclei stain very intensely. Blood vessels also abound in the lamina propria, as well as large, blindly ending lymphatic channels, known as **lacteals** (l), recognizable by their large size and lack of red blood cells. Frequently, these lacteals are collapsed. The deeper aspect of the lamina propria houses glands, the **crypts of Lieberkühn** (CL). These simple tubular glands deliver their secretions into the intervillar spaces. The bases of these crypts reach the **muscularis mucosae** (MM), composed of inner circular and outer longitudinal layers of smooth muscle. Deep to this muscle layer is the submucosa, which, in the duodenum, is occupied by compound tubular **glands of Brunner** (GB). These glands deliver their mucous secretion via **ducts** (D), which pierce the muscularis mucosae, into the crypts of Lieberkühn. A region similar to the boxed area is presented at a higher magnification in Figure 1b.

FIGURE 1B ▨ *Epithelium and core of villus. Monkey. Plastic section.* × 540.

This higher magnification of a region similar to the boxed area presents the epithelium and part of the connective tissue core of a villus. Note that the **surface absorptive cells** (SA) display a **brush border** (BB), terminal bars (arrow), and **goblet cells** (GC). Although APUD cells are also present, they constitute only a small percentage of the cell population. The **lamina propria** (LP) core of the villus is highly cellular, housing **lymphoid cells** (LC), **smooth muscle cells** (SM), mast cells, **macrophages** (Ma), and fibroblasts, among others.

FIGURE 2 ▨ *Duodenum. l.s. Monkey. Plastic section.* × 132.

This photomicrograph is a continuation of the montage presented in Figure 1a (compare asterisks). Note that the **submucosa** (Sm), occupied by **glands of Brunner** (GB), is a **vascular** structure (BV) and also houses Meissner's submucosal plexus. The submucosa extends to the **muscularis externa** (ME), composed of an **inner circular** (IC) and **outer longitudinal** (OL) smooth muscle layer. Note the presence of **Auerbach's myenteric plexus** (AP) between these two muscle layers. The duodenum, in part, is covered by a **serosa** (Se), whose mesothelium provides this organ with a smooth, moist surface.

FIGURE 3A ▨ *Duodenum. x.s. Monkey. Plastic section.* × 540.

The base of the crypt of Lieberkühn displays the several types of cells that compose this gland. **Paneth cells** (Pc) are readily recognizable due to the large granules in their apical cytoplasm. **DNES cells** (APD) are clear cells with fine granules usually located basally. **Goblet cells** (GC), **columnar cells** (Cc), and **stem cells** (Sc) constitute the remaining cell population.

FIGURE 3B ▨ *Duodenum. x.s. Monkey. Plastic section.* × 540.

The submucosa of the intestinal tract displays small parasympathetic ganglia, Meissner's submucosal plexus. Note the large, **postganglionic cell bodies** (PB) surrounded by elements of **connective tissue** (CT).

▨ KEY

AP	Auerbach's plexus	GC	goblet cell	OL	outer longitudinal muscle
APD	DNES cell	IC	inner circular muscle	PB	postganglionic cell body
BB	brush border	I	lacteal	Pc	Paneth cell
BV	blood vessels	L	lumen	SA	surface absorptive cell
Cc	columnar cell	LC	lymphoid cell	Sc	stem cell
CL	crypts of Lieberkühn	LP	lamina propria	Se	serosa
CT	connective tissue	Ma	macrophage	Sm	submucosa
D	duct	ME	muscularis externa	SM	smooth muscle cell
GB	glands of Brunner	MM	muscularis mucosae	V	villi

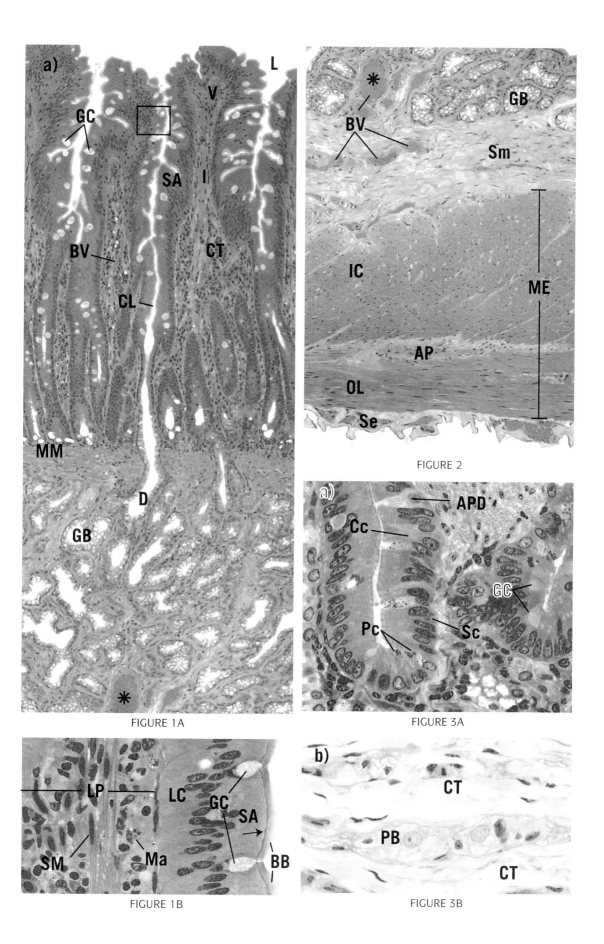

a)

L

V

GC

SA   I

BV   CT

CL

MM

D

GB

*

FIGURE 1A

*

BV

GB

Sm

IC

ME

AP

OL

Se

FIGURE 2

a)

APD

Cc

GC

Pc   Sc

FIGURE 3A

LP   LC

GC

SM   Ma   SA   BB

FIGURE 1B

b)

CT

PB

CT

FIGURE 3B

PLATE 14-5 ■ *Jejunum, Ileum*

FIGURE 1 ▒ *Jejunum. x.s. Monkey. Plastic section.* × 132.

The **mucosa** (M) and **submucosa** (Sm) of the jejunum are presented in this photomicrograph. The **villi** (V) of this region possess more **goblet cells** (GC) than those of the duodenum. Observe that the **crypts of Lieberkühn** (CL) open into the intervillar spaces (arrow) and that the lamina propria displays numerous dense nuclei, evidence of lymphatic infiltration. The flimsy **muscularis mucosae** (MM) separates the lamina propria from the submucosa. Large **blood vessels** (BV) occupy the submucosa, which is composed of a loose type of collagenous connective tissue. The **inner circular** (IC) layer of the muscularis externa is evident at the bottom of the photomicrograph. The boxed region is presented at a higher magnification in Figure 2.

FIGURE 3 ▒ *Ileum. l.s. Human. Paraffin section.* × 14.

The entire wall of the ileum is presented, displaying spiral folds of the submucosa that partially encircle the lumen. These folds, known as **plicae circulares** (Pci) increase the surface area of the small intestines. Note that the lamina propria is clearly delineated from the **submucosa** (Sm) by the muscularis mucosae. The lamina propria forms numerous **villi** (V) that protrude into the **lumen** (L), and glands, known as **crypts of Lieberkühn** (CL), deliver their secretions into the intervillar spaces. The submucosa abuts the **inner circular** (IC) layer of smooth muscle that, in turn, is surrounded by the **outer longitudinal** (OL) smooth muscle layer of the muscularis externa. Observe the **serosa** (Se) investing the ileum. A region similar to the boxed area is presented at a higher magnification in Figure 4.

FIGURE 2 ▒ *Jejunum. x.s. Monkey. Plastic section.* × 540.

This photomicrograph is a higher magnification of the boxed area of Figure 1. The crypts of Lieberkühn are composed of several cell types, some of which are evident in this figure. **Goblet cells** (GC) that manufacture mucus may be noted in various degrees of mucus production. Narrow **stem cells** (Sc) undergo mitotic activity (arrowhead), and newly formed cells reconstitute the cell population of the crypt and villus. **Paneth cells** (PC) are located at the base of crypts and may be recognized by their large granules. **DNES cells** (APD) appear as clear cells, with fine granules usually basally located. The lamina propria displays numerous **plasma cells** (PIC).

FIGURE 4 ▒ *Ileum. x.s. Monkey. Plastic section.* × 132.

This is a higher magnification of a region similar to the boxed area of Figure 3. Note that the **villi** (V) are covered by a simple columnar epithelium, whose cellular constituents include numerous **goblet cells** (GC). The core of the villus displays **blood vessels** (BV), as well as a large lymphatic vessel, known as a **lacteal** (l). The **crypts of Lieberkühn** (CL) open into the intervillar spaces (arrow). The group of lymphatic nodules of the ileum are known as **Peyer's patches** (PP).

Inset a. **Crypt of Lieberkühn. l.s. Monkey. Plastic section.** × 540.

The crypts of Lieberkühn also possess **DNES cells** (APD), recognizable by their clear appearance and usually basally oriented fine granules.

Inset b. **Crypt of Lieberkühn. l.s. Monkey. Plastic section.** × 540.

The base of the crypt of Lieberkühn displays cells with large granules. These cells are **Paneth cells** (PC) that produce the bacteriocidal agent lysozyme.

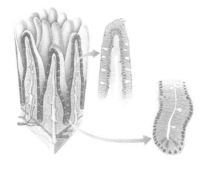

Small intestine

■ KEY

APD	DNES cell	L	lumen	PP	Peyer's patch
BV	blood vessels	M	mucosa	OL	outer longitudinal muscle
CL	crypts of Lieberkühn	MM	muscularis mucosae	Sc	stem cell
GC	goblet cell	PC	Paneth cell	Se	serosa
IC	inner circular muscle	Pci	plicae circulares	Sm	submucosa
l	lacteal	PIC	plasma cell	V	villi

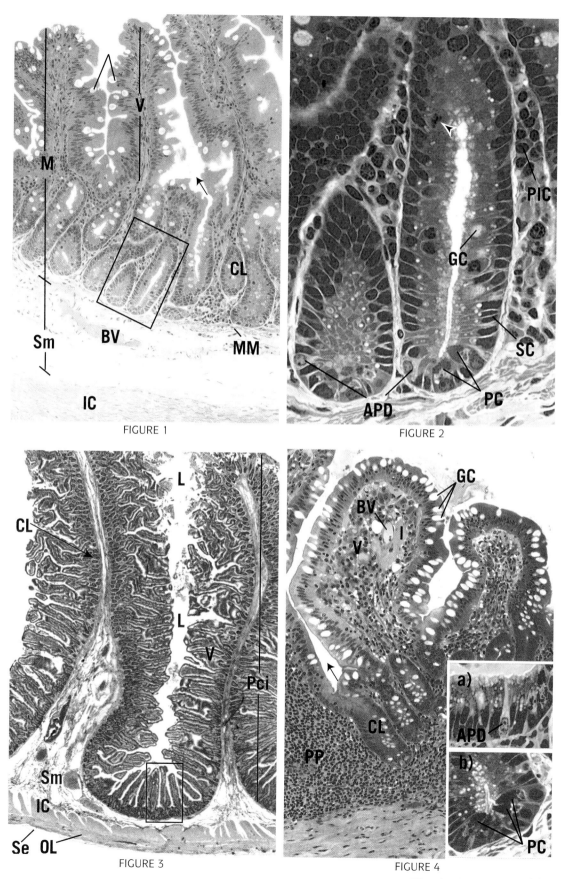

FIGURE 1

FIGURE 2

FIGURE 3

FIGURE 4

a)

b)

Digestive System II ■ 297

PLATE 14-6 ■ *Colon, Appendix*

FIGURE 1 ■ *Colon. l.s. Monkey. Plastic section.* × 132.

This photomicrograph depicts the mucosa and part of the submucosa of the colon. Note the absence of surface modifications such as pits and villi, which indicate that this section is not of the stomach or small intestines. The epithelium (Ep) lining the lumen (L) is simple columnar with numerous goblet cells (GC). The straight tubular glands are crypts of Lieberkühn (CL), which extend down to the muscularis mucosae (MM). The inner circular (IC) and outer longitudinal (OL) layers of smooth muscle comprising this region of the mucosa are clearly evident. The submucosa (Sm) is very vascular (BV) and houses numerous fat cells (FC). The boxed area is presented at a higher magnification in Figure 2.

FIGURE 2 ■ *Colon. l.s. Monkey. Plastic section.* × 540.

This photomicrograph is a higher magnification of the boxed area of Figure 1. The cell population of the crypts of Lieberkühn (CL) is composed of numerous goblet cells (GC), which deliver their mucus into the lumen (L) of the crypt. Surface epithelial cells (SEC), as well as undifferentiated stem cells are also present. The latter undergo mitosis (arrow) to repopulate the epithelial lining. DNES cells (APD) constitute a small percentage of the cell population. Note that Paneth cells are not present in the colon. The lamina propria (LP) is very cellular, housing many lymphoid cells (LC). The inner circular (IC) and outer longitudinal (OL) smooth muscle layers of the muscularis mucosae (MM) are clearly evident.

FIGURE 3 ■ *Appendix. x.s. Paraffin section.* × 132.

The cross-section of the appendix displays a lumen (L) that frequently contains debris (arrow). The lumen is lined by a simple columnar epithelium (Ep), consisting of many goblet cells (GC). Crypts of Lieberkühn (CL) are relatively shallow in comparison with those of the colon. The lamina propria (LP) is highly infiltrated with lymphoid cells (LC), derived from lymphatic nodules (LN) of the submucosa (Sm) and lamina propria. The muscularis mucosae (MM) delineates the border between the lamina propria and the submucosa.

FIGURE 4 ■ *Anorectal junction. l.s. Human. Paraffin section.* × 132.

The anorectal junction presents a superficial similarity to the esophagogastric junction because of the abrupt epithelial transition. The simple columnar epithelium (CE) of the rectum is replaced by the stratified squamous epithelium of the anal canal (AC). The crypts of Lieberkühn (CL) of the anal canal are shorter than those of the colon and the lamina propria (LP) is infiltrated by lymphoid cells (LC).

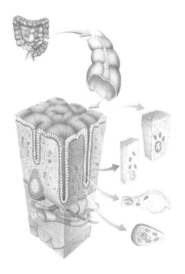

Large intestine and cells

■ **KEY**

AC	anal canal	FC	fat cell	MM	muscularis mucosae
APD	DNES cell	GC	goblet cell	OL	outer longitudinal muscle
BV	blood vessels	IC	inner circular muscle	SE	stratified squamous epithelium
CE	simple columnar epithelium	L	lumen	SEC	surface epithelial cell
CL	crypts of Lieberkühn	LC	lymphoid cell	Sm	submucosa
EP	epithelium	LN	lymphatic nodule		
		LP	lamina propria		

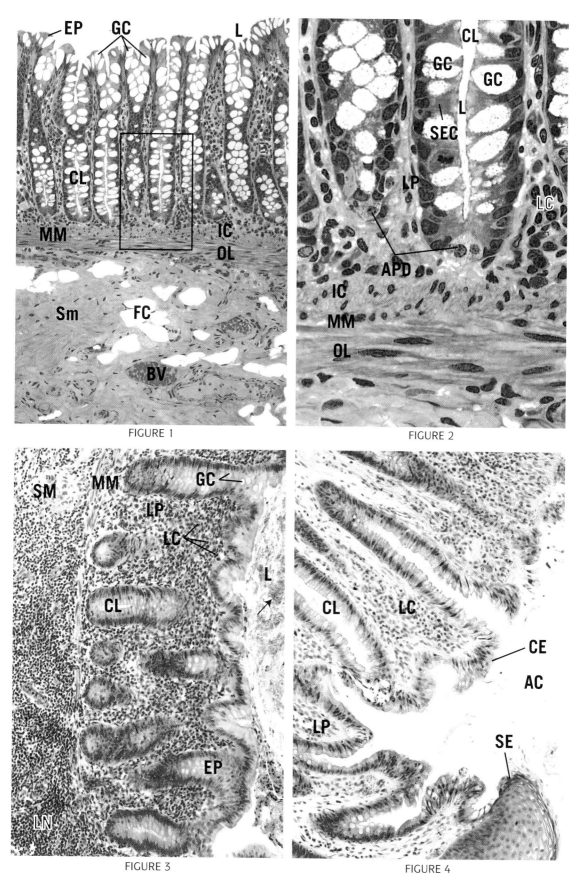

FIGURE 1

FIGURE 2

FIGURE 3

FIGURE 4

Digestive System II ■ 299

PLATE 14-7 ■ *Colon, Electron Microscopy*

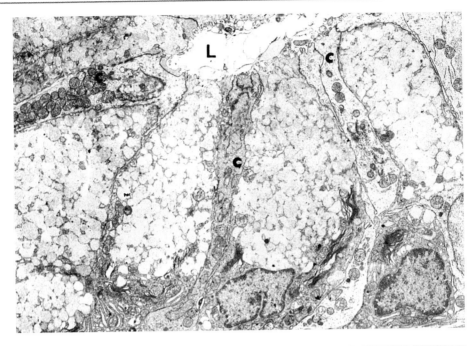

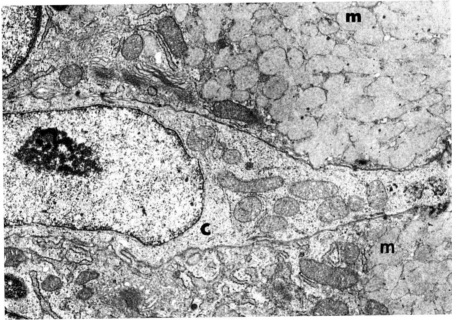

FIGURE 1 ■ *Colon. Rat. Electron microscopy.* × 3780.

The deep aspect of the crypt of Lieberkühn presents **columnar cells** (c) and deep crypt cells that produce a mucous type of secretion that is delivered into the **lumen** (L) of the crypt. (From Altmann GG: *Am J Anat* 167:95–117, 1983.)

FIGURE 2 ■ *Colon. Rat. Electron microscopy.* × 12,600.

At a higher magnification of the deep aspect of the crypt of Lieberkühn, the deep crypt cells present somewhat electron-dense **vacuoles** (m). Note that many of these vacuoles coalesce, forming amorphous vacuolar profiles. The slender **columnar cell** (C) displays no vacuoles, but does possess numerous mitochondria and occasional profiles of rough endoplasmic reticulum. Observe the large, oval nucleus and clearly evident nucleolus. (From Altmann GG: *Am J Anat* 167:95–117, 1983.)

PLATE 14-8 ■ *Colon, Scanning Electron Microscopy*

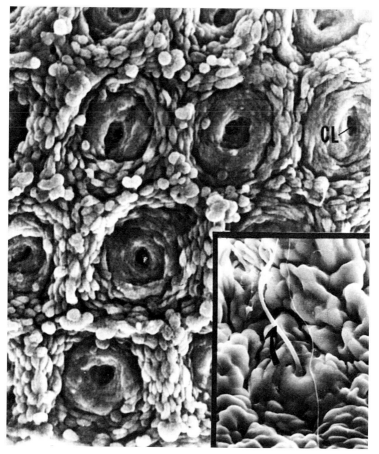

FIGURE 1 ■ *Colon. Monkey. Scanning electron microscopy.* × 614.

This scanning electron micrograph displays the openings of the **crypts of Lieberkühn** (CL), as well as the cells lining the mucosal surface. (From Specian RD, Neutra MR: *Am J Anat* 160:461–472, 1981.)

Inset. Colon. Rabbit. Scanning electron microscopy. × 778.

The openings of the crypts of Lieberkühn are not as regularly arranged in the rabbit as in the monkey. Observe the mucus arising from the crypt opening (arrow). (From Specian RD, Neutra MR: *Am J Anat* 160:461–472, 1981.)

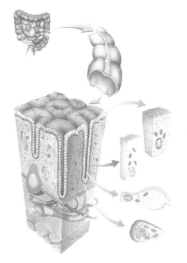

Large intestine and cells

15

Digestive System III

The major **glands of the digestive system** are located outside the wall of the alimentary canal but are connected to its lumen of via ducts. These glands include the major salivary glands, pancreas, and liver.

MAJOR SALIVARY GLANDS

The three **major salivary glands, parotid, submandibular**, and **sublingual**, deliver their secretory product, saliva, into the oral cavity. **Saliva** is composed of a thin watery suspension of enzymes, mucus, inorganic ions, and antibodies. The parotid gland produces **serous secretions**, whereas the submandibular and sublingual glands manufacture **mixed secretions**.

PANCREAS

The **pancreas** is a mixed gland, in that it has exocrine and endocrine functions (see Graphic 15-1). The **exocrine pancreas** produces an alkaline fluid rich in digestive enzymes, which is delivered to the duodenum via the pancreatic duct. The release of the enzymes and alkaline fluid is intermittent and is controlled by the hormones **cholecystokinin** and **secretin**, respectively and the two types of secretions may be delivered independent of each other. These hormones are produced by the **DNES cells** of the epithelial lining of the alimentary tract mucosa. The **endocrine** pancreas is composed of scattered spherical aggregates of richly vascularized cords of endocrine cells, known as **islets of Langerhans**. Five cell types are present in these structures: α (**A**) **cells**, producing **glucagon**; β (**B**) **cells**, manufacturing **insulin**; **G cells**, producing **gastrin**; δ (**D**) **cells**, manufacturing **somatostatin**; and **PP cells**, secreting **pancreatic polypeptide**.

LIVER

The **liver** is the largest gland of the body. It performs a myriad of functions, many of which are not glandular in nature (see Graphic 15-2). The parenchymal cells of the liver, known as **hepatocytes**, perform each of the tasks of the liver. The exocrine by-product, **bile**, is delivered into a system of bile ducts, which then directs the bile into the **gallbladder**, a storage organ associated with the liver. The release of concentrated bile into the duodenum via the cystic and common bile ducts is regulated by hormones of the DNES cells in the alimentary tract. Since each hepatocyte is bordered by a vascular sinusoid, liver cells can absorb toxic materials and by-products of digestion, which they detoxify and store for future use. Additionally, hepatocytes can release various biosynthetic molecules into the bloodstream to be utilized throughout the body. Moreover, foreign particulate matter is phagocytosed in the liver by **Kupffer cells**, macrophages derived from monocytes.

GALLBLADDER

The **gallbladder** is a small, pear-shaped organ that receives bile from the liver. It not only stores but also concentrates bile and, in response to the **cholecystokinin** released by the DNES cells of the alimentary tract, forces the bile into the lumen of the duodenum via the cystic and common bile ducts. The **bile** emulsifies fats, facilitating the action of the enzyme **pancreatic lipase**. The lamina propria, lined by a simple columnar epithelium, is thrown into highly convoluted folds in the empty gallbladder. These folds disappear on distention. Occasionally, tubuloalveolar mucous glands are present.

Histophysiology

I. MAJOR SALIVARY GLANDS

The major salivary glands are the **parotid, submandibular**, and **sublingual glands**. These produce about 1 L of saliva per day, approximately 95% of the daily salivary secretion. These glands possess a secretory component that is responsible for the formation of **primary saliva**, which is modified by the initial portion of the **duct** system (**striated ducts**) to form the **secondary saliva**. Saliva is a **hypotonic** solution whose functions include lubrication and cleansing of the oral cavity (and reducing bacterial flora by **lysozyme, lactoferrin**, and **immunoglobulin A [IgA]**), initial digestion of carbohydrates by **salivary amylase**, and assisting in the process of **taste** (by dissolving food substances).

II. PANCREAS

Acinar cells of the **exocrine pancreas** secrete digestive enzymes in response to the hormone **cholecystokinin**, released by the **enteroendocrine cells** of the small intestine. Some of these enzymes are released as proenzymes (chymotrypsin, trypsin, elastase, and carboxypeptidase), and others are released as active enzymes (DNase, RNase, pancreatic lipase, and pancreatic amylase). In response to **secretin** (released by **enteroendocrine cells** of the small intestine), **centroacinar cells** and cells of **intercalated ducts** release a copious amount of an alkaline fluid that is believed to help neutralize and buffer the acidic chyme entering the duodenum from the stomach.

Islets of Langerhans are composed of five different types of cells, each of which is responsible for the secretion of a hormone.

III. LIVER AND GALLBLADDER

A. Hepatocytes

It is believed that each **hepatocyte** is capable of performing each of the approximately 100 functions of the liver.

Bile formation and secretion are the **exocrine** functions of the liver. Bile is a green, somewhat viscous fluid composed of water, ions, cholesterol, phospholipids, bilirubin glucuronide, and bile acids. One of these components, **bilirubin glucuronide**, is a water-soluble conjugate of nonsoluble **bilirubin**, a toxic breakdown product of **hemoglobin**. It is in the **smooth endoplasmic reticulum (sER)** of the hepatocytes that detoxification of bilirubin occurs.

Detoxification of various drugs, toxins, metabolic by-products, and chemicals occurs either by the **microsomal mixed-function oxidase** system of the sER or by **peroxidases** of peroxisomes.

Endocrine functions of the liver include the synthesis and release of numerous plasma proteins and components, such as fibrinogen, urea, albumin, prothrombin, and lipoproteins; **storage** of glycogen and lipids for release during intervals between eating; synthesis of glucose; **gluconeogenesis** from noncarbohydrate sources (amino acids and lipids); and **transport** of IgA into the bile and, subsequently, into the lumen of the small intestine.

B. Kupffer Cells and Ito Cells

Kupffer cells of the liver participate in removing defunct red blood cells and other undesirable particulate matter from the bloodstream. **Fat-storing (Ito) cells** are believed to function in the accumulation and storage of **vitamin A**.

C. Gallbladder

The **gallbladder** stores and concentrates bile. It releases bile in response to the enteroendocrine cell hormone **cholecystokinin**.

Gastrinoma

Gastrinoma is a disease where the **G cells** of the pancreas undergo **excess proliferation** (frequently cancerous) resulting in an **overproduction of the hormone gastrin**. This hormone is responsible for binding to parietal cells of the stomach causing them to over-secrete hydrochloric acid with a resultant formation of peptic ulcers in the stomach and the duodenum. Antiulcer drugs may alleviate the hyperacidity and resolve the ulcerations; otherwise surgical intervention may be indicated.

Type I Diabetes

Type I (**insulin-dependent**) diabetes is characterized by **polyphagia** (insatiable hunger), **polydipsia** (unquenchable thirst), and **polyuria** (excessive urination). It usually has a sudden onset before 20 years of age, is distinguished by damage to and destruction of beta cells, results from a **low level of plasma insulin**, and is treated with a combination of insulin therapy and diet.

Type II Diabetes Mellitus

Type II (**non-insulin-dependent**) diabetes mellitus commonly occurs in overweight individuals over 40 years of age. It does not result from low levels of plasma insulin and is **insulin resistant**, which is a major factor in its pathogenesis. The resistance to insulin is due to decreased binding of insulin to its plasmalemma receptors and to defects in postreceptor insulin action. Type II diabetes is usually controlled by diet.

Jaundice (Icterus)

Jaundice (icterus) is characterized by excess bilirubin in the blood and deposition of **bile pigment** in the skin and sclera of the eyes, resulting in a yellowish appearance. It may be hereditary or due to pathologic conditions such as excess destruction of red blood cells (**hemolytic jaundice**), liver dysfunction, and obstruction of the biliary passages (**obstructive jaundice**).

Gallstones (Biliary Calculi)

Gallstones (biliary calculi) are concretions, usually of fused crystals of **cholesterol** that form in gallbladder or bile duct. They may accumulate to such an extent that the cystic duct is blocked, thus preventing emptying of the gallbladder, and they may require surgical removal if less invasive methods fail to dissolve or pulverize them.

Summary of Histological Organization

I. MAJOR SALIVARY GLANDS

Three **major salivary glands** are associated with the oral cavity. These are the **parotid, submandibular**, and **sublingual glands**.

A. Parotid Gland

The **parotid gland** is a purely serous **compound tubuloalveolar gland** whose **capsule** sends **septa** (frequently containing adipose cells) into the substance of the gland, dividing it into **lobes** and **lobules**. **Serous acini**, surrounded by **myoepithelial cells**, deliver their secretions into **intercalated ducts**.

B. Submandibular Gland

This compound **tubuloalveolar gland** is mostly **serous**, although it contains enough **mucous units**, capped by **serous demilunes**, to manufacture a mixed secretion. **Acini** are surrounded by **myoepithelial (basket) cells**. The **capsule** sends **septa** into the substance of the gland, subdividing it into **lobes** and **lobules**. The **duct** system is extensive.

C. Sublingual Gland

The **sublingual gland** is a **compound tubuloalveolar gland** whose capsule is not very definite. The gland produces a **mixed** secretion, possessing mostly **mucous acini** capped by **serous demilunes** and surrounded by **myoepithelial (basket) cells**. The **intralobular duct** system is not very extensive.

II. PANCREAS

The **exocrine pancreas** is a **compound tubuloalveolar serous gland** whose connective tissue **capsule** sends **septa** to divide the parenchyma into lobules. **Acini** present **centroacinar cells**, the beginning of the ducts that empty into **intercalated ducts**, which lead to **intralobular**, then **interlobular ducts**. The **main duct** receives secretory products from the interlobular ducts. The **endocrine pancreas** with its **islets of Langerhans** (composed of **A, B, G**, and **D cells**) are scattered among the serous acini.

III. LIVER

A. Capsule

Glisson's capsule invests the liver and sends **septa** into the substance of the liver at the **porta hepatis** to subdivide the parenchyma into lobules.

B. Lobules

1. Classical Lobule
Classical lobules are hexagonal with **portal areas (triads)** at the periphery and a **central vein** in the center. **Trabeculae (plates)** of liver cells anastomose. **Sinusoids** are lined by **sinusoidal lining cells** and **Kupffer cells** (macrophages). Within the **space of Disse**, **fat-accumulating cells** may be noted. **Portal areas** housing **bile ducts, lymph vessels**, and branches of the **hepatic artery** and the **portal vein** are surrounded by **terminal plates** composed of **hepatocytes**. Bile passes peripherally within **bile canaliculi**, intercellular spaces between liver cells, to enter **bile ductules**, then **canals of Hering** (and **cholangioles**), to be delivered to **bile ducts** at the portal areas.

2. Portal Lobule
The apices of triangular cross-sections of **portal lobules** are **central veins**. Thus, **portal areas** form the centers of these lobules. The portal lobule is based on bile flow.

3. Acinus of Rappaport (Liver Acinus)
The **acinus of Rappaport** in section is a diamond-shaped area of the liver whose long axis is the straight line between neighboring **central veins** and whose short axis is the intersecting line between neighboring portal areas. The liver acinus is based on **blood flow**.

IV. GALLBLADDER

The **gallbladder** is connected to the liver via its **cystic duct**, which joins the **common hepatic duct**.

A. Epithelium

The gallbladder is lined by a **simple columnar epithelium**.

B. Lamina Propria

The **lamina propria** is thrown into intricate folds that disappear in the distended gallbladder. **Rokitansky-Aschoff sinuses** (epithelial diverticula) may be present.

C. Muscularis Externa

The **muscularis externa** is composed of an obliquely oriented **smooth muscle** layer.

D. Serosa

Adventitia attaches the gallbladder to the capsule of the liver, while **serosa** covers the remaining surface.

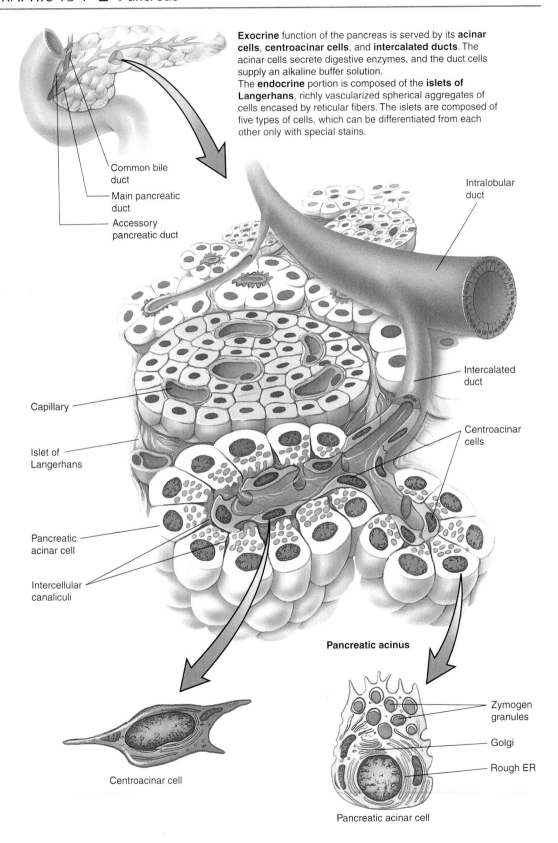

Exocrine function of the pancreas is served by its **acinar cells**, **centroacinar cells**, and **intercalated ducts**. The acinar cells secrete digestive enzymes, and the duct cells supply an alkaline buffer solution.

The **endocrine** portion is composed of the **islets of Langerhans**, richly vascularized spherical aggregates of cells encased by reticular fibers. The islets are composed of five types of cells, which can be differentiated from each other only with special stains.

Common bile duct

Main pancreatic duct

Accessory pancreatic duct

Intralobular duct

Intercalated duct

Capillary

Centroacinar cells

Islet of Langerhans

Pancreatic acinar cell

Intercellular canaliculi

Pancreatic acinus

Centroacinar cell

Zymogen granules

Golgi

Rough ER

Pancreatic acinar cell

GRAPHIC 15-2 ■ *Liver*

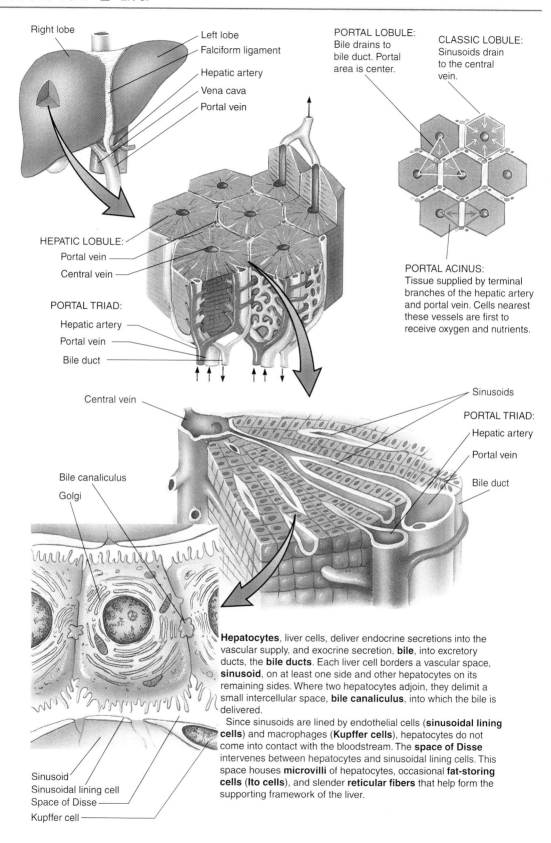

Right lobe

Left lobe

Falciform ligament

Hepatic artery

Vena cava

Portal vein

PORTAL LOBULE:
Bile drains to
bile duct. Portal
area is center.

CLASSIC LOBULE:
Sinusoids drain
to the central
vein.

HEPATIC LOBULE:
Portal vein
Central vein

PORTAL TRIAD:
Hepatic artery
Portal vein
Bile duct

PORTAL ACINUS:
Tissue supplied by terminal
branches of the hepatic artery
and portal vein. Cells nearest
these vessels are first to
receive oxygen and nutrients.

Central vein

Sinusoids

PORTAL TRIAD:
Hepatic artery
Portal vein
Bile duct

Bile canaliculus
Golgi

Sinusoid
Sinusoidal lining cell
Space of Disse
Kupffer cell

Hepatocytes, liver cells, deliver endocrine secretions into the
vascular supply, and exocrine secretion, **bile**, into excretory
ducts, the **bile ducts**. Each liver cell borders a vascular space,
sinusoid, on at least one side and other hepatocytes on its
remaining sides. Where two hepatocytes adjoin, they delimit a
small intercellular space, **bile canaliculus**, into which the bile is
delivered.

Since sinusoids are lined by endothelial cells (**sinusoidal lining
cells**) and macrophages (**Kupffer cells**), hepatocytes do not
come into contact with the bloodstream. The **space of Disse**
intervenes between hepatocytes and sinusoidal lining cells. This
space houses **microvilli** of hepatocytes, occasional **fat-storing
cells (Ito cells)**, and slender **reticular fibers** that help form the
supporting framework of the liver.

PLATE 15-1 ■ *Salivary Glands*

FIGURE 1 ■ *Parotid gland. Monkey. Plastic section.* × 132.

The parotid gland is purely serous with a connective tissue capsule sending **trabeculae** (T) into the substance of the gland, subdividing it into **lobules** (Lo). Slender connective tissue sheets penetrate the lobules, surrounding small **blood vessels** (BV) and **intralobular ducts** (iD). **Interlobular ducts** (ID) are surrounded by increased amounts of **connective tissue** (CT) and large blood vessels. Observe that the **acini** (Ac) are closely packed within each lobule.

Inset. **Parotid gland. Monkey. Plastic section.** × 540.

Note that the round **nuclei** (N) of these serous acini are basally located. The lateral cell membranes (arrows) are not clearly visible, nor are the lumina of the acini. Observe the slender sheets of connective tissue (arrowheads) investing each acinus.

FIGURE 2 ■ *Sublingual gland. Monkey. Plastic section.* × 270.

The sublingual gland is a mixed gland in that it produces both serous and mucous secretory products. The **mucous acini** (MA) possess dark **nuclei** (N) that are flattened against the basal cell membrane. Moreover, the cytoplasm is filled with a "frothy" appearing material, representing the viscous secretory product. Many of the mucous acini are capped by serous cells, forming a crescent-shaped cap, the **serous demilune** (SD). The sublingual gland is subdivided into lobes and lobules by **connective tissue septa** (CT) that act as the supporting network for the nerves, vessels, and ducts of the gland. The boxed area is presented at a higher magnification in Figure 3.

FIGURE 3 ■ *Sublingual gland. Monkey. Plastic section.* × 540.

This photomicrograph is a higher magnification of the boxed area of Figure 2. The flattened, dark **nuclei** (N) of the mucous acini are clearly evident as they appear to be pressed against the basal cell membrane. Observe that much of the cytoplasm is occupied by small, mucin-containing vesicles (arrows), that the lateral cell membrane (arrowheads) are clearly evident, and that the **lumen** (L) is usually identifiable. **Serous demilunes** (SD) are composed of serous-producing cells whose **nuclei** (N) are round to oval in morphology. Note also that the lateral cell membranes are not distinguishable in serous cells.

FIGURE 4 ■ *Submandibular gland. Monkey. Plastic section.* × 132.

The submandibular gland also produces a mixed type of secretion; however, unlike in the sublingual gland, serous acini predominate. **Serous** (SA) and **mucous acini** (MA) are easily distinguishable from each other, but most mucous units display a cap of serous demilunes. Moreover, the submandibular gland is characterized by an extensive system of **ducts** (D), recognizable by their pale cytoplasm, comparatively large **lumina** (L), and round nuclei. This gland is also subdivided into lobes and lobules by **connective tissue septa** (CT).

Inset. **Submandibular gland. Monkey. Plastic section.** × 540.

Note the granular appearance of the cells comprising the **serous demilune** (SD) in contrast with the "frothy" appearing cytoplasm of the **mucous acinus** (MA).

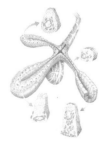

Salivary glands

■ KEY

Ac	acinus	ID	interlobular duct	N	nucleus
BV	blood vessel	L	lumen	SA	serous acini
CT	connective tissue	Lo	lobule	SD	serous demilune
D	duct	MA	mucous acini	T	trabeculae
iD	intralobular duct				

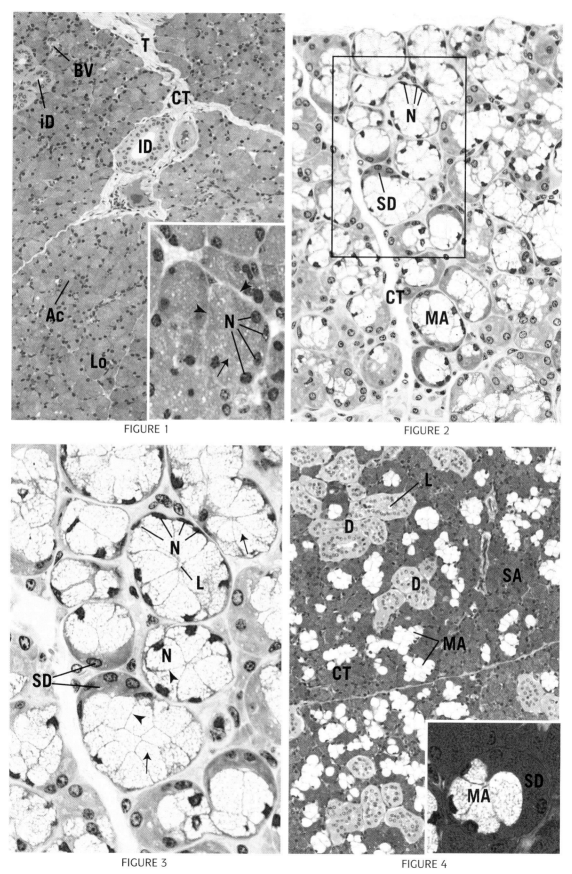

FIGURE 1

FIGURE 2

FIGURE 3

FIGURE 4

PLATE 15-2 ■ *Pancreas*

FIGURE 1 ▦ *Pancreas. Human. Paraffin section.* × 132.

The pancreas is a complex gland since it has both exocrine and endocrine components. The exocrine portion comprises the bulk of the organ as a compound tubuloaveolar gland, secreting a serous fluid. The gland is subdivided into lobules by **connective tissue septa** (CT). Each **acinus** (Ac) is composed of several pyramid-shaped cells, possessing round nuclei. Cells located in the center of the acinus, **centroacinar cells** (CA), form the smallest ducts of the gland. The endocrine portion of the pancreas is composed of small, spherical clumps of cells, **islets of Langerhans** (IL), which are richly endowed by capillaries. These islets of Langerhans are haphazardly scattered among the serous acini of the pancreas. The boxed area is presented at a higher magnification in Figure 2.

FIGURE 3 ▦ *Pancreas. Monkey. Plastic section.* × 540.

With the use of plastic sections, the morphology of the pancreatic acinus is well defined. Observe that in fortuitous sections the acinus resembles a pie, with the individual cells clearly delineated (arrows). The **nucleus** (N) of each trapezoid-shaped cell is round and the basal cytoplasm (arrowhead) is relatively homogeneous, while the apical cytoplasm is packed with **zymogen granules** (ZG). **Centroacinar cells** (CA) may be recognized both by their locations, as well as by the pale appearance of their nuclei.

Inset. **Pancreas. Monkey. Plastic section.** × 540.

Observe the **centroacinar cell** (CA), whose pale nucleus is readily differentiated from the surrounding acinar cell nuclei.

FIGURE 2 ▦ *Pancreas. Human. Paraffin section.* × 270.

This photomicrograph is a higher magnification of the boxed area of Figure 1. Note that the **connective tissue septa** (CT), while fairly extensive in certain regions, are quite slender in the interlobular areas. The trapezoidal morphologies of individual cells of the serous acini are clearly evident in fortuitous sections (arrow). Observe also the **centroacinar cells** (CA), located in the center of acini, which represent the smallest units of the pancreatic duct system.

FIGURE 4 ▦ *Islets of Langerhans. Monkey. Plastic section.* × 270.

The **islets of Langerhans** (IL), the endocrine portion of the pancreas, is a more or less spherical configuration of cells randomly scattered throughout the exocrine portion of the gland. As such, each islet is surrounded by serous **acini** (Ac). The islets receive their rich **blood supply** (BV) from the **connective tissue elements** (CT) of the exocrine pancreas.

Inset. Islets of Langerhans. Monkey. Plastic section. × 540.

Observe the rich vascularity of the islets of Langerhans, as evidenced by the presence of **erythrocyte** (RBC)-engorged blood vessels. Although each islet is composed of A, B, C, and D cells, they can only be distinguished from each other by the use of special stains. However, it should be noted that in the human, B cells are the most populous and are usually located in the center of the islet, while A cells are generally found at the periphery. This situation is reversed in the monkey.

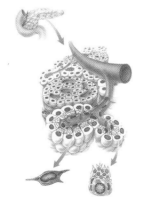

Pancreas and cells

■ **KEY**

Ac	acinus		CT	connective tissue septa		RBC	erythrocyte
BV	blood vessel		IL	islets of Langerhans		ZG	zymogen granule
CA	centroacinar cell		N	nucleus			

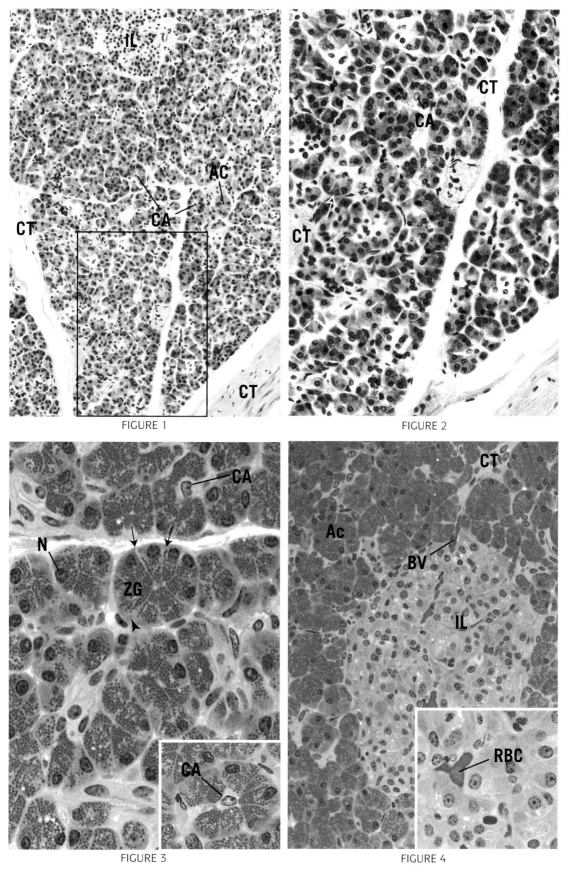

FIGURE 1

FIGURE 2

FIGURE 3

FIGURE 4

PLATE 15-3 ■ *Liver*

FIGURE 1 ▪ *Liver. Pig. Paraffin section.* × 14.

Note that the liver is invested by a connective tissue capsule, **Glisson's capsule** (GC), from which, in the pig, **septa** (S) extend to subdivide the gland into more or less hexagon-shaped classical **lobules** (Lo). Blood vessels, lymph vessels, and bile ducts travel within the connective tissue septa to reach the apices of the classic lobules, which are known as the **portal areas** (PA). Bile reaches the portal areas from within the lobules, while blood enters the substance of the lobules from the portal areas. Within each lobule, the blood flows through tortuous channels, the liver sinusoids, to enter the **central vein** (CV) in the middle of the classical lobule.

FIGURE 2 ▪ *Liver. Dog. Paraffin section.* × 132.

The portal area of the liver houses terminal branches of the **hepatic artery** (HA) and **portal vein** (PV). Note that the vein is much larger than the artery and its wall is very thin in comparison to the size of its lumen. Branches of **lymph vessels** (LV) and **bile ducts** (BD) are also present in the portal area. Bile ducts may be recognized by their cuboidal-to-columnar epithelium. Observe that unlike in the pig, connective tissue septa do not demarcate the boundaries of classic liver lobules, although the various structures of the portal area are invested by connective tissue elements. **Plates of liver cells** (PL) and **sinusoids** (Si) extend from the portal areas.

FIGURE 3 ▪ *Liver. Monkey. Plastic section.* × 132.

The **central vein** (CV) of the liver lobule (a terminal radix of the hepatic vein) collects blood from the **sinusoids** (Si) and delivers it to sublobular veins. The **plates of liver cells** (PL) and hepatic sinusoids appear to radiate, as spokes of a wheel, from the central vein. The boxed area is presented at a higher magnification in Figure 4.

FIGURE 4 ▪ *Liver. Monkey. Plastic section.* × 270.

This photomicrograph is a higher magnification of the boxed area of the previous figure. Note that the lumen of the **central vein** (CV) is lined by a simple squamous **epithelium** (Ep), which is continuous with the endothelial lining of the hepatic **sinusoids** (Si), tortuous vascular channels that freely communicate with each other. Observe also that the **liver plates** (LP) are composed of **hepatocytes** (H), one to two cell layers thick, and that each plate is bordered by sinusoids.

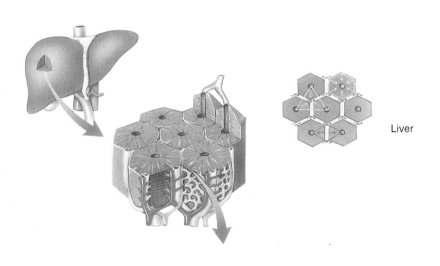

Liver

■ **KEY**

BD	bile duct	HA	hepatic artery	PL	plates of liver cells
CV	central vein	Lo	lobule	PV	portal vein
Ep	epithelium	LP	liver plates	S	septa
GC	Glisson's capsule	LV	lymph vessel	Si	sinusoid
H	hepatocyte	PA	portal area		

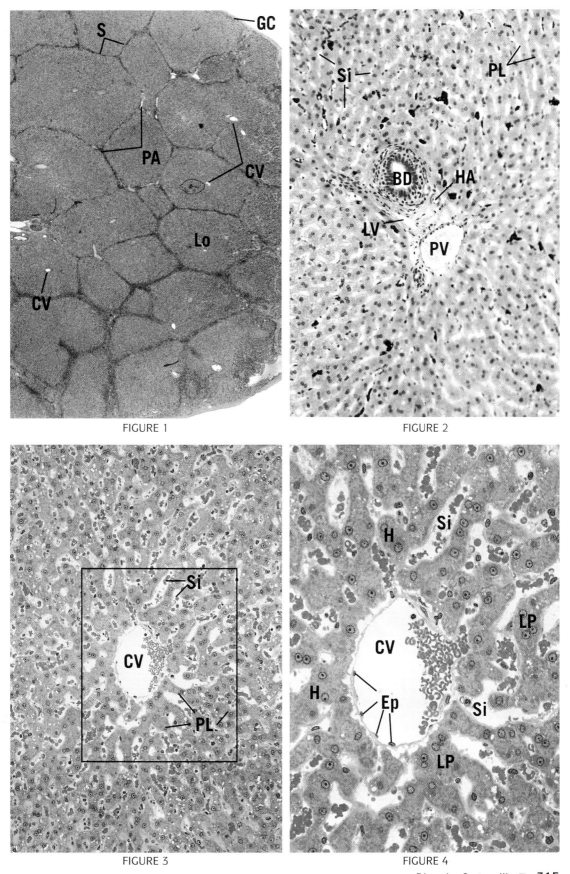

FIGURE 1

FIGURE 2

FIGURE 3

FIGURE 4

PLATE 15-4 ■ *Liver, Gallbladder*

FIGURE 1 ■ *Liver. Monkey. Plastic section.* × 540.

This photomicrograph is a high magnification of **liver plates** (LP). Observe that individual **hepatocytes** (H) are polygonal in shape. Each hepatocyte possesses one or two nuclei, although occasionally some have three nuclei. Plates of hepatocytes enclose hepatic **sinusoids** (Si) that are lined by **sinusoidal lining cells** (SC); therefore, hepatocytes do not come into direct contact with the bloodstream. The space between the sinusoidal lining cells and the hepatocytes, the space of Disse, is at the limit of resolution of the light microscope.

Inset. **Liver. Human. Paraffin section.** × 540.

The hepatocyte cell membranes are clearly evident in this photomicrograph. Note that in fortuitous sections small intercellular spaces (arrows) are recognizable. These are bile canaliculi through which bile flows to the periphery of the lobule.

FIGURE 2 ■ *Liver. Paraffin section.* × 540.

A system of macrophages, known as **Kupffer cells** (KC), are found interspersed among the endothelial lining cells of liver **sinusoids** (Si). These macrophages are larger than the epithelial cells and may be recognized by the presence of phagocytosed material within them. Kupffer cells may be demonstrated by injecting an animal intravenously with India ink, as in this specimen. Observe that some cells appear as large black smudges since they are filled with phagocytosed ink (asterisk) while other cells possess only small quantities of the phagocytosed material (arrowheads). Note also that much of the sinusoidal lining is devoid of ink, indicating that the endothelial cells are probably not phagocytic.

FIGURE 3 ■ *Gallbladder. Human. Paraffin section.* × 132.

The gallbladder is a pear-shaped, hollow organ that functions in storing and concentrating bile. Its histologic structure is relatively simple, but its appearance may be deceiving. The mucosa of an empty gallbladder, as in this photomicrograph, is thrown into numerous folds (arrows), providing it with a glandular morphology. However, close observation of the **epithelium** (Ep) demonstrates that all of the simple columnar cells of the mucous membrane are identical. A loose **connective tissue** (CT), sometimes referred to as a lamina propria, lies deep to the epithelium. Observe that a muscularis mucosae is lacking, and the **smooth muscle** (SM) surrounding the connective tissue is the muscularis externa. The outermost coat of the gallbladder is a serosa or adventitia. A region similar to the boxed area is presented in Figure 4.

FIGURE 4 ■ *Gallbladder. Human. Paraffin section.* × 540.

This photomicrograph is a higher magnification of a region similar to the boxed area of Figure 3. Note that the **epithelium** (Ep) is composed of identical-appearing tall columnar cells, whose **nuclei** (N) are basally oriented. The lateral cell membranes are evident in certain regions (arrows), while the apical brush border is usually not visible in hematoxylin and eosin stained specimens. Observe that a relatively thick **basal membrane** (BM) separates the epithelium from the underlying loose **connective tissue** (CT).

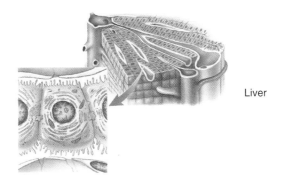

Liver

■ **KEY**

BM	basal membrane	KC	Kupffer cell	Si	sinusoid
CT	connective tissue	LP	liver plate	SM	smooth muscle
Ep	epithelium	N	nucleus		
H	hepatocyte	SC	sinusoidal lining cell		

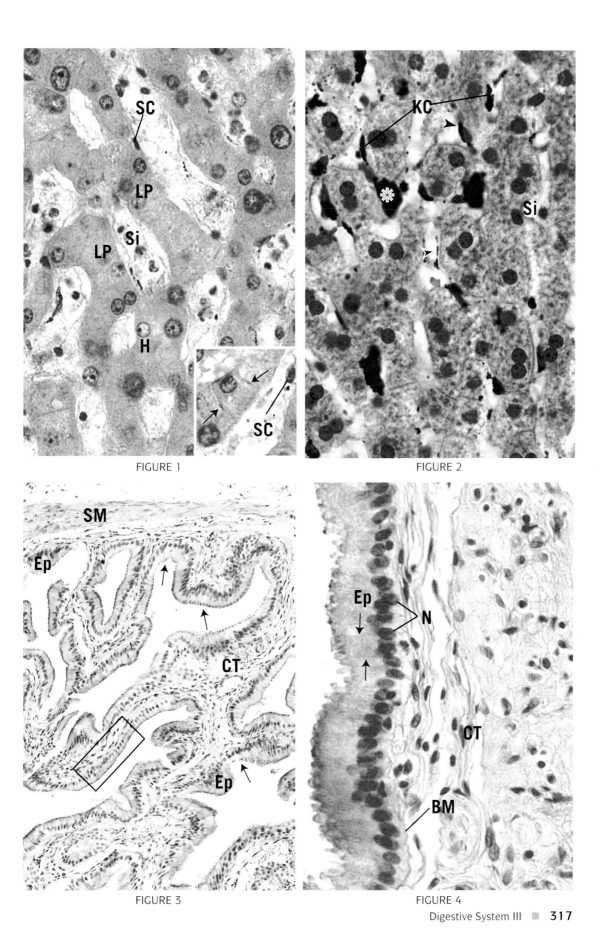

FIGURE 1

FIGURE 2

FIGURE 3

FIGURE 4

Digestive System III ■ **317**

PLATE 15-5 ■ *Salivary Gland, Electron Microscopy*

FIGURE 1 ■ *Sublingual gland. Human. Electron microscopy.* × 4050.

The human sublingual gland is composed mostly of mucous acini capped by serous demilunes. The **mucous cells** (mc) display numerous **filamentous bodies** (f) and secretory granules, which appear to be empty (asterisks). The **serous cells** (dc) may be recognized by their paler cytoplasm and the presence of secretory granules (arrows) housing electron-dense materials. Note also the presence of **myoepithelial cells** (myo), whose processes (arrowheads) encircle the acinus. (Courtesy of Dr. A. Riva.)

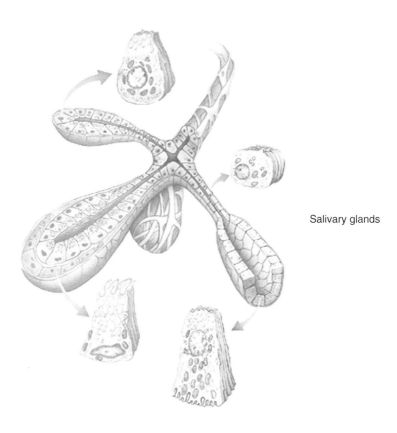

Salivary glands

■ **KEY**

dc	serous cells	mc	mucous cells	myo	myoepithelial cells
f	filamentous bodies				

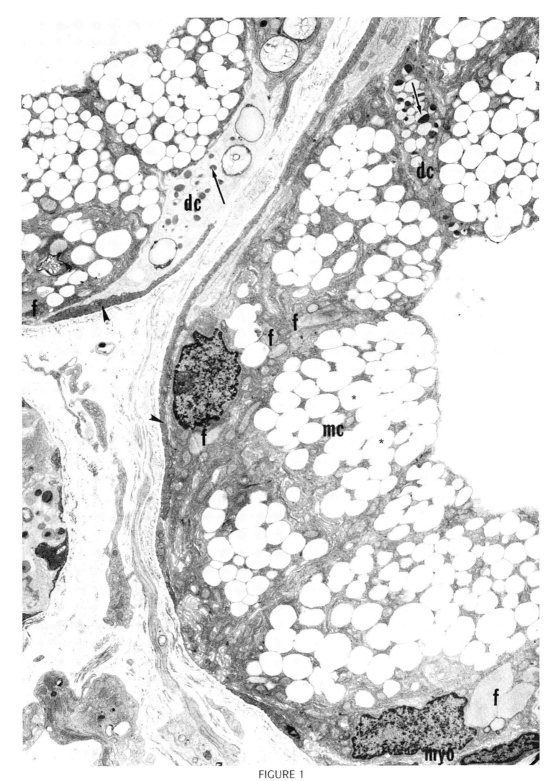

FIGURE 1

PLATE 15-6 ■ *Liver, Electron Microscopy*

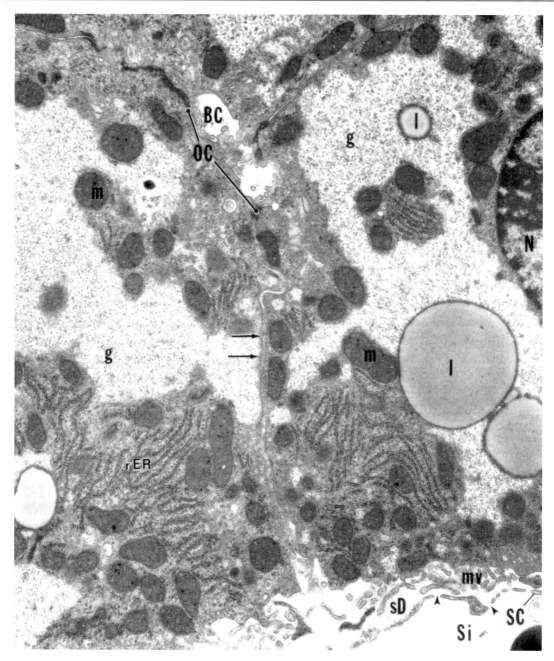

FIGURE 1 ▓ *Liver. Mouse. Electron microscopy.*
× 11,255.

The hepatocytes of this electron micrograph display two of their surfaces, one bordering a **sinusoid** (Si) and the other where two parenchymal cells contact each other (arrows). The sinusoidal surface displays **microvilli** (mv) that extend into the **space of Disse** (sD). They almost contact **sinusoidal lining cells** (SC) that present numerous fenestrae (arrowheads). The parenchymal contacts are characterized by the presence of **bile canaliculi** (BC), intercellular spaces that are isolated by the formation of **occluding junctions** (OC). The cytoplasm of hepatocytes houses the normal cellular complements, such as numerous **mitochondria** (m), elements of **rough endoplasmic reticulum** (rER), Golgi apparatus, smooth endoplasmic reticulum, lysosomes, and inclusions such as **glycogen** (g) and **lipid droplets** (l). The **nucleus** (N) of one of the hepatocytes is clearly evident.

PLATE 15-7 ■ *Islet of Langerhans, Electron Microscopy*

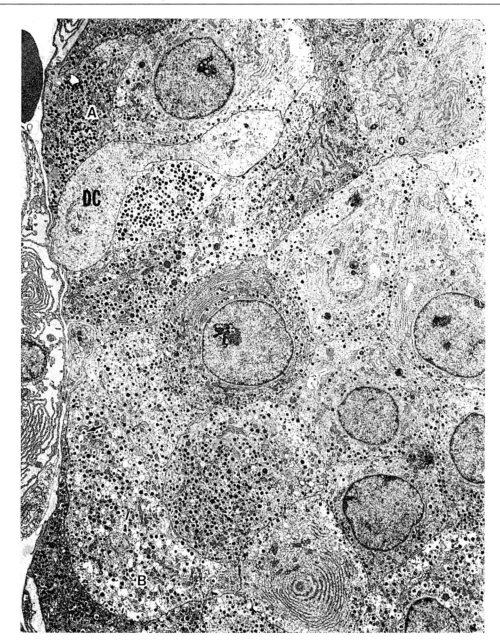

FIGURE 1 ■ *Islet of Langerhans. Rabbit. Electron microscopy.* × 3578.

The islets of Langerhans house four types of parenchymal cells, namely A, B, C, and D cells. **B cells** (B) are the most numerous and may be recognized by the presence of secretory granules whose electron-dense core is surrounded by a clear zone (arrows). **A cells** (A), the second most numerous secretory cell, also house many secretory granules; however, these lack an electron-lucent periphery. **D cells** (DC) are the least numerous and are characterized by secretory granules that are much less electron-dense than those of the other two cell types. (From Sato T, Herman L: *Am J Anat* 161:71–84, 1981.)

Urinary System

The urinary system, composed of the kidneys, ureters, urinary bladder, and urethra, functions in the formation of urine, regulation of blood pressure and fluid volume of the body, acid-base balance, and formation and release of certain hormones.

The functional unit of the kidney is the **uriniferous tubule (see Graphic 16-1)**, consisting of the **nephron** and the **collecting tubule**, each of which is derived from a different embryologic primordium.

KIDNEY

The **kidneys** possess a convex and a concave border, the latter of which is known as the **hilum**. It is here that arteries enter and the ureter and veins leave the kidney. Each kidney is divided into a **cortex** and a **medulla**.

The cortical region is subdivided into the **cortical labyrinth** and the **medullary rays**. The medulla is composed of 10–18 **renal pyramids**, each of whose apex is perforated by 15–20 **papillary ducts** (of Bellini) at the **area cribrosa**. Each renal pyramid is said to constitute a **lobe** of the kidney. The region of the medulla between neighboring renal pyramids is occupied by cortical-like material known as **renal columns** (of Bertin). Each medullary ray is an extension of the renal medulla into the cortex, where it forms the core of a kidney **lobule**.

To understand the histophysiology of the kidney, its vascular supply must be appreciated. Each kidney is supplied by the renal artery, a direct branch of the abdominal aorta. This vessel subdivides into several major branches as it enters the hilum of the kidney. Each branch subsequently divides to give rise to two or more interlobar arteries.

Interlobar arteries pass between neighboring pyramids toward the cortex and, at the corticomedullary junction, give rise to **arcuate arteries** that follow the base of the pyramid. Small, **interlobular arteries** derived from arcuate arteries enter the cortical labyrinth (equidistant from neighboring medullary rays) to reach the **renal capsule**. Along the extent of the interlobular arteries, smaller vessels, **afferent glomerular arterioles**, arise, become enveloped by **Bowman's capsule,** and form a capillary plexus known as the **glomerulus.**

Collectively, Bowman's capsule and the glomerulus are referred to as the **renal corpuscle** (see Graphic 16-2). Efferent glomerular arterioles drain the glomerulus, passing into the cortex, where they form the **peritubular capillary network,** or into the medulla as **arteriolae rectae spuriae,** a part of the vasa recta.

The interstitium of the cortical labyrinth and the capsule are drained by **interlobular veins**, most of which enter the **arcuate veins**, tributaries of the **interlobar veins**. Blood from the interlobar veins enters the **renal vein**, which delivers its contents to the inferior vena cava.

Uriniferous Tubule

The functional unit of the kidney is the **uriniferous tubule**, consisting of the **nephron** and the **collecting tubule**, each of which is derived from a different embryologic primordium.

Nephron

There are two types of nephrons, classified by the location of their renal corpuscles in the kidney cortex: **juxtamedullary,** possessing long thin limbs of Henle's loop, and **cortical**. It is the long thin limbs of Henle's loop that assist in the establishment of a concentration gradient in the renal medulla, permitting the formation of hypertonic urine.

The nephron begins as a distended, blindly ending invaginated region of the tubule, known as **Bowman's capsule.** The modified cells of the inner, **visceral layer** are known as **podocytes.** Some of their **primary (major)** processes but mainly their secondary processes and terminal **pedicels** wrap around the glomerular capillaries. These capillaries are fenestrated with large pores (60–90 nm in diameter) lacking diaphragms.

A thick **basal lamina** is derived from and is interposed between the podocytes and the endothelial cells of the capillary. The spaces between adjoining pedicels, known as **filtration slits**, are bridged by thin **slit diaphragms** that extend from one pedicel to the next. Interstitial tissue composed of **intraglomerular mesangial cells** and the extracellular matrix they manufacture is also associated with the glomerulus.

The ultrafiltrate from the capillaries enters **Bowman's (urinary) space** and is drained from there by the **neck** of the **proximal tubule**. The simple cuboidal epithelium of the proximal tubule adjoins the simple squamous epithelium of the parietal layer of Bowman's capsule.

The cells of the next portion, the **proximal convoluted tubule**, possess an extensive **brush border** (microvilli) on their luminal surface. Their lateral and basal plasma membranes are considerably convoluted, forming numerous interdigitations with membranes of adjoining cells. The exaggerated folding of the basal plasmalemma presents a region rich in mitochondria and provides a striated appearance when viewed with the light microscope.

The straight portion, or **pars recta**, of the proximal tubules is also referred to as the **descending thick limb of Henle's loop**. It is histologically similar to the convoluted portion; however, its brush border becomes shorter at its distal terminus, where it joins the descending thin limb of Henle's loop.

The **descending thin limb** of juxtaglomerular nephrons extends to the apex of the medullary pyramid, where it forms a hairpin loop and continues toward the cortex as the **ascending thin limb of Henle's loop**. The thin limbs of Henle's loop are composed of simple squamous epithelial cells (types I–IV) whose structure varies according to their permeability to water, organelle content, and complexity of tight junctions. Type I cells are present only in cortical nephrons, whereas type II, III, and IV cells are present in juxtaglomerular nephrons.

The **ascending thick limb of Henle's loop** is also known as the **pars recta of the distal tubule**. It is composed of simple cuboidal cells that resemble the cells of the **distal convoluted tubule**. Cells of the distal tubule that contact the afferent (and efferent) glomerular arteriole are modified, in that they are thin, tall cuboidal cells whose nuclei are close to one another. This region is referred to as the macula densa of the distal tubule.

Cells of the **macula densa** communicate with modified smooth muscle cells, **juxtaglomerular (JG) cells**, of the afferent (and efferent) glomerular arterioles. The macula densa and the JG cells together form the **juxtaglomerular apparatus**. Frequently, the extraglomerular mesangial cells, also known as lacis cells, are likewise considered to belong to the juxtaglomerular apparatus.

Collecting Duct

Several distal convoluted tubules join each **collecting duct**, which is composed of a simple cuboidal epithelium whose lateral cell membranes are clearly evident with the light microscope. The collecting ducts descend from the medullary rays of the cortex through the renal pyramids. As they descend, several collecting ducts merge to form the ducts of Bellini, which terminate at the area cribrosa.

The **ducts of Bellini** then deliver the urine formed by the uriniferous tubule to the intrarenal passage, namely, the **minor calyx**, to be drained into a **major calyx** and then into the **pelvis** of the **ureter**. These excretory passages, lined by **transitional epithelium**, possess a fibroelastic subepithelial connective tissue, a smooth muscle tunic composed of **inner longitudinal** and **outer circular** layers, as well as a fibroelastic adventitia.

EXTRARENAL EXCRETORY PASSAGES

The **extrarenal excretory passages** consist of the ureters, urinary bladder, and urethra. The ureters and bladder are also lined by transitional epithelia. The **ureters** possess a fibroelastic lamina propria and two to three layers of smooth muscle, arranged as above. The third muscle layer, the **outermost longitudinal layer**, appears in the lower one-third of the ureter.

The **transitional epithelial lining** of the **bladder** and of the other urinary passages offers an impermeable barrier to urine. To be able to perform its function, the plasma membrane of the surfacemost cells is thicker than the average plasma membrane and is composed of a lattice structure consisting of hexagonally arrayed elements. Furthermore, since cells of the transitional epithelium must line an ever larger surface as the urinary bladder distends, the plasma membrane is folded in a mosaic-like fashion. Folding occurs at the **interplaque regions**, whereas the thickened **plaque regions** present **vesicular profiles**, which probably become unfolded as urine accumulates in the bladder.

The subepithelial connective tissue of the bladder is composed, according to most, of a lamina propria and a submucosa. The three smooth muscle layers are extensively interlaced, making them indistinguishable in some areas.

The **urethra** of the male differs from that of the female not only in its length but also in its function and epithelial lining. The lamina propria of both sexes contain mucous **glands of Littré** and **intraepithelial glands**, which lubricate the lining of the urethra, facilitating the passage of urine to the outside.

Histophysiology

I. FORMATION OF THE ULTRAFILTRATE

Since the renal artery is a direct branch of the abdominal aorta, the two kidneys receive 20% of the total blood volume per minute. Most of this blood enters the glomeruli, where the high arterial pressure expresses approximately 10% of its fluid volume, 125 mL/min, into Bowman's spaces. Vascular pressure is opposed by two forces, the **colloid osmotic pressure** of the blood and the pressure exerted by the ultrafiltrate present in Bowman's space.

The renal **filtration barrier**, composed of the fenestrated endothelial cell, the fused **basal laminae** of the podocyte and capillary, and the diaphragm-bridged filtration slits between pedicels, permits only the passage of water, ions, and small molecules into Bowman's space. The presence of the polyanionic **heparan sulfate** in the **lamina rara** of the basal lamina impedes the passage of large and negatively charged proteins through the barrier. Moreover, type IV collagen of the **lamina densa** acts as a molecular sieve and traps proteins larger than 69,000 MW.

To maintain the efficiency of the filtering system, **intraglomerular mesangial cells** phagocytose the lamina densa, which then is renewed by the combined actions of the podocytes and endothelial cells. The modified plasma that enters Bowman's space is known as the **ultrafiltrate**.

II. FUNCTION OF THE PROXIMAL TUBULE

The **proximal tubule** resorbs approximately 80% of the water, sodium, and chloride, as well as 100% of the proteins, amino acids, and glucose from the ultrafiltrate.

The resorbed materials are eventually returned into the **peritubular capillary network** of the cortical labyrinth for distribution to the remainder of the body. The movement of sodium is via an active transport mechanism utilizing a **sodium pump** in the basal plasmalemma, with chloride and water following passively. Since salt and water are resorbed in equimolar concentrations, the **osmolarity** of the ultrafiltrate is **not** altered in the proximal tubule, but remains the same as that of blood. The endocytosed proteins are degraded into amino acids that are also released into the renal interstitium for distribution by the vascular system. The proximal tubule also secretes organic acids, bases, and other substances into the ultrafiltrate.

III. FUNCTIONS OF THE THIN LIMBS OF HENLE'S LOOP

The **descending thin limb of Henle's loop** is completely permeable to water and salts, hence the ultrafiltrate in the lumen will attempt to equilibrate its osmolarity with the renal interstitium in its vicinity.

The **ascending thin limb** is mostly impermeable to water but is relatively permeable to salts; thus the movement of water is impeded, but that of sodium and chloride is not. The ultrafiltrate will maintain the same osmolarity as the renal interstitium in its immediate surroundings as the concentration gradient decreases approaching the cortex.

IV. FUNCTIONS OF THE DISTAL TUBULE

The **pars recta** of the distal tubule (ascending thick limb of Henle's loop) is impermeable to water but possesses a chloride pump (and possibly sodium pump) that actively pumps chloride out into the renal interstitium. To maintain electrical neutrality, sodium follows passively. However, water cannot enter or leave the ultrafiltrate, which consequently loses its osmotic pressure, becoming **hypoosmotic** by the time it reaches the macula densa region.

The distal convoluted tubule, whose cells possess **aldosterone receptors**, resorbs sodium ions from and secretes hydrogen, potassium, and ammonium ions into the ultrafiltrate, which it then delivers to the collecting duct.

V. FUNCTION OF THE JUXTAGLOMERULAR APPARATUS

It is believed that the **macula densa cells** monitor the osmolarity and volume of the ultrafiltrate. If either of these is elevated, the macula densa cells, via gap junctions, instruct the **juxtaglomerular cells** to release their stored proteolytic enzyme, **renin**, into the bloodstream. Renin cleaves two amino acids from the circulating decapeptide **angiotensinogen**, changing it to **angiotensin I**, which, in turn, is cleaved by **converting enzyme** located on the luminal surfaces of capillaries (especially in the lungs), forming **angiotensin II**. This powerful vasoconstrictor also prompts the release of the mineralocorticoid aldosterone from the suprarenal cortex.

Aldosterone binds to receptors on cells of the distal convoluted tubules, prompting them to resorb sodium (and chloride) from the ultrafiltrate. The addition of sodium to the extracellular compartment causes the retention of fluid with the subsequent elevation in blood pressure.

VI. CONCENTRATION OF URINE

A. Nephron (Countercurrent Multiplier System)

The concentration of urine occurs only in juxtamedullary nephrons, whose long thin limbs of Henle's loop function in the establishment of an **osmotic concentration gradient**. This gradient gradually increases from about 300 mOsm/L in the interstitium of the outer medulla to as much as 1200 mOsm/L at the renal papilla.

The **chloride pump** of the ascending thick limb of Henle's loop transfers chloride ions from the lumen into the renal interstitium. Sodium follows passively, and water is not permitted to leave; hence the salt concentration of the interstitium increases. Since the supply of chloride inside the ascending thick limb decreases as the ultrafiltrate proceeds toward the cortex (because it is constantly being removed from the lumen), less and less chloride is available for transport; consequently, the interstitial salt concentration decreases closer to the cortex.

The osmotic concentration gradient of the inner medulla, deep to the junction of the thin and thick ascending limbs of Henle's loop, is controlled by urea rather than sodium and chloride.

As the ultrafiltrate passes down the descending thin limb of Henle's loop, it reacts to the increasing gradient of osmotic concentration in the interstitium. Water leaves and salts enter the lumen, **reducing the volume** and **increasing the salt concentration** of the ultrafiltrate (which becomes **hypertonic**).

In the ascending thin limb of Henle's loop, water is conserved but salts are permitted to leave the ultrafiltrate, decreasing its osmolarity and contributing to the maintenance of the osmotic concentration gradient.

B. Collecting Duct

The ultrafiltrate that enters the collecting duct is **hypoosmotic**. As it passes down the collecting duct it is subject to the increasing osmotic gradient of the renal interstitium.

If **antidiuretic hormone (ADH)** is released from the pars nervosa of the pituitary, the cells of the collecting ducts become permeable to water, which leaves the lumen of the collecting duct, increasing the concentration of the urine. In the absence of ADH the cells of the collecting duct are impermeable to water, and the urine remains **hypotonic**.

The collecting duct is also responsible for permitting **urea** to diffuse into the interstitium of the **inner medulla**. The high interstitial osmolarity of this region is attributed to the urea concentration.

C. Vasa Recta (Countercurrent Exchange System)

The **vasa recta** assists in the maintenance of the osmotic concentration gradient of the renal medulla, since these capillary loops are completely permeable to salts and water. Thus, as the blood descends in the arteria recta, it becomes hyperosmotic, but as it ascends in the vena recta, its osmolarity returns to normal.

It is also important to realize that the arteria recta carries a smaller volume than the vena recta, permitting the removal of the fluid and salts transported into the renal interstitium by the uriniferous tubules.

Tubular Necrosis

Tubular necrosis may result in **acute renal failure**. Cells of the renal tubules die either by being poisoned due to exposure to toxic chemicals, such as mercury or carbon tetrachloride, or die because of severe cardiovascular shock that reduces blood flow to the kidneys. The dead cells become sloughed off and occlude the lumina of their tubules. If the basal laminae remain intact, epithelial cell division may be able to repair the damage in less than three weeks.

Acute Glomerulonephritis

Acute glomerulonephritis is usually the result of a localized beta Streptococcal infection in a region of the body other than the kidney (e.g., strep throat). Plasma cells secrete antibodies that complex with streptococcal antigens, forming an insoluble antigen-antibody complex that is filtered by the basal lamina between the podocytes and the endothelial cells of the glomerulus. As the immune complex builds up in the glomerular basal lamina, the epithelial cells and mesangial cells proliferate. Additionally, leukocytes accumulate in the glomerulus, congesting and blocking it. Moreover, pharmacologic agents released at the site of damage cause the glomerulus to become leaky and proteins, platelets, and even erythrocytes may enter the glomerular filtrate. Usually after the acute inflammation abates the glomeruli repair themselves and the normal kidney function returns. Occasionally, however, the damage is extensive and kidney function becomes permanently impaired.

Diabetes Insipidus

Diabetes insipidus occurs because of damage to the cells of the hypothalamus that manufacture ADH (antidiuretic hormone). The low levels of ADH interfere with the ability of the collecting tubules of the kidney to concentrate urine. The excess fluid loss in the formation of copious quantities of dilute urine results in **polydipsia** (excessive thirst) and dehydration.

Kidney Stones

Kidney stones usually form due to the condition known as **hyperparathyroidism**, where the formation of excess parathyroid hormone (PTH) by the parathyroid glands results in an increased level of osteoclastic activity. The resorption of bone, as well as the increased absorption of calcium and phosphates from the gastrointestinal tract, eventuate higher than normal blood calcium levels. As the kidneys excrete higher than normal concentration of calcium and phosphates, their presence in the urine, especially under alkaline conditions, causes their precipitation in the kidney tubules. Continued accretion of these ions onto the crystal surface causes an increase in the size of the crystals and they become known as **kidney stones**.

Cancers of the Kidney

Cancers of the kidney are usually solid tumors, whereas cysts of the kidney are usually benign. The most common symptom of kidney cancer is **blood in the urine**, although the amount of blood may be undetectable without a microscopic examination of the urine. Usually, kidney cancers are accompanied by pain and fever, but frequently they are discovered by abdominal palpation during routine physicals when the physician detects a lump in the region of the kidney. If the cancer did not metastasize the treatment of choice is removal of the affected kidney and regional lymph nodes. Since kidney cancers spread early and usually to the lung the prognosis is poor but interleukine-2 therapy has been shown to be promising.

Summary of Histological Organization

I. KIDNEY

A. Capsule

The **capsule** is composed of dense irregular collagenous connective tissue. Occasional **fibroblasts** and blood vessels may be seen.

B. Cortex

The **cortex** consists of parts of **nephrons** and **collecting tubules** arranged in **cortical labyrinths** and **medullary rays**. Additionally, blood vessels and associated connective tissue (**renal interstitium**) are also present.

1. Cortical Labyrinth

The **cortical labyrinth** is composed of **renal corpuscles** and cross-sections of **proximal convoluted tubules**, **distal convoluted tubules**, and the **macula densa** region of **distal tubules**. Renal corpuscles consist of **mesangial cells**, **parietal** (simple squamous) and **visceral** (modified to **podocytes**) **layers** of **Bowman's capsule**, and an associated capillary bed, the **glomerulus**, as well as the intervening **Bowman's space**, which receives the ultrafiltrate. The **afferent** and **efferent glomerular arterioles** supply and drain the glomerulus, respectively, at its vascular pole. **Bowman's space** is drained at the **urinary pole** into the **proximal convoluted tubule** composed of eosinophilic simple cuboidal epithelium with a brush border. The **distal convoluted tubule** profiles are fewer in number and may be recognized by the pale cuboidal epithelial cells. The **macula densa** region of the distal tubule is associated with the **juxtaglomerular** (modified smooth muscle) **cells** of the afferent (and sometimes efferent) glomerular arterioles.

2. Medullary Rays

Medullary rays are continuations of medullary tissue extending into the cortex. They are composed mostly of **collecting tubules, pars recta of proximal tubules, ascending thick limbs of Henle's loop**, and blood vessels.

C. Medulla

The **medulla** is composed of **renal pyramids** that are bordered by **cortical columns**. The renal pyramids consist of **collecting tubules** whose simple cuboidal epithelium displays 1) clearly defined lateral cell membranes; 2) **thick descending limbs of Henle's loop**, whose cells resemble those of the proximal tubule; 3) **thin limbs of Henle's loop**, resembling capillaries but containing no blood; and 4) **ascending thick limbs of Henle's loop**, whose cells are similar to those of the distal tubule. Additionally, numerous blood vessels, the **vasa recta**, are also present, as well as slight connective tissue elements, the **renal interstitium**. The apex of the renal pyramid is the **renal papilla**, whose perforated tip is the **area cribrosa**, where the large **collecting ducts (of Bellini)** open to deliver the urine into the **minor calyx**.

D. Pelvis

The **renal pelvis**, subdivided into the **minor** and **major calyces**, constitutes the beginning of the main excretory duct of the kidney. The **transitional epithelium** of the minor calyx is reflected onto the renal papilla. The calyces are lined by transitional epithelium. The subepithelial connective tissue of both is loosely arranged and abuts the **muscularis**, composed of **inner longitudinal** and **outer circular** layers of **smooth muscle**. An **adventitia** of loose connective tissue surrounds the muscularis.

II. EXTRARENAL PASSAGES

A. Ureter

The **ureter** possesses a stellate-shaped lumen that is lined by **transitional epithelium**. The subepithelial connective tissue (sometimes said to be subdivided into **lamina propria** and **submucosa**) is composed of a fibroelastic connective tissue. The **muscularis** is again composed of **inner longitudinal** and **outer circular** layers of **smooth muscle**, although in its lower portion near the bladder a third, **outermost longitudinal** layer of **smooth muscle** is present. The muscularis is surrounded by a fibroelastic **adventitia**.

B. Bladder

The **urinary bladder** resembles the ureter except that it is a much larger structure and does not possess a stellate lumen, although the mucosa of the empty bladder is thrown into folds. The **lamina propria** is fibroelastic in character and may contain occasional **mucous glands** at the internal orifice of the urethra. The **muscularis** is composed of three indefinite layers of smooth muscle: **inner longitudinal, middle circular,** and **outer longitudinal.** The circular muscle coat forms the **internal sphincter** at the neck of the bladder. An **adventitia** or **serosa** surrounds the bladder. The urethra is described in Chapter 17, "Female Reproductive System," and Chapter 18, "Male Reproductive System."

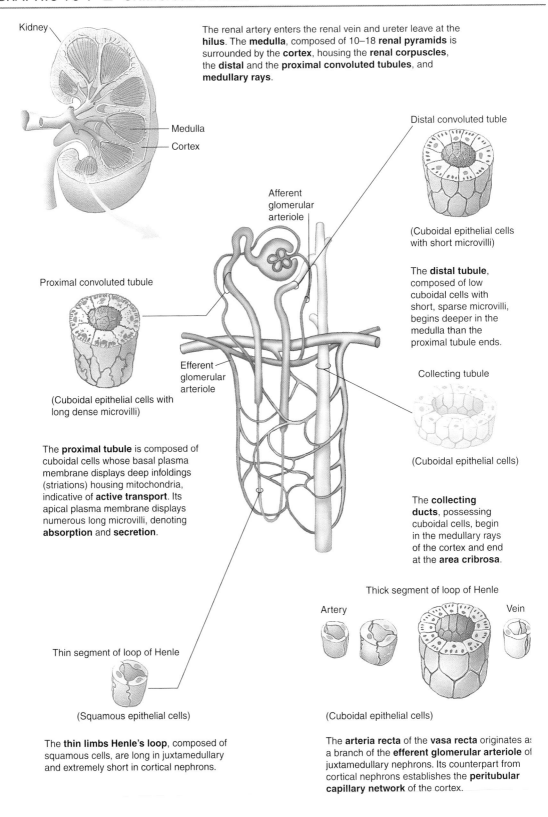

Kidney

The renal artery enters the renal vein and ureter leave at the **hilus**. The **medulla**, composed of 10–18 **renal pyramids** is surrounded by the **cortex**, housing the **renal corpuscles**, the **distal** and the **proximal convoluted tubules**, and **medullary rays**.

Medulla

Cortex

Distal convoluted tuble

(Cuboidal epithelial cells with short microvilli)

The **distal tubule**, composed of low cuboidal cells with short, sparse microvilli, begins deeper in the medulla than the proximal tubule ends.

Afferent glomerular arteriole

Proximal convoluted tubule

Efferent glomerular arteriole

(Cuboidal epithelial cells with long dense microvilli)

The **proximal tubule** is composed of cuboidal cells whose basal plasma membrane displays deep infoldings (striations) housing mitochondria, indicative of **active transport**. Its apical plasma membrane displays numerous long microvilli, denoting **absorption** and **secretion**.

Collecting tubule

(Cuboidal epithelial cells)

The **collecting ducts**, possessing cuboidal cells, begin in the medullary rays of the cortex and end at the **area cribrosa**.

Thick segment of loop of Henle

Artery

Vein

Thin segment of loop of Henle

(Squamous epithelial cells)

The **thin limbs Henle's loop**, composed of squamous cells, are long in juxtamedullary and extremely short in cortical nephrons.

(Cuboidal epithelial cells)

The **arteria recta** of the **vasa recta** originates as a branch of the **efferent glomerular arteriole** of juxtamedullary nephrons. Its counterpart from cortical nephrons establishes the **peritubular capillary network** of the cortex.

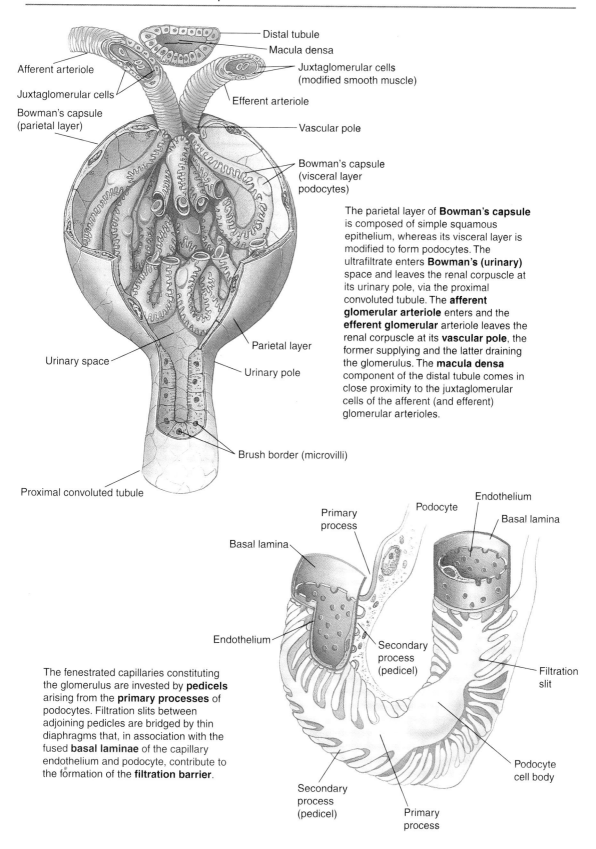

Distal tubule

Macula densa

Juxtaglomerular cells
(modified smooth muscle)

Afferent arteriole

Juxtaglomerular cells

Efferent arteriole

Bowman's capsule
(parietal layer)

Vascular pole

Bowman's capsule
(visceral layer
podocytes)

The parietal layer of **Bowman's capsule** is composed of simple squamous epithelium, whereas its visceral layer is modified to form podocytes. The ultrafiltrate enters **Bowman's (urinary) space** and leaves the renal corpuscle at its urinary pole, via the proximal convoluted tubule. The **afferent glomerular arteriole** enters and the **efferent glomerular** arteriole leaves the renal corpuscle at its **vascular pole**, the former supplying and the latter draining the glomerulus. The **macula densa** component of the distal tubule comes in close proximity to the juxtaglomerular cells of the afferent (and efferent) glomerular arterioles.

Parietal layer

Urinary space

Urinary pole

Brush border (microvilli)

Proximal convoluted tubule

Endothelium

Podocyte

Basal lamina

Primary process

Basal lamina

Endothelium

Secondary process
(pedicel)

Filtration slit

The fenestrated capillaries constituting the glomerulus are invested by **pedicels** arising from the **primary processes** of podocytes. Filtration slits between adjoining pedicels are bridged by thin diaphragms that, in association with the fused **basal laminae** of the capillary endothelium and podocyte, contribute to the formation of the **filtration barrier**.

Podocyte cell body

Secondary process
(pedicel)

Primary process

PLATE 16-1 ■ *Kidney, Survey and General Morphology*

FIGURE 1 ■ *Kidney cortex and medulla. Human. Paraffin section.* × 14.

The kidney cortex and part of the medulla are presented at a low magnification to provide an insight into the cortical architecture. The **capsule** (Ca) appears as a thin, light line at the top of the photomicrograph. The darker area below it, occupying the top half of the photomicrograph, is the **cortex** (C), whereas the lower lighter region is the **medulla** (M). Note that longitudinal rays of the medulla appear to invade the cortex; these are known as **medullary rays** (MR). The tissue between medullary rays appears convoluted and is referred to as the **cortical labyrinth** (CL). It is occupied by dense, round structures, the **renal corpuscles** (RC). These are the first part of the nephrons, and their location in the cortex is indicative of their time of development, as well as of their function. They are referred to as **superficial** (1), **midcortical** (2), or **juxta-medullary nephrons** (3). Each medullary ray and one-half of the cortical labyrinth on either side of it constitutes a lobule of the kidney. The lobule extends into the medulla, but its borders are undefinable histologically (approximated by vertical lines). The large vessels at the corticomedullary junction are **arcuate vessels** (AV), whereas those in the cortical labyrinth are **interlobular vessels** (IV).

FIGURE 2 ■ *Kidney capsule. Monkey. Plastic section.* × 540.

The kidney is invested by a **capsule** (Ca) composed of dense collagenous connective tissue containing occasional **fibroblasts** (Fb). Although this structure is not highly vascular, it does possess some **capsular vessels** (CV). Observe the numerous red blood cells in the lumina of these vessels. The deeper aspect of the capsule possesses a rich **capillary network** (CN) that is supplied by the terminal branches of the interlobular arteries and is drained by the stellate veins, tributaries of the interlobular veins. Note the cross-sections of the **proximal convoluted tubules** (PT).

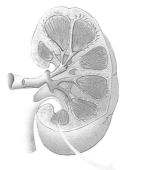

Kidney

FIGURE 3 ■ *Kidney cortex. Human. Paraffin section.* × 132.

The various component parts of the cortical labyrinth and portions of two medullary rays are evident. The orientation of this photomicrograph is perpendicular to that of Figure 1. Note that two **renal corpuscles** (RC) in the center of the photomicrograph display a slight shrinkage artifact and thus clearly demonstrate **Bowman's space** (BS). The renal corpuscles are surrounded by cross-sections of **proximal convoluted tubules** (PT), **distal convoluted tubules** (DT), and **macula densa** (MD). Since the proximal convoluted tubule is much longer than the convoluted portion of the distal tubule, the number of proximal convoluted tubule profiles around a renal corpuscle outnumber the distal convoluted tubule profiles by approximately 7 to 1. The medullary rays contain the **pars recta** (PR) of the **proximal tubule**, the **ascending thick limbs of Henle's loop** (AT), and **collecting tubules** (CT).

FIGURE 4 ■ *Colored colloidin-injected kidney. Paraffin section.* × 132.

This specimen was prepared by injecting the renal artery with colored colloidin, and a thick section was taken to demonstrate the vascular supply of the renal corpuscle. Each renal corpuscle contains tufts of capillaries, the **glomerulus** (G), which is supplied by the **afferent glomerular arteriole** (AA) and drained by the **efferent glomerular arteriole** (EA). Note that the outer diameter of the afferent glomerular arteriole is greater than that of the efferent glomerular arteriole: however, the diameters of the two lumina are about equal. It is important to realize that the glomerulus is an arterial capillary network; therefore, the pressure within these vessels is greater than that of normal capillary beds. This results in more effective filtration pressure. The large vessel on the lower right is an **interlobular artery** (IA), and it is the parent vessel of the afferent glomerular arterioles.

■ KEY

AA	afferent arteriole	CN	capillary network	IV	interlobular vessel
AT	ascending thick limb	CT	collecting tubule	M	medulla
	of Henle's loop	CV	capsular vessel	MD	macula densa
AV	arcuate vessel	DT	distal convoluted tubule	MR	medullary ray
BS	Bowman's space	EA	efferent arteriole	PR	pars recta
C	cortex	Fb	fibroblast	PT	proximal convoluted tubule
Ca	capsule	G	glomerulus	RC	renal corpuscle
CL	cortical labyrinth	IA	interlobular artery		

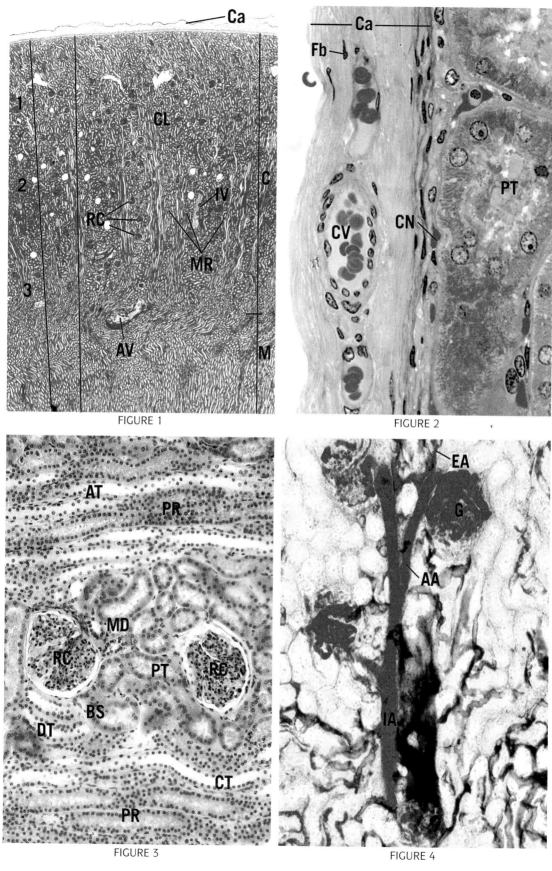

FIGURE 1

FIGURE 2

FIGURE 3

FIGURE 4

PLATE 16-2 ■ *Renal Cortex*

FIGURE 1 ■ *Kidney cortical labyrinth. Monkey. Plastic section.* × 270.

The center of this photomicrograph is occupied by a renal corpuscle. The urinary pole is evident as the short neck empties into the convoluted portion of the **proximal tubule** (PT). The renal corpuscle is composed of the **glomerulus** (G), tufts of capillaries, the visceral layer of Bowman's capsule (podocytes) that is intimately associated with the glomerulus, **Bowman's space** (BS), into which the ultrafiltrate is expressed from the capillaries, and the **parietal layer** (PL) of Bowman's capsule, consisting of a simple squamous epithelium. Additionally, mesangial cells are also present in the renal corpuscle. Most of the tubular profiles surrounding the renal corpuscle are transverse sections of the darker staining **proximal tubules** (PT), which outnumber the cross-sections of the lighter staining **distal tubules** (DT).

FIGURE 2 ■ *Kidney cortical labyrinth. Monkey. Plastic section.* × 270.

The renal corpuscle in the center of the photomicrograph displays all of the characteristics identified in Figure 1, except that instead of the urinary pole, the **vascular pole** (VP) is presented. That is the region where the afferent and efferent glomerular arterioles enter and leave the renal corpuscle, respectively. Some of the smooth muscle cells of the afferent (and sometimes efferent) glomerular arterioles are modified in that they contain renin granules. These modified cells are known as **juxtaglomerular cells** (JC). They are closely associated with the **macula densa** (MD) region of the distal tubule. Again, note that most of the cross-sectional profiles of tubules surrounding the renal corpuscle belong to the convoluted portion of the **proximal tubules** (PT) while only one or two are distal tubules. Observe the rich **vascularity** (BV) of the renal cortex, as well as the scant amount of connective tissue elements (arrows) associated with these vessels.

FIGURE 3 ■ *Kidney cortical labyrinth. Monkey. Plastic section.* × 270.

The vascular pole of this renal corpuscle is very clearly represented. It is in this region that the **afferent glomerular arteriole** (AA) enters the renal corpuscle and the **efferent glomerular arteriole** (EA) leaves, draining the glomerulus. Observe that these two vessels and their capillaries are supported by **mesangial cells** (Mg). Note that although the outer diameter of the afferent glomerular arteriole is greater than that of the efferent glomerular arteriole, their luminal diameters are approximately the same. The renal corpuscle is surrounded by cross-sectional profiles of **distal** (DT) and **proximal** (PT) **tubules.** The boxed area is presented at a higher magnification in Figure 4.

Inset. **Glomerulus. Kidney. Monkey. Plastic section.** × 720.

The glomerulus is composed of capillaries whose **endothelial cell** (En) nuclei bulge into the lumen. The endothelial cells are separated from **podocytes** (P), modified visceral cell layer of Bowman's capsule, by a thick basal lamina (arrows). **Mesangial cells** (Mg) from both supporting and phagocytic elements of the renal corpuscle. Note that major processes (asterisks) of the podocytes are also distinguishable in this photomicrograph.

FIGURE 4 ■ *Juxtaglomerular apparatus. Kidney. Monkey. Plastic section.* × 1325.

The boxed area of Figure 3 is magnified to present the juxtaglomerular apparatus. This is composed of the **macula densa** (MD) region of the distal tubule and apparent **juxtaglomerular cells** (JC), modified smooth muscle cells of the **afferent glomerular arteriole** (AA). Observe the granules (arrowheads) in the juxtaglomerular cells, which are believed to be the enzyme renin. Note the nuclei (asterisks) of the endothelial cells lining the afferent glomerular arteriole.

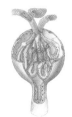

Renal corpuscle

■ KEY

AA	afferent arteriole	En	endothelial cell	P	podocyte
BS	Bowman's space	G	glomerulus	PL	parietal layer
BV	blood vessel	JC	juxtaglomerular cell	PT	proximal tubule
DT	distal tubule	MD	macula densa	VP	vascular pole
EA	efferent arteriole	Mg	mesangial cell		

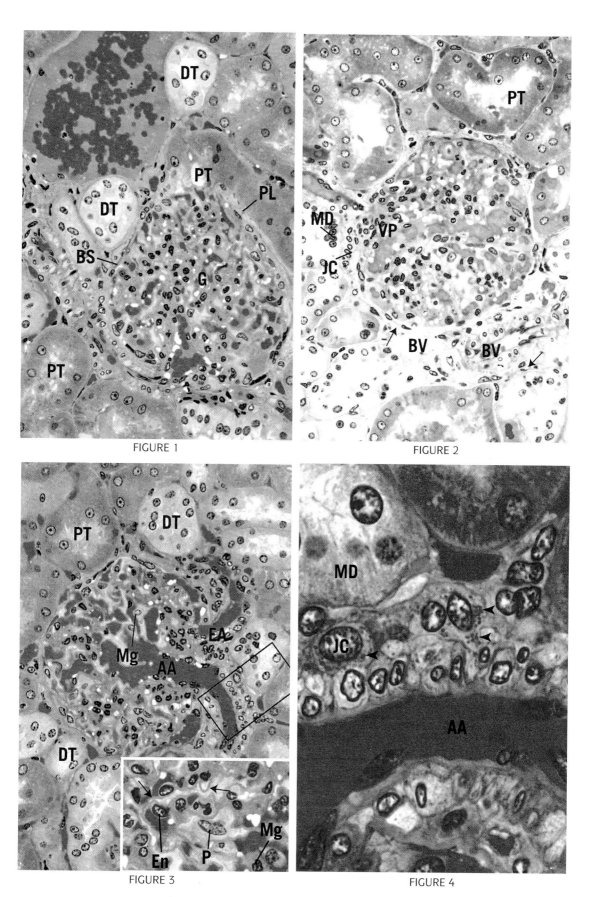

FIGURE 1

FIGURE 2

FIGURE 3

FIGURE 4

PLATE 16-3 ■ *Glomerulus, Scanning Electron Microscopy*

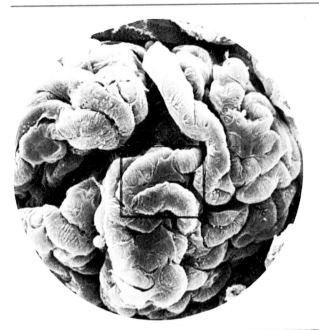

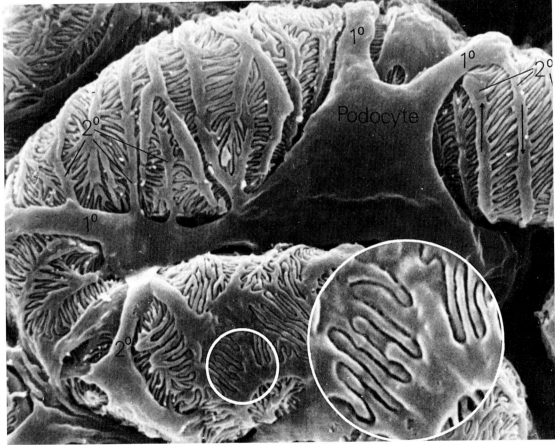

FIGURE 1 ■ *Scanning electron micrograph of a glomerulus, displaying the primary and secondary processes and pedicels of podocytes. Top,* × 700; *bottom,* × 4000; *and inset,* × 6000. *(From Ross MH, Reith EJ, Romrell LJ: Histology: A Text and Atlas. 2nd ed. Baltimore: Williams & Wilkins, 1989:536.)*

PLATE 16-4 ■ *Renal Corpuscle, Electron Microscopy*

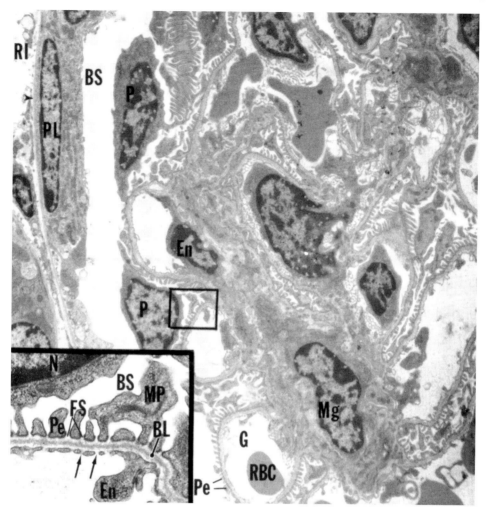

FIGURE 1 ■ *Kidney cortex. Renal corpuscle.*
Mouse. Electron microscopy. × 3780.

Various components of the renal corpuscle are displayed in this electron micrograph. Note the basal lamina (arrowhead) separating the simple squamous cells of the **parietal layer** (PL) of Bowman's capsule from the **renal interstitium** (RI). **Bowman's space** (BS) and the **podocytes** (P) are shown to advantage, as are the **glomeruli** (G) and surrounding **pedicels** (Pe). **Mesangial cells** (Mg) occupy the space between capillary loops, and several **red blood cells** (RBC) and **endothelial cells** (En) are also evident.

Inset. **Podocyte and glomerulus. Mouse. Electron microscopy.** × 6300.

This is a higher magnification of the boxed area, presenting a portion of a podocyte. Observe its **nucleus** (N), **major process** (MP), and **pedicels** (Pe). Note that the pedicels lie on a **basal lamina** (BL) that is composed of a lamina rara externa, lamina densa, and lamina rara interna. Observe the fenestrations (arrows) in the **endothelial lining** (En) of the glomerulus. The spaces between the pedicels, known as **filtration slits** (FS), lead into **Bowman's space** (BS).

PLATE 16-5 ■ *Renal Medulla*

FIGURE 1 ■ *Renal medulla. Monkey. Plastic section.* × 270.

This photomicrograph of the renal medulla demonstrates the arrangement of the various tubular and vascular structures. The formed connective tissue elements among the tubules and vessels are very sparse and constitute mainly fibroblasts, macrophages, and fibers (asterisks). The major tubular elements in evidence are the **collecting tubules** (CT), recognizable by the conspicuous lateral plasma membranes of their tall cuboidal (or low columnar) cells, **thick limbs of Henle's loop** (TH), and occasional **thin limbs of Henle's loop** (TL). Many vascular elements are noted; these are the vasa recta spuria whose thicker walled descending limbs are the **arteriolae rectae spuriae** (AR) and thinner walled ascending limbs are the **venulae rectae spuriae** (VR).

FIGURE 2 ■ *Renal papilla. x.s. Human. Paraffin section.* × 270.

The most conspicuous tubular elements of the renal papilla are the **collecting tubules** (CT) with their cuboidal cells, whose lateral plasma membranes are clearly evident. The numerous thin-walled structures are the **thin limbs of Henle's loop** (TL), as well as the **arteriolae rectae spuriae** (AR) and **venulae rectae spuriae** (VR) that may be identified by the presence of blood in their lumina. The formed connective tissue elements (asterisks) may be discerned in the interstitium among the various tubules of the kidney. An occasional thick limb of Henle's loop (TH) may also be observed.

FIGURE 3 ■ *Renal papilla. x.s. Monkey. Plastic section.* × 540.

In the deeper aspect of the medulla collecting tubules merge with each other, forming larger and larger structures. The largest of these ducts are known as **papillary ducts** (PD) or ducts of Bellini that may be recognized by their tall, pale columnar cells and their easily discernible lateral plasma membranes (arrows). These ducts open at the apex of the renal papilla, in the region known as the area cribrosa. The **thin limbs of Henle's loop** (TL) are clearly evident. These structures form the hairpin-like loops of Henle in this region, where the ascending thin limbs recur to ascend in the medulla, eventually to become thicker, forming the straight portion of the distal tubule. Note that the **arteriolae rectae spuriae** (AR) and the **venulae rectae spuriae** (VR) follow the thin limbs of Henle's loop deep into the renal papilla. Some of the connective tissue elements are marked by asterisks.

FIGURE 4 ■ *Renal medulla. l.s. Monkey. Plastic section.* × 270.

This photomicrograph is similar to Figure 1, except that it is a longitudinal rather than a transverse section of the renal medulla. The center is occupied by a **collecting tubule** (CT), as is distinguished by the tall cuboidal cells whose lateral plasma membranes are clearly evident. The collecting tubule is flanked by **thick limbs of Henle's loop** (TH). The vasa recta are filled with blood, and the thickness of their walls identifies whether they are **arteriolae rectae spuriae** (AR) or **venulae rectae spuriae** (VR). A thin limb of Henle's loop (TL) is also identifiable.

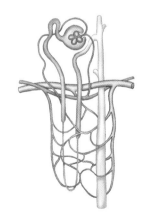

Uriniferous tubule

■ **KEY**

AR	arteriolae rectae spuriae	PD	papillary duct	TL	thin limb of Henle's loop
CT	collecting tubule	TH	thick limb of Henle's loop	VR	venulae rectae spuriae

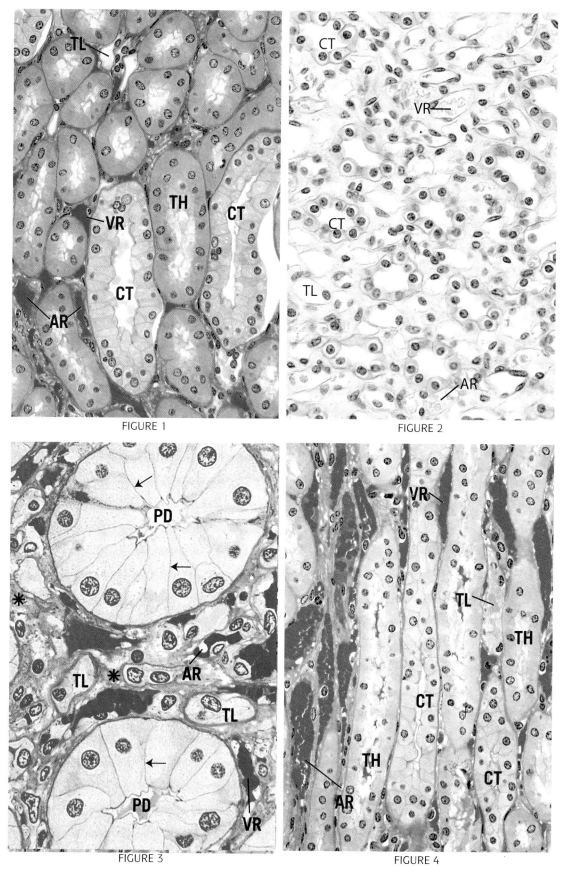

FIGURE 1

FIGURE 2

FIGURE 3

FIGURE 4

PLATE 16-6 ■ *Ureter and Urinary Bladder*

FIGURE 1 ▒ *Ureter. x.s. Human. Paraffin section.* × 14.

This low power photomicrograph of the ureter displays its stellate-shaped **lumen** (L) and thick lining **epithelium** (E). The interface between the **subepithelial connective tissue** (SCT) and the **smooth muscle coat** (SM) is indicated by arrows. The muscle coat is surrounded by a fibrous **adventitia** (Ad), which houses the numerous vascular channels and nerve fibers that travel with the ureter. Thus, the wall of the ureter consists of the mucosa (epithelium and underlying connective tissue), muscularis, and adventitia.

FIGURE 2 ■ *Ureter. x.s. Monkey. Plastic section.* × 132.

The mucosa is highly convoluted and consists of a thick, transitional epithelium whose free surface possesses characteristic **dome-shaped cells** (D). The basal cell layer sits on a basal lamina (arrows), which separates the epithelium from the underlying fibrous connective tissue. The **muscularis** consists of three layers of smooth muscle: **inner longitudinal** (IL), **middle circular** (MC), and **outer longitudinal** (OL). These three layers are not always present, for the outer longitudinal layer is found only in the inferior one-third of the ureter, that is, the portion nearest the urinary bladder. The **adventitia** (Ad) is composed of fibrous connective tissue that anchors the ureter to the posterior body wall and adjacent structures.

FIGURE 3 ■ *Urinary bladder. Monkey. Plastic section.* × 14.

The urinary bladder stores urine until it is ready to be voided. Since the volume of the bladder changes with the amount of urine it contains, its mucosa may or may not display folds. This particular specimen is not distended, hence the numerous folds (arrows). Moreover, the **transitional epithelium** (TE) of this preparation is also thick, while in the distended phase, the epithelium would be much thinner. Note also that the thick **muscularis** is composed of three layers of smooth muscle: **inner longitudinal** (IL), **middle circular** (MC), and **outer longitudinal** (OL). The muscle layers are surrounded either by an adventitia composed of loose connective tissue—as is the case in this photomicrograph—or by a serosa, depending on the region of the bladder being examined.

FIGURE 4 ■ *Urinary bladder. Monkey. Plastic section.* × 132.

The bladder is lined by **transitional epithelium** (TE), whose typical surface dome-shaped cells are shown to advantage. Some of these cells are binucleated. The epithelium is separated from the underlying connective tissue by a basal lamina (arrows). This subepithelial connective tissue is frequently said to be divided into a **lamina propria** (LP) and a **submucosa** (Sm). The vascularity of this region is demonstrated by the numerous **venules** (V) and **arterioles** (A). These vessels possess smaller tributaries and branches that supply the regions closer to the epithelium.

Inset. **Transitional epithelium. Monkey. Plastic section.** × 540.

The boxed region of the transitional epithelium is presented at a higher magnification to demonstrate the large dome-shaped cells (arrow) at the free surface. These cells are characteristic of the empty bladder. When that structure is distended with urine, the dome-shaped cells assume a flattened morphology and the entire epithelium becomes thinner (being reduced from five to seven to only three cell layers thick). Note that occasional cells may be binucleated.

■ **KEY**

A	arteriole	L	lumen	SM	smooth muscle coat
Ad	adventitia	LP	lamina propria	Sm	submucosa
D	dome-shaped cell	MC	middle circular muscularis	TE	transitional epithelium
E	epithelium	OL	outer longitudinal muscularis	V	venule
IL	inner longitudinal muscularis	SCT	subepithelial connective tissue		

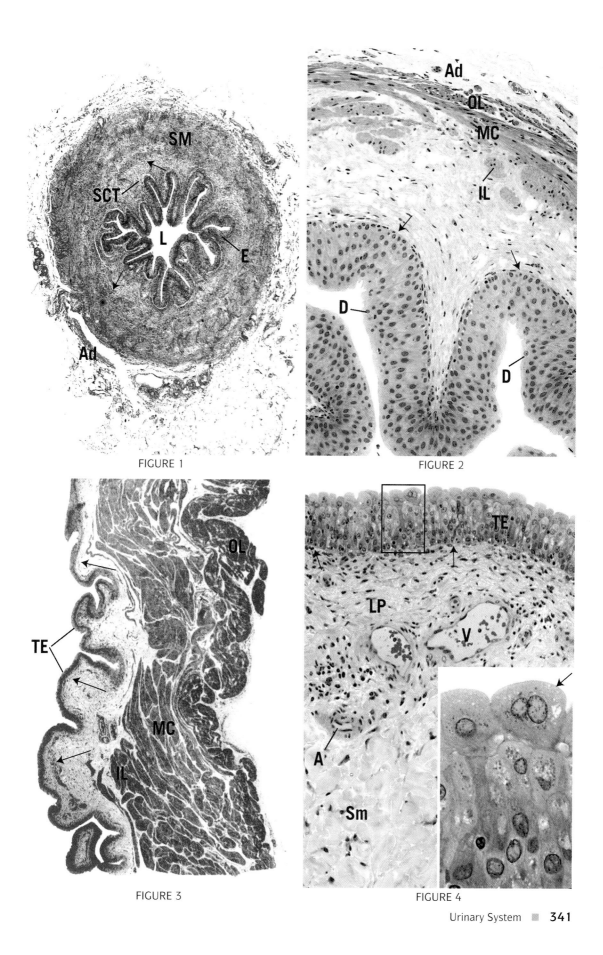

FIGURE 1

FIGURE 2

FIGURE 3

FIGURE 4

Female Reproductive System

The female reproductive system (**see Graphic 17-1**) is composed of the ovaries, genital ducts, external genitalia, and the mammary glands, although, in a strict sense, the mammary glands are not genital organs. The reproductive system functions in the propagation of the species and is under the control of a complex interplay of hormonal, neural and, in the human, psychologic factors.

OVARY

Each **ovary** is a small, almond-shaped structure whose thick connective tissue capsule, the **tunica albuginea**, is covered by a **simple squamous** to **cuboidal mesothelium** known as the **germinal epithelium**. The ovary is divisible into a **cortex** rich in ovarian follicles and a highly vascular **medulla**.

The **cortex**, located just deep to the tunica albuginea, houses the female germ cells, **oogonia**, which have undergone cell divisions to form numerous oocytes. Each **oocyte** is surrounded by a layer of epithelial cells, and these two structures together constitute an **ovarian follicle**. Under the influence of **follicle stimulating hormone**, follicles enlarge, are modified, become encapsulated by the ovarian **stroma** (connective tissue), and mature.

Ovarian Follicles

The follicle passes through various maturational stages, from the primordial follicle, to the primary, the secondary, and, finally, the Graafian (mature) follicle. The **primordial follicle** is composed of a **primary oocyte** surrounded by a single layer of flattened follicular cells. As maturation progresses, the follicular cells become cuboidal in shape, and the follicle is referred to as a **unilaminar primary follicle**. Multilaminar primary follicles display an oocyte surrounded by several layers of follicular cells and an intervening **zona pellucida**, as well as an externally positioned **theca interna**.

With further growth of the follicle, accumulations of follicular fluid in the intercellular spaces of the follicular cells form. At this point the entire structure is known as a **secondary follicle**, and it presents a well-developed zona pellucida, a clearly distinguishable basal membrane, and a theca interna and a **theca externa**.

As maturation progresses, the **Graafian follicle** stage is reached. This large structure is characterized by a follicular fluid containing the central antrum whose wall is composed of the **membrana granulosa**. Jutting into the antrum is the **cumulus oophorus** housing the primary oocyte and its attendant zona pellucida and **corona radiata**. The membrana granulosa is separated from the theca interna by the basal membrane. The theca externa merges imperceptibly with the surrounding ovarian stroma. The Graafian follicle, mostly because of the activity of **luteinizing hormone**, ruptures, thus releasing the oocyte with its attendant follicular cells.

Corpus Luteum

Once the Graafian follicle loses its oocyte, it becomes transformed into the **corpus hemorrhagicum**. Within a couple of days the corpus hemorrhagicum is transformed into the **corpus luteum**, a yellow structure that produces **estrogens** and **progesterone**. When the corpus luteum degenerates it becomes the fibrotic **corpus albicans**.

GENITAL DUCTS

Oviduct

Each **oviduct** (**fallopian tube**) is a short muscular tube leading from the vicinity of the ovary to the uterine lumen. The oviduct is subdivided into four regions: the **infundibulum** (whose **fimbriae** approximate the ovary), the **ampulla**, the **isthmus**, and the **intramural portion**, which pierces the wall of the uterus. The mucosa of the oviduct is extensively folded in the infundibulum and ampulla, but the folding is reduced in the isthmus and intramural portions.

Uterus

The **uterus**, a pear-shaped viscus, is divisible into a **fundus**, a **body**, and a **cervix**. During pregnancy it is this organ that houses and supports the developing embryo and fetus. The uterus is composed of a thick, muscular **myometrium** (covered by serosa and/or adventitia) and a spongy mucosal layer, the **endometrium**. The endometrium, composed of an epithelially lined lamina propria, with its superficial functional and deep basal layers, undergoes hormonally modulated cyclic changes during the menstrual cycle. The three stages of the endometrium are:

a. **Follicular (proliferative) phase,** during which the free surface of the endometrium is reepithelialized, and the glands, connective tissue elements, and vascular supply of the endometrium are reestablished.

b. **Luteal (secretory) phase,** occurring within a few days after ovulation, during which the glands further enlarge and become tortuous and their lumina become filled with secretory products. Additionally, the helical arteries become more coiled, and fibroblasts of the stroma accumulate glycogen and fat.

c. **Menstrual phase,** during which the functional layer of the endometrium is desquamated, resulting in menstrual flow, while the basal layer remains more or less undisturbed.

PLACENTA

During pregnancy the uterus participates in the formation of the **placenta**, a highly vascular structure that permits the exchange of various materials between the maternal and fetal circulatory systems (see Graphic 17-2). It must be stressed that the exchange occurs without the commingling of the maternal and fetal bloods and that the placenta is derived from both maternal and fetal tissues.

VAGINA

The **vagina** is a muscular sheath adapted for the reception of the penis during copulation and for the passage of the fetus from the uterus during birth. The wall of the vagina is composed of three layers: an **outer fibrous layer**, a **middle muscular layer**, and an **inner mucosal layer**. The lamina propria of the mucosa possesses no glands. A stratified squamous nonkeratinized epithelium lines the vagina.

EXTERNAL GENITALIA

The **external genitalia**, composed of **labia majora**, **labia minora**, **clitoris**, and **vestibular glands**, are also referred to as the **vulva**. These structures are richly innervated and function during sexual arousal and copulation.

MAMMARY GLANDS

Mammary Gland

The **mammary glands**, highly modified **sweat glands**, are identical in males and females until the onset of puberty, when under hormonal influences the female breasts develop. The mammary gland is composed of numerous individual compound glands, each of which is considered a lobe. Each lobe is drained by a **lactiferous duct** that delivers the secretion onto the surface of the nipple.

Areola

The pigmented region of the skin surrounding the nipple, known as the **areola**, is richly endowed by sweat, sebaceous, and areolar glands. The mammary glands undergo cyclic changes and, subsequent to pregnancy, produce milk to nourish the newborn.

Histophysiology

I. REGULATION OF FOLLICLE MATURATION AND OVULATION

Gonadotropin-releasing hormones from the hypothalamus activate gonadotrophs of the adenohypophysis to release follicle-stimulating hormone (FSH) and luteinizing hormone (LH).

FSH not only induces secondary follicles to mature into Graafian follicles but also causes cells of the **theca interna** to secrete **androgens**. Additionally, FSH prompts **granulosa cells** to develop **LH receptors**, to convert androgens to **estrogens**, and to secrete **inhibin, activin,** and **folliculostatin**. These hormones assist in the feedback regulation of FSH release. Moreover, as estrogen reaches a threshold level, it causes a surge of LH release.

The **LH** surge results not only in resumption of meiosis I in the primary oocyte and initiation of meiosis II in the (now) secondary oocyte but also in **ovulation**. Additionally, LH induces the development of the **corpus luteum** from the theca interna and membrana granulosa.

II. FUNCTION AND FATE OF THE CORPUS LUTEUM

The **corpus luteum** secretes **progesterone**, a hormone that suppresses LH release by inhibiting gonadotropin-releasing hormone (GnRH) and facilitates the thickening of the uterine **endometrium**. Additionally, **estrogen** (inhibitor of FSH) and **relaxin** (which causes the fibrocartilage of the pubic symphysis to become more pliable) are also released by the corpus luteum.

In case pregnancy does not occur, the corpus luteum **atrophies**, and the absence of estrogen and progesterone will once again permit the release of FSH and LH from the adenohypophysis.

In case pregnancy does occur, the **syncytiotrophoblasts** of the forming placenta release **human chorionic gonadotropin** (hCG), a hormone that maintains the placenta well into the second trimester. These cells also secrete **human chorionic mammotropin** (facilitates milk production and growth), **thyrotropin, corticotropin, relaxin,** and **estrogen**.

III. UTERINE RESPONSE TO HORMONES

A. Endometrium

The **endometrium** is separated into a deeper basal and a more superficial functional layer, each with its own blood supply. The **basal layer**, which remains intact during menstruation, is served by short **straight arteries** and is occupied by the base of the **uterine glands**. The **functional layer**, served by the **helicine (coiled) arteries**, undergoes hormonally modulated cyclic changes.

FSH facilitates the **proliferative phase**, a thickening of the endometrium and the renewal of the connective tissue, glandular structures and blood vessels (**helicine arteries**) subsequent to the menstrual phase.

LH facilitates the **secretory phase**, characterized by the further thickening of the endometrium, coiling of the endometrial glands, accumulation of glandular secretions, and further coiling and lengthening of the **helicine arteries**.

Decreased levels of LH and progesterone are responsible for the **menstrual phase**, which begins with long-term, intermittent **vasoconstriction** of the helicine arteries, with subsequent necrosis of the vessel walls and endometrial tissue of the functional layer. It should be understood that the basal layer is unaffected because it is being supplied by the straight arteries. During relaxation (between events of vasoconstriction), the helicine arteries rupture, and the rapid blood flow dislodges the blood-filled necrotic functional layer, so that only the basal layer remains.

B. Myometrium

During pregnancy the smooth muscle cells of the **myometrium** undergo both **hypertrophy** and **hyperplasia**, increasing the thickness of the muscle wall. Additionally, these smooth muscle cells also acquire **gap junctions** that facilitate their coordinated contractile actions. At parturition, **oxytocin** and **prostaglandins** cause the uterine muscles to undergo rhythmic contractions that assist in expelling the fetus.

IV. HORMONAL EFFECTS ON THE MAMMARY GLAND

During pregnancy, several hormones interact to promote the development of the secretory units of the mammary gland. Cells of the **terminal interalveolar ducts** proliferate to form secretory **alveoli**. The hormones involved in promoting this process are **progesterone, estrogen,** and **human chorionic mammotropin** from the placenta and **lactogenic hormone (prolactin)** from the **acidophils** of the adenohypophysis.

Alveoli and terminal interalveolar ducts are surrounded by **myoepithelial cells** that contract as result of the release of **oxytocin** from the neurohypophysis (in response to suckling), forcing milk out of the breast (**milk ejection reflex**).

V. MILK

Milk is composed of water, proteins, lipids, and lactose. However, milk secreted during the first few days (**colostrum**) is different. It is rich in vitamins, minerals, **lymphoid cells**, and proteins, especially **immunoglobulin A**, providing antibodies for the neonate for the first few months of life.

Clinical Considerations ▨ ▨ ■

Papanicolaou (Pap) Smear
Papanicolaou (Pap) smear is performed as part of routine gynecological examination to examine stained exfoliative cells of the lining of the cervix and vagina. Evaluation of the smeared cells permits the recognition of precancerous conditions, as well as cancer of the cervix. An annual smear test is recommended since cervical cancer is relatively slow growing and the Pap smear is an extremely cost-effective procedure that has been responsible for the early detection of cervical cancer and for saving lives of affected individuals.

Gonorrhea
Gonorrhea is a sexually transmitted bacterial infection caused by the gram negative diplococcus, *Neisseria gonorrhoeae*. In the United States over a million cases of gonorrhea occur annually. Frequently, this sexually transmitted disease (STD) is responsible for pelvic inflammatory disease and for acute salpingitis.

Pelvic Inflammatory Disease (PID)
Pelvic inflammatory disease (PID) is infection of the cervix, uterus, fallopian tubes, and/or ovary, usually a sequel to microbial infection. Individuals suffering from PID exhibit tenderness and pain in the lower abdominal region, fever, unpleasant-smelling vaginal discharge, and episodes of abnormal bleeding. In severe conditions the pain may be debilitating, requiring bed rest and the administration of powerful analgesics.

Endometriosis
Endometriosis is distinguished by the presence of ectopic endometrial tissue dispersed to various sites along the peritoneal cavity. Occasionally the tissues may migrate to extraperitoneal areas, including the eyes and brain. The etiology of this disease is not known, but possibly during the menstrual cycle some of the endometrial cells may migrate along the oviducts and thus enter the peritoneal cavity. In most cases the lesions of endometriosis involve small cysts attached separately or in small clumps on the visceral or parietal peritoneum.

Endometrial Cancer
Endometrial cancer is a malignancy of the uterine endometrium usually occurring in postmenopausal women. The most common type of endometrial cancer is adenocarcinoma. Since during the early stages the cancer cells do not invade the cervix, Pap smears are not very effective in diagnosing this disease until it has entered its later stages. The major symptom of the endometrial cancer is abnormal uterine bleeding.

Paget's Disease of the Nipple
Paget's disease of the nipple usually occurs in elderly women and is associated with breast cancer of ductal origin. Initially the disease manifests as scaly or crusty nipple frequently accompanied by a fluid discharge from the nipple. Usually the patient has no other symptoms and frequently neglects the condition. The treatment of choice is a mastectomy with removal of regional lymph nodes.

Summary of Histological Organization

I. OVARY

A. Cortex

The **cortex** of the **ovary** is covered by a modified mesothelium, the **germinal epithelium**. Deep to this simple cuboidal to simple squamous epithelium is the **tunica albuginea**, the fibrous connective tissue capsule of the ovary. The remainder of the ovarian connective tissue is more cellular and is referred to as the **stroma**. The cortex houses ovarian **follicles** in various stages of development.

1. Primordial Follicles
Primordial follicles consist of a **primary oocyte** surrounded by a single layer of flattened **follicular (granulosa) cells**.

2. Primary Follicles
a. Unilaminar Primary Follicles
Consist of a **primary oocyte** surrounded by a single layer of cuboidal **follicular cells**.
b. Multilaminar Primary Follicles
Consist of a **primary oocyte** surrounded by several layers of **follicular cells**. The **zona pellucida** is visible. The **theca interna** is beginning to be organized.

3. Secondary (Vesicular) Follicle
The **secondary follicle** is distinguished from the primary multilaminar follicle by its larger size, by a well-established **theca interna** and **theca externa**, and especially by the presence of **follicular fluid** in small cavities formed from intercellular spaces of the **follicular cells**. These fluid-filled cavities are known as **Call-Exner bodies**.

4. Graafian (Mature) Follicles
The **Graafian follicle** is very large, the Call-Exner bodies have coalesced into a single space, the **antrum,** filled with **follicular fluid**. The wall of the antrum is referred to as the **membrana granulosa**, and the region of the oocyte and follicular cells jutting into the antrum is the **cumulus oophorus**. The single layer of follicular cells immediately surrounding the oocyte is the **corona radiata**. Long apical processes of these cells extend into the **zona pellucida**. The **theca interna** and **theca externa** are well developed; the former displays numerous cells and capillaries, whereas the latter is less cellular and more fibrous.

5. Atretic Follicles
Atretic follicles are in the state of degeneration. They are characterized in later stages by the presence of **fibroblasts** in the follicle and a degenerated oocyte.

B. Medulla

The **medulla** of the ovary is composed of a relatively loose fibroelastic connective tissue housing an extensive **vascular** supply including spiral arteries and convoluted veins.

C. Corpus Luteum

Subsequent to the extrusion of the **secondary oocyte** with its attendant **follicular cells**, the remnant of the Graafian follicle becomes partly filled with blood and is known as the **corpus hemorrhagicum**. Cells of the **membrana granulosa** are transformed into large **granulosa lutein cells**. Moreover, the cells of the **theca interna** also increase in size to become **theca lutein cells**, although they remain smaller than the **granulosa lutein cells**.

D. Corpus Albicans

The **corpus albicans** is a **corpus luteum** that is in the process of involution and hyalinization. It becomes fibrotic with few **fibroblasts** among the intercellular materials. Eventually, the corpus albicans will become **scar tissue** on the ovarian surface.

II. GENITAL DUCTS

A. Oviduct

1. Mucosa
The **mucosa** of the oviduct is highly folded in the **infundibulum** and **ampulla**. It is composed of a loose, cellular connective tissue **lamina propria** and a **simple columnar epithelial** lining. The epithelium is composed of **peg cells** and **ciliated cells**.

2. Muscularis
The **muscle coat** is composed of an **inner circular** and an **outer longitudinal smooth muscle layer**.

3. Serosa
The oviduct is invested by a **serosa**.

B. Uterus

1. Endometrium

The **endometrium** is subdivided into a **basal** and a **functional layer**. It is lined by a **simple columnar epithelium**. The **lamina propria** varies with the phases of the menstrual cycle.

a. Follicular Phase

The **glands** are straight and display mitotic figures, and the helical arteries grow into the functional layer.

b. Luteal Phase

Glands become tortuous, and the **helical arteries** become coiled. The **lumina** of the glands accumulate **secretory products**. Fibroblasts enlarge and accumulate glycogen.

c. Menstrual Phase

The **functional layer** is desquamated, and the lamina propria displays extravasated blood.

2. Myometrium

The **myometrium** is thick and consists of three poorly delineated **smooth muscle** layers: **inner longitudinal, middle circular**, and **outer longitudinal**. During pregnancy the myometrium increases in size as a result of hypertrophy of existing muscle cells and the accumulation of new smooth muscle cells.

3. Serosa

Most of the uterus is covered by a **serosa**; the remainder is attached to surrounding tissues by an **adventitia**.

C. Placenta

1. Decidua Basalis

The **decidua basalis**, the maternally derived **endometrial layer**, is characterized by the presence of large, glycogen-rich **decidual cells**. **Coiled arteries** and straight **veins** open into the labyrinth-like **intervillous spaces**.

2. Chorionic Plate and Villi

The **chorionic plate** is a region of the **chorionic sac** of the fetus from which **chorionic villi** extend into the intervillous spaces of the **decidua basalis**. Each villus has a core of **fibromuscular connective tissue** surrounding **capillaries** (derived from the umbilical vessels). The villus is covered by **trophoblast cells**. During the first half of pregnancy, there are two layers of trophoblast cells, an inner cuboidal layer of **cytotrophoblasts** and an outer layer of **syncytiotrophoblasts**. During the second half of pregnancy, only the **syncytiotrophoblasts** remain. However, at points where chorionic villi are anchored into the decidua basalis, **cytotrophoblasts** are present.

D. Vagina

1. Mucosa

The vagina is lined by a **stratified squamous nonkeratinized epithelium**. The **lamina propria**, composed of a **fibroelastic connective tissue**, possesses no glands. The **mucosa** is thrown into longitudinal folds known as **rugae**.

2. Submucosa

The **submucosa** is also composed of a fibroelastic type of connective tissue housing numerous blood vessels.

3. Muscularis

The **muscularis** is composed of interlacing bundles of **smooth muscle** fibers. Near its external orifice, the vagina is equipped with a **skeletal muscle sphincter**.

4. Adventitia

The vagina is connected to surrounding structures via its **adventitia**.

E. Mammary Glands

1. Inactive Gland

The **inactive gland** is composed mainly of **dense irregular collagenous connective tissue** interspersed with lobules of **adipose tissue** and numerous **ducts**. Frequently, at the blind ends of ducts, **buds of alveoli** and attendant **myoepithelial cells** are present.

2. Lactating Gland

The **mammary gland** becomes active during pregnancy and lactation. The expanded **alveoli** that form numerous **lobules** are composed of **simple cuboidal cells**, resembling the thyroid gland. However, the presence of **ducts** and **myoepithelial cells** provides distinguishing characteristics. **Alveoli** and the **lumen** of the ducts may contain a fatty secretory product.

3. Areola and Nipple

The **areola** is composed of thin, **pigmented epidermis** displaying large **apocrine areolar glands**. Additionally, **sweat** and large **sebaceous glands** are also present. The **dermis** presents numerous **smooth muscle fibers**. The **nipple** possesses several minute pores representing the distal ends of **lactiferous ducts**. These ducts arise from **lactiferous sinuses**, enlarged reservoirs at the base of the nipple. The **epidermis** covering the nipple is thin, and the dermis is richly supplied by **smooth muscle fibers** and **nerve endings**. Although the nipple possesses no hair follicles or sweat glands, it is richly endowed with **sebaceous glands**.

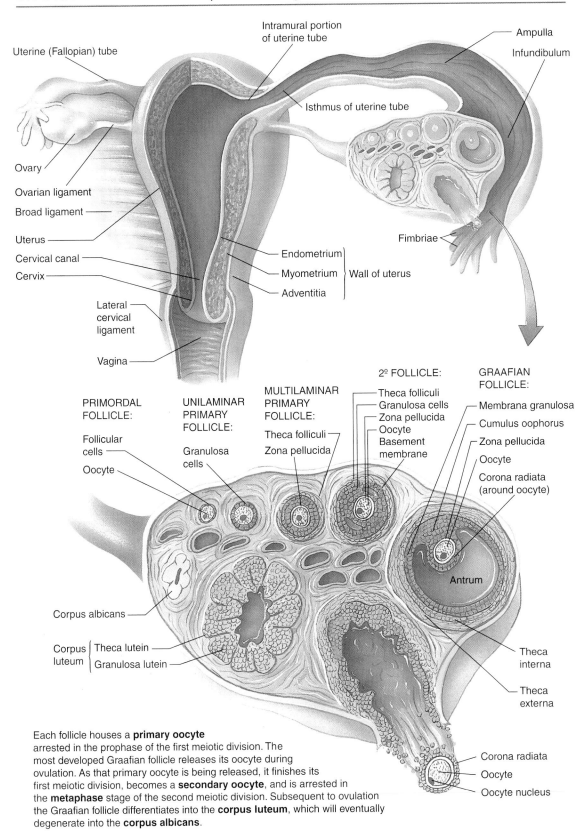

Each follicle houses a **primary oocyte** arrested in the prophase of the first meiotic division. The most developed Graafian follicle releases its oocyte during ovulation. As that primary oocyte is being released, it finishes its first meiotic division, becomes a **secondary oocyte**, and is arrested in the **metaphase** stage of the second meiotic division. Subsequent to ovulation the Graafian follicle differentiates into the **corpus luteum**, which will eventually degenerate into the **corpus albicans**.

Placental Structure

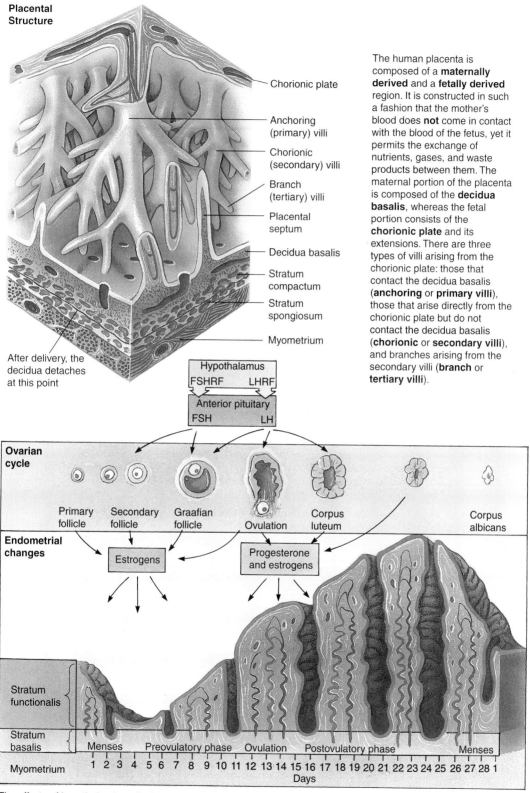

Chorionic plate

Anchoring (primary) villi

Chorionic (secondary) villi

Branch (tertiary) villi

Placental septum

Decidua basalis

Stratum compactum

Stratum spongiosum

Myometrium

After delivery, the decidua detaches at this point

The human placenta is composed of a **maternally derived** and a **fetally derived** region. It is constructed in such a fashion that the mother's blood does **not** come in contact with the blood of the fetus, yet it permits the exchange of nutrients, gases, and waste products between them. The maternal portion of the placenta is composed of the **decidua basalis**, whereas the fetal portion consists of the **chorionic plate** and its extensions. There are three types of villi arising from the chorionic plate: those that contact the decidua basalis (**anchoring** or **primary villi**), those that arise directly from the chorionic plate but do not contact the decidua basalis (**chorionic** or **secondary villi**), and branches arising from the secondary villi (**branch** or **tertiary villi**).

Hypothalamus

FSHRF LHRF

Anterior pituitary

FSH LH

Ovarian cycle

Primary follicle Secondary follicle Graafian follicle Ovulation Corpus luteum Corpus albicans

Endometrial changes

Estrogens Progesterone and estrogens

Stratum functionalis

Stratum basalis

Myometrium

Menses Preovulatory phase Ovulation Postovulatory phase Menses

1 2 3 4 5 6 7 8 9 10 11 12 13 14 15 16 17 18 19 20 21 22 23 24 25 26 27 28 1

Days

The effects of hypothalamic and adenohypohyseal hormones on the ovarian cortex and uterine endometrium.

PLATE 17-1 ■ *Ovary*

FIGURE 1 ▧ *Ovary. Monkey. Plastic section.* × 14.

The ovary is subdivided into a **medulla** (Me) and a **cortex** (Co). The medulla houses large **blood vessels** (BV) from which the cortical vascular supply is derived. The cortex of the ovary contains numerous ovarian follicles, most of which are very small (arrows) while a few maturing follicles have reached the **Graafian follicle** (GF) stage. The thick fibrous connective tissue capsule, **tunica albuginea** (TA), is shown to advantage, while the **germinal epithelium** (GE) is evident occasionally. Observe that the **mesovarium** (Mo) not only suspends the ovary but also conveys the vascular supply to the medulla. A region similar to the boxed area is presented at a higher magnification in Figure 2.

FIGURE 2 ▧ *Ovary. Monkey. Plastic section.* × 132.

This photomicrograph is a higher magnification of a region similar to the boxed area of Figure 1. Observe that the **germinal epithelium** (GE) covers the collagenous capsule, the **tunica albuginea** (TA). This region of the **cortex** (Co) houses numerous **primordial follicles** (PF). Observe that the connective tissue of the ovary is highly cellular and is referred to as the **stroma** (St).

Inset. **Ovary. Cortex. Monkey. Plastic section.** × 540.

The primordial follicle is composed of a **primary oocyte** (PO) whose **nucleus** (N) and **nucleolus** (arrow) are clearly evident. Observe the single layer of flat **follicular cells** (FC) surrounding the oocyte. The **tunica albuginea** (TA) and the **germinal epithelium** (GE) are also shown to advantage in this photomicrograph.

FIGURE 3 ▧ *Primary follicles. Monkey. Plastic section.* × 270.

Primary follicles differ from primordial follicles not only in size but also in morphology and number of follicular cells. The unilaminar primary follicle of the *inset* (× 270) displays a single layer of **cuboidal follicular cells** (FC) that surround the relatively small **primary oocyte** (PO), whose **nucleus** (N) is clearly evident. The multilaminar primary follicle displays a **primary oocyte** (PO) that has increased in size. The **follicular cells** (FC) now form a stratified layer around the oocyte, being separated from it by the intervening **zona pellucida** (ZP). The **stroma** (St) is being reorganized around the follicle to form the **theca interna** (TI). Note the presence of a **basal membrane** (BM) between the follicular cells and the theca interna.

FIGURE 4 ▧ *Secondary follicle. Rabbit. Paraffin section.* × 132.

Secondary follicles are very similar to primary multilaminar follicles, the major difference being their larger size. Moreover, the stratification of the **follicular cells** (FC) has increased, displaying more layers and, more important, a **follicular fluid** (FF) begins to appear in the intercellular spaces, which coalesces into several Call-Exner bodies. Note also that the stroma immediately surrounding the follicular cells is rearranged to form a cellular **theca interna** (TI) and a more fibrous **theca externa** (TE).

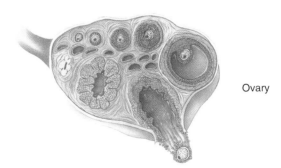

Ovary

■ **KEY**

BM	basal membrane	GF	Graafian follicle	St	stroma
BV	blood vessel	Me	medulla	TA	tunica albuginea
Co	cortex	Mo	mesovarium	TE	theca externa
FC	follicular cell	N	nucleus	TI	theca interna
FF	follicular fluid	PF	primordial follicle	ZP	zona pellucida
GE	germinal epithelium	PO	primary oocyte		

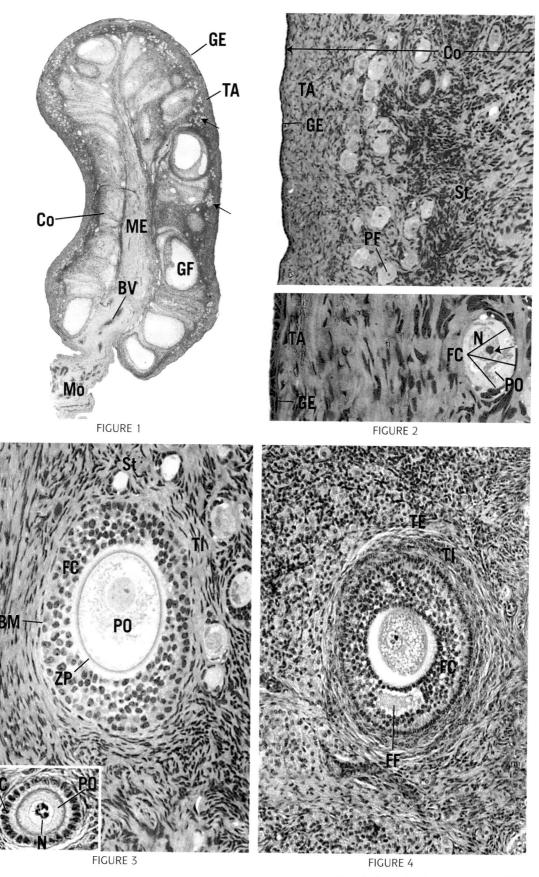

FIGURE 1

FIGURE 2

FIGURE 3

FIGURE 4

PLATE 17-2 ■ *Ovary and Corpus Luteum*

FIGURE 1 ■ *Graafian follicle. Paraffin section.* × 132.

The Graafian follicle is the most mature of all ovarian follicles, and is ready to release its primary oocyte in the process of ovulation. The **follicular fluid** (FL) fills a single chamber, the antrum, which is surrounded by a wall of granulosa (follicular) cells, known as the **membrana granulosa** (MG). Some of the granulosa cells, which surround the **primary oocyte** (PO), jut into the antrum as the **cumulus oophorus** (CO). Observe the **basal membrane** (BM), which separates the granulosa cells from the **theca interna** (TI). The fibrous **theca externa** (TE) merges almost imperceptibly with the surrounding stroma. The boxed area is presented at a higher magnification in Figure 2.

FIGURE 2 ■ *Graafian follicle. Cumulus oophorus. Paraffin section.* × 270.

This photomicrograph is a higher magnification of the boxed area of Figure 1. Observe that the cumulus oophorus houses the **primary oocyte** (PO) whose **nucleus** (N) is just visible in this section. The **zona pellucida** (ZP) surrounds the oocyte, and processes (arrows) of the surrounding follicular cells extend into this acellular region. The single layer of follicular cells appears to radiate as a crown at the periphery of the primary oocyte and is referred to as the **corona radiata** (CR). Note the **basal membrane** (BM), as well as the **theca interna** (TI) and the **theca externa** (TE).

FIGURE 3 ■ *Corpus luteum. Human. Paraffin section.* × 14.

Subsequent to ovulation the Graafian follicle becomes modified to form a temporary structure, the corpus hemorrhagicum, which will become the corpus luteum. The cells comprising the membrana granulosa enlarge, become vesicular in appearance, and are referred to as **granulosa lutein cells** (GL), which become folded, and the spaces between the folds are occupied by connective tissue elements, blood vessels, and cells of the theca interna (arrows). These theca interna cells also enlarge, become glandular, and are referred to as the theca lutein cells. The remnants of the antrum are filled with fibrin and serous exudate that will be replaced by connective tissue elements. A region similar to the boxed area is presented at a higher magnification in Figure 4.

FIGURE 4 ■ *Corpus luteum. Human. Paraffin section.* × 132.

This photomicrograph is a higher magnification of a region similar to the boxed area of Figure 3. The **granulosa lutein cells** (GL) of the corpus luteum are easily distinguished from the **connective tissue** (CT) elements, since the former display round **nuclei** (N) mostly in the center of large round cells (arrowheads). The center of the field is occupied by a fold, housing **theca lutein cells** (TL) amid numerous **connective tissue** (CT) and **vascular** (BV) elements. A region similar to the boxed area is presented at a higher magnification in Figure 1 of the next plate.

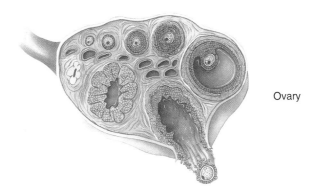

Ovary

■ **KEY**

BM	basal membrane	FL	follicular fluid	TE	theca externa
BV	vascular elements	GL	granulosa lutein cells	TI	theca interna
CO	cumulus oophorus	MG	membrana granulosa	TL	theca lutein cells
CR	corona radiata	N	nucleus	ZP	zona pellucida
CT	connective tissue	PO	primary oocyte		

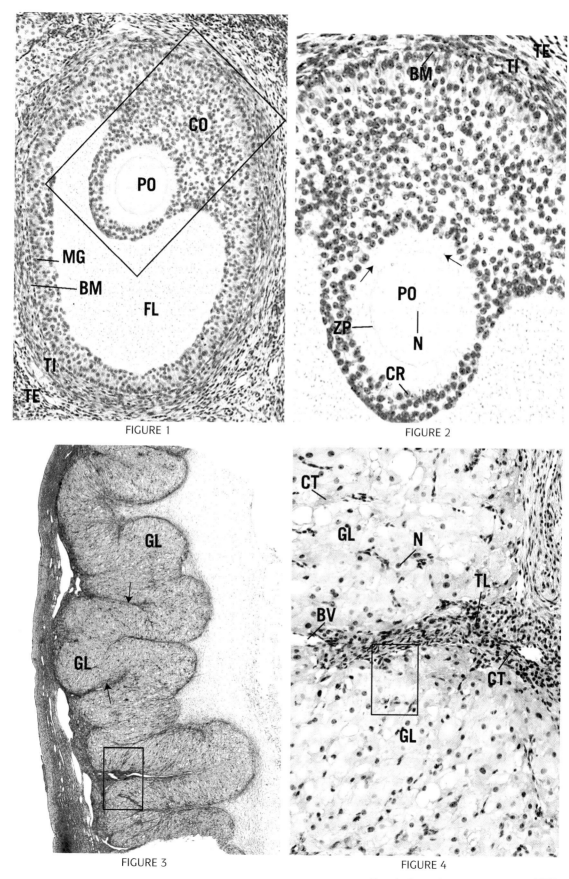

FIGURE 1

FIGURE 2

FIGURE 3

FIGURE 4

PLATE 17-3 ■ *Ovary and Oviduct*

FIGURE 1 ■ *Corpus luteum. Human. Paraffin section.* × 540.

This photomicrograph is similar to the boxed area of Figure 4 of the previous plate. Observe the large **granulosa lutein cells** (GL) whose cytoplasm appears vesicular, representing the spaces occupied by lipids in the living tissue. Note that the **nuclei** (N) of these cells are farther away from each other than the nuclei of the smaller **theca lutein cells** (TL), which also appear to be darker staining (arrowheads). The flattened nuclei (arrows) belong to various connective tissue cells.

FIGURE 3 ■ *Oviduct. x.s. Human. Paraffin section.* × 14.

The oviduct, also referred to as the fallopian or uterine tube, extends from the ovary to the uterine cavity. It is suspended from the body wall by the **broad ligament** (BL), which conveys a rich **vascular supply** (BV) to the **serosa** (S) of the oviduct. The thick **muscularis** (M) is composed of ill-defined inner circular and outer longitudinal muscle layers. The **mucosa** (Mu) is thrown into longitudinal folds, which are so highly exaggerated in the infundibulum and ampulla that they subdivide the **lumen** (L) into labyrinthine spaces. A region similar to the boxed area is presented at a higher magnification in Figure 4.

FIGURE 2 ■ *Corpus albicans. Human. Paraffin section.* × 132.

As the corpus luteum involutes, its cellular elements degenerate, and undergo autolysis. The corpus luteum becomes invaded by macrophages that phagocytose the dead cells, leaving behind relatively acellular **fibrous tissue** (FT). The previously rich **vascular supply** (BV) also regressed, and the entire corpus albicans appears pale in comparison to the relatively dark staining of the surrounding ovarian **stroma** (St). The corpus albican will regress until it becomes a small scar on the surface of the ovary.

FIGURE 4 ■ *Oviduct. x.s. Monkey. Plastic section.* × 132.

This photomicrograph is a higher magnification of a region similar to the boxed area of Figure 3. The entire thickness of the wall of the oviduct displays its **vascular** (BV) **serosa** (S) that envelops the thick muscularis, whose **outer longitudinal** (OL) and **inner circular** (IC) layers are not very well delineated. The **mucosa** (Mu) is highly folded and is lined by a simple columnar **epithelium** (Ep). The loose connective tissue of the **lamina propria** (LP) is richly vascularized (arrows). The boxed area is presented in a higher magnification in Figure 1 in the following plate.

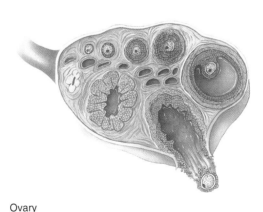

Ovary

■ **KEY**

BL	broad ligament	IC	inner circular muscle	N	nucleus
BV	vascular supply	L	lumen	OL	outer longitudinal muscle
Ep	epithelium	LP	lamina propria	S	serosa
FT	fibrous tissue	M	muscularis	St	stroma
GL	granulosa lutein cell	Mu	mucosa	TL	theca lutein cell

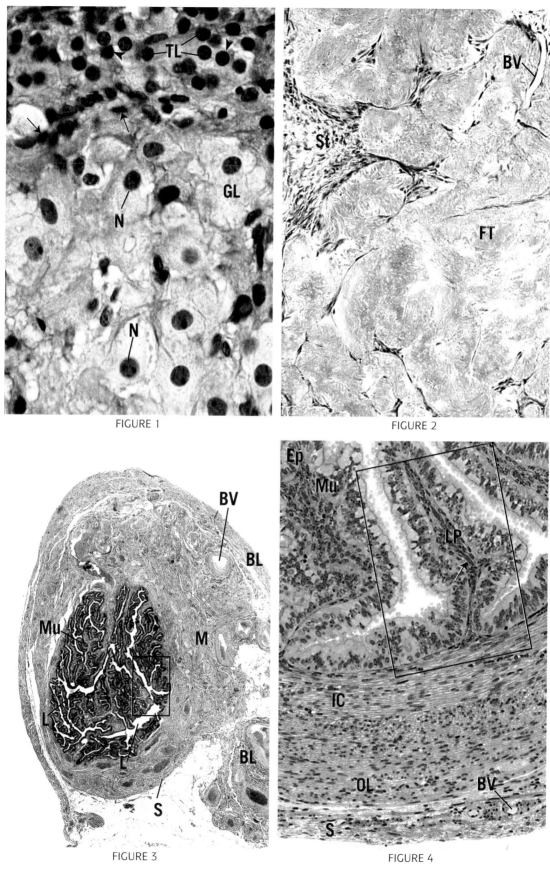

FIGURE 1

FIGURE 2

FIGURE 3

FIGURE 4

PLATE 17-4 ■ *Oviduct, Light and Electron Microscopy*

FIGURE 1 ■ *Oviduct. x.s. Monkey. Plastic section.* × 270.

This photomicrograph is a higher magnification of the boxed area of Figure 4 of the previous plate. Observe the **inner circular muscle** (IC) layer of the muscularis. The **lamina propria** (LP) is very narrow in this region (arrows), but presents longitudinal epithelially lined folds. The core of these folds is composed of a **vascular** (BV), loose, but highly cellular **connective tissue** (CT). The simple columnar **epithelium** (Ep) lines the labyrinthine **lumen** (L) of the oviduct. A region similar to the boxed area is presented at a higher magnification in Figure 2.

FIGURE 2 ■ *Oviduct. x.s. Monkey. Plastic section.* × 540.

This photomicrograph is a higher magnification of a region similar to the boxed area of Figure 1. The **lamina propria** (LP) is a highly cellular, loose connective tissue that is richly **vascularized**. The **basal membrane** (BM) separating the connective tissue from the epithelial lining is clearly evident. Note that the epithelium is composed of two different cell types, a thinner **peg cell** (PC), which bears no cilia, but whose apical extent bulges above the ciliated cells. These bulges (arrowheads) contain nutritive materials that nourishes gametes. The second cell type of the oviduct epithelium is a **ciliated cell** (CL), whose cilia move in unison with those of neighboring cells, propelling the nutrient material toward the uterine lumen.

FIGURE 3 ■ *Oviduct epithelium. Human. Electron microscopy.* × 4553.

The human oviduct at midcycle (day 14) presents two types of epithelial cells, the **peg cell** (PC) and the **ciliated cell** (CC). The former are secretory cells as indicated by their extensive **Golgi apparatus** (GA) situated in the region of the cell apical to the **nucleus** (N). Observe the electron-dense secretory products (arrows) in the expanded, apical free ends of these cells. Note also that some ciliated cells display large accumulations of **glycogen** (Gl) at either pole of the nucleus. (From Verhage H, Bareither M, Jaffe R, Akbar M: *Am J Anat* 156:505–522, 1979.)

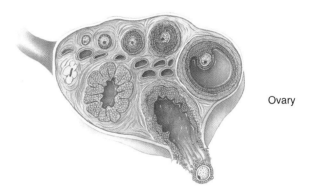

Ovary

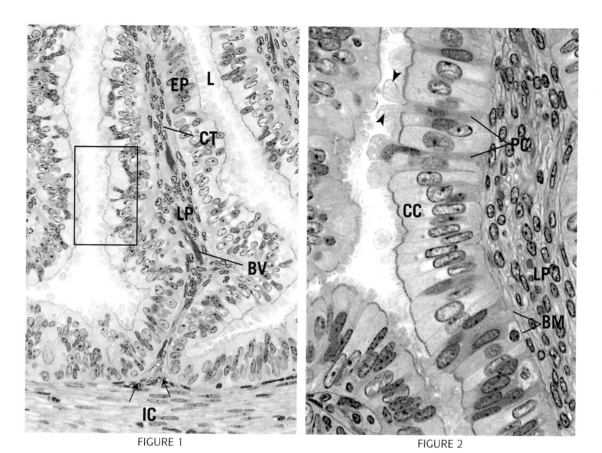

FIGURE 1

FIGURE 2

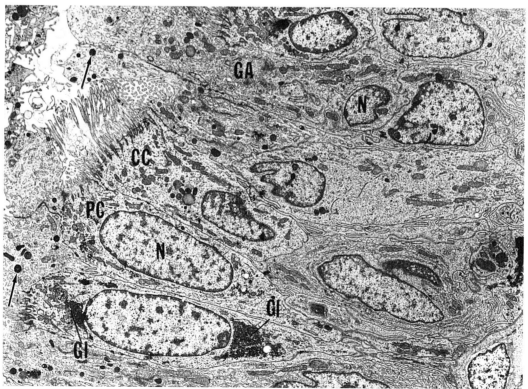

FIGURE 3

PLATE 17-5 ■ *Uterus*

FIGURE 1 ■ *Uterus. Follicular phase. Human. Paraffin section.* × 14.

The uterus is a thick-walled organ, whose wall consists of three layers. The external serosa (or in certain regions, adventitia) is unremarkable and is not presented in this photomicrograph. The thick **myometrium** (My) is composed of smooth muscle, subdivided into three poorly delineated layers: **outer longitudinal** (OL), **middle circular** (MC), and **inner longitudinal** (IL). The **endometrium** (En) is subdivided into a **basal layer** (B) and a **functional layer** (F). The functional layer varies in thickness and constitution and passes through a sequence of phases during the menstrual cycle. Note that the functional layer is in the process of being built-up and that the forming **glands** (GL) are straight. The deeper aspects of some of these glands display branching (arrow). The boxed area is presented at a higher magnification in Figure 2.

FIGURE 2 ■ *Uterus. Follicular phase. Human. Paraffin section.* × 132.

This photomicrograph is a higher magnification of the boxed area of Figure 1. Note that the **functional layer** (F) of the endometrium is lined by a simple columnar **epithelium** (Ep) that is displaying mitotic activity (arrows). The forming **glands** (GL) also consist of a simple columnar **epithelium** (Ep) whose cells are actively dividing. The **stroma** (St) is highly cellular, as evidenced by the numerous connective tissue cell nuclei visible in this field. Note also the rich **vascular supply** (BV) of the endometrial stroma.

FIGURE 3 ■ *Uterus. Luteal phase. Human. Paraffin section.* × 14.

The **myometrium** (My) of the uterus remains constant during the various endometrial phases. Observe its three layers, noting especially that the middle circular layer of smooth muscle is richly vascularized and is, therefore, frequently referred to as the **stratum vasculare** (SV). The **endometrium** (En) is richly endowed with **glands** (GL) that become highly tortuous in anticipation of the blastocyst that will be nourished by secretions of these glands subsequent to implantation. A region similar to the boxed area is presented at a higher magnification in Figure 4.

FIGURE 4 ■ *Uterus. Early luteal phase. Human. Paraffin section.* × 132.

This photomicrograph is a higher magnification of a region similar to the boxed area of Figure 3. The functional layer of the endometrium is covered by a simple columnar **epithelium** (Ep), separating the endometrial **stroma** (St) from the uterine **lumen** (L). Note that the **glands** (GL), also composed of simple columnar epithelium, are more abundant than those in the follicular phase (Figure 2, above). Observe also that these glands appear more tortuous and are dilated and their lumina contain a slight amount of secretory product (arrow).

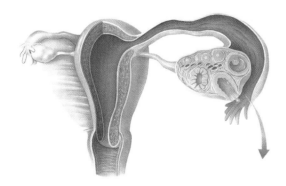

Female reproductive system

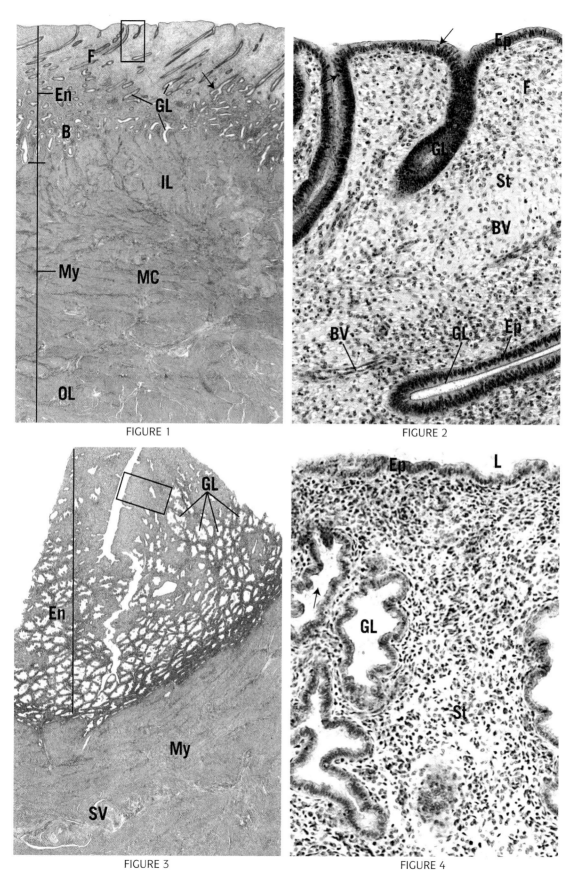

FIGURE 1

FIGURE 2

FIGURE 3

FIGURE 4

PLATE 17-6 ■ *Uterus*

FIGURE 1 ■ *Uterus. Midluteal phase. Human. Paraffin section.* × 270.

During the midluteal phase the endometrial **glands** (GL) become quite tortuous and corkscrew-shaped, and the simple **columnar cells** (CC) accumulate glycogen (arrow). Observe that during this phase of the endometrium, the glycogen is basally located, displacing the **nucleus** (N) toward the center of the cell. Note also that the **stroma** (St) is undergoing a decidual reaction in that some of the connective tissue cells enlarge as they become engorged with lipid and glycogen. A **helical artery** (HA) is evident as several cross-sections.

FIGURE 2 ■ *Uterus. Late luteal phase. Human. Paraffin section.* × 132.

During the late luteal phase of the endometrium, the glands assume a characteristic ladder (or sawtooth) shape (arrows). The simple columnar **epithelial cells** (CC) appear pale and, interestingly, the position of the glycogen is now apical (arrowheads) rather than basal. The apical location of the glycogen imparts a ragged, torn appearance to the free surface of these cells. Note that the **lumina** (L) of the glands are filled with a glycogen-rich, viscous fluid. Observe also that the **stroma** (St) is infiltrated by numerous **leukocytes** (Le).

FIGURE 3 ■ *Uterus. Menstrual phase. Human. Paraffin section.* × 132.

The menstrual phase of the endometrium is characterized by periodic constriction and sequential opening of **helical arteries** (HA), resulting in ischemia with subsequent necrosis of the superficial aspect of the functional layer. Due to these spasmodic contractions sudden spurts of arterial blood detach **necrotic fragments** (NF) of the superficial layers of the endometrium that are then discharged as menstrual flow. The endometrial stroma becomes engorged with blood, increasing the degree of ischemia, and eventually the entire functional layer is desquamated. Observe that the **lumen** (L) no longer possesses a complete epithelial lining (arrowheads). The boxed area is presented at a higher magnification in Figure 4.

FIGURE 4 ■ *Uterus. Menstrual phase. Human. Paraffin section.* × 270.

This photomicrograph is a higher magnification of the boxed area of Figure 3. Observe that some of the endometrial **glands** (GL) are torn and a **necrotic fragment** (NF) has been detached from the **functional layer** (F) of the endometrium. The **stroma** (St) is infiltrated by leukocytes, whose dense **nuclei** (N) mask most of the endometrial cells. Note that some of the endometrial cells are still enlarged, indicative of the decidual reaction.

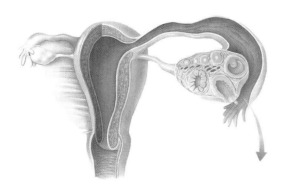

Female reproductive system

■ **KEY**

CC	columnar cell	HA	helical artery	N	nucleus
F	functional layer	L	lumen	NF	necrotic fragment
GL	gland	Le	leukocyte	St	stroma

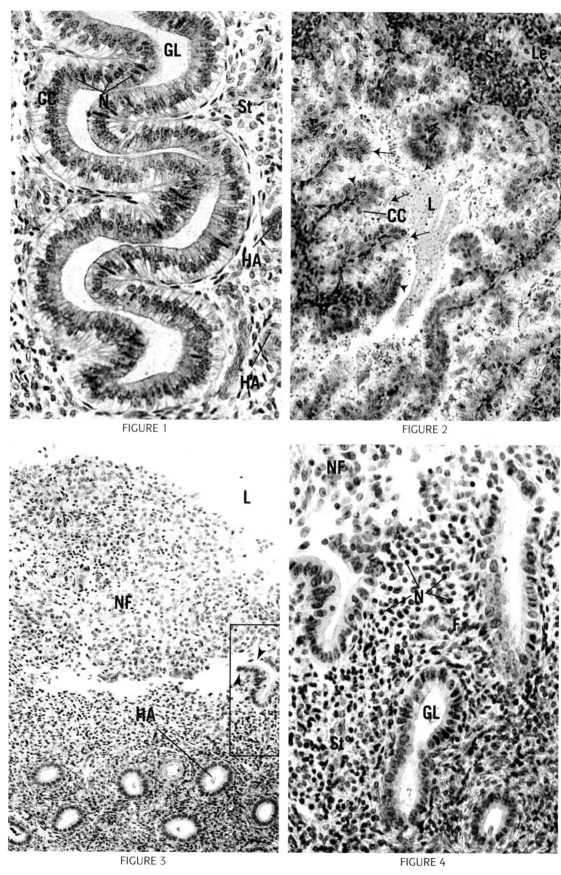

FIGURE 1

FIGURE 2

FIGURE 3

FIGURE 4

PLATE 17-7 ■ *Placenta and Vagina*

FIGURE 1 ■ *Placenta. Human. Paraffin section.* × 132.

The human placenta is intimately associated with the uterine endometrium. At this junction, the **decidua basalis** (DB) is rich in clumps of large, round to polygonal **decidual cells** (DC), whose distended cytoplasm is filled with lipid and glycogen. Anchoring **chorionic villi** (AV) are attached to the decidua basalis, while other villi are blindly ending in the **intervillous space** (IS). These are the most numerous and are referred to as **terminal villi** (TV), most of which are cut in cross or oblique sections. These villi are freely branching and, in the mature placenta, are smaller in diameter than in the immature placenta.

Inset. **Placenta. Human. Paraffin section.** × 270.

Note that the **decidual cells** (DC) are round to polygonal in shape. Their **nuclei** (N) are more or less centrally located, and their cytoplasm appears vacuolated due to the extraction of glycogen and lipids during histologic preparation.

FIGURE 3 ■ *Vagina. l.s. Monkey. Plastic section* × 14.

The vagina is a fibromuscular tube, whose **vaginal space** (VS) is mostly obliterated since its walls are normally in contact with each other. This wall is composed of four layers: mucosa (Mu), **submucosa** (SM), **muscularis** (M), and **adventitia** (A). The mucosa consists of an **epithelium** (Ep) and underlying **lamina propria** (LP). Deep to the mucosa is the submucosa, whose numerous large blood vessels impart to it an erectile tissue appearance. The smooth muscle of the muscularis is arranged in two layers, an **inner circular** (IC) and a thicker **outer longitudinal** (OL). A region similar to the boxed area is presented at a higher magnification in Figure 4.

FIGURE 2 ■ *Placenta. Human. Paraffin section.* × 270.

Cross-sections of **terminal villi** (TV) are very simple in the mature placenta. They are surrounded by the **intervillous space** (IS) that, in the functional placenta, is filled with maternal blood. Hence, the cells of the villus act as a placental barrier. This barrier is greatly reduced in the mature placenta, as presented in this photomicrograph. The external layer of the terminal villus is composed of **syncytial trophoblasts** (ST), whose numerous **nuclei** (N) are frequently clustered together as **syncytial knots** (SK). The core of the villus houses numerous fetal **capillaries** (Ca) that are located usually in regions of the villus void of syncytial nuclei (arrowheads). Larger fetal **blood vessels** (BV) are also found in the core, surrounded by **mesoderm** (Me). The cytotrophoblasts and phagocytic Hofbauer cells of the immature placenta mostly disappear by the end of the pregnancy.

FIGURE 4 ■ *Vagina. l.s. Human. Paraffin section.* × 132.

This photomicrograph is a higher magnification of a region similar to the boxed area in Figure 3. The stratified squamous nonkeratinized **epithelium** (Ep) of the vagina is characterized by the empty appearance of the cells comprising most of its thickness. This is due to the extraction lipids and glycogen during histologic preparation. Observe that the cells in the deeper aspect of the epithelium possess fewer inclusions; therefore, their cytoplasm appears normal. Note also that the **lamina propria** (LP) is richly **vascularized** (BV) and always possesses numerous **leukocytes** (Le) (arrows). Finally, note the absence of glands and muscularis mucosae.

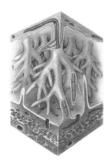

Placenta

■ KEY

A	adventitia	IC	inner circular muscle	N	nucleus
AV	anchoring chorionic villus	IS	intervillous space	OL	outer longitudinal muscle
BV	blood vessel	Mu	mucosa	SK	syncytial knot
Ca	capillary	Le	leukocyte	SM	submucosa
DB	decidua basalis	LP	lamina propria	ST	syncytial trophoblast
DC	decidual cell	M	muscularis	TV	terminal villus
Ep	epithelium	Me	mesoderm	VS	vaginal space

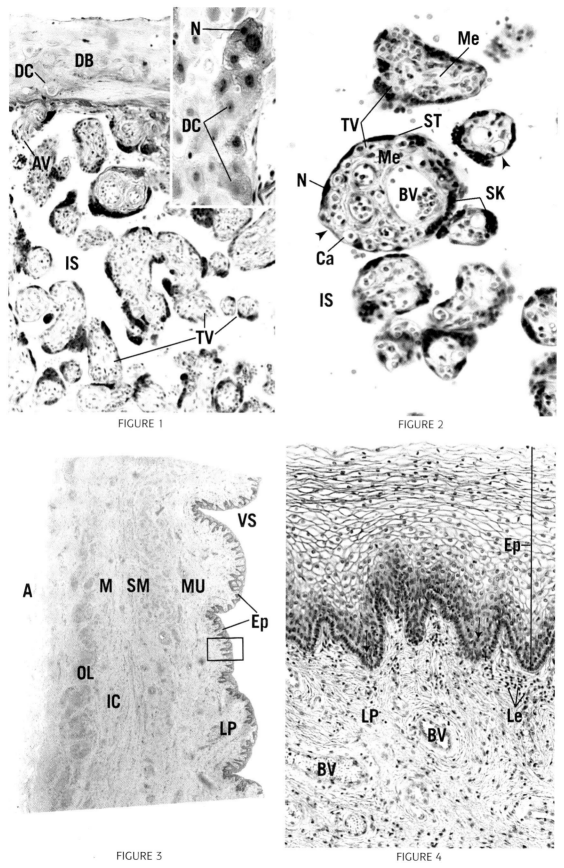

FIGURE 1

FIGURE 2

FIGURE 3

FIGURE 4

Female Reproductive System ▪ 365

PLATE 17-8 ■ *Mammary Gland*

FIGURE 1 ■ *Mammary gland. Inactive. Human. Paraffin section.* × 132.

The mammary gland is a modified sweat gland that, in the resting stage, presents **ducts** (D) with occasional **buds of alveoli** (BA) branching from the blind ends of the duct. The remainder of the breast is composed of **dense collagenous connective tissue** (dCT) interspersed with lobules of fat. However, in the immediate vicinity of the ducts and buds of alveoli the **connective tissue** (CT) is more loosely arranged. It is believed that this looser connective tissue is derived from the papillary layer of the dermis. Compare this photomicrograph with Figure 2.

FIGURE 2 ■ *Mammary gland. Lactating. Human. Paraffin section.* × 132.

During pregnancy the **ducts** (D) of the mammary gland undergo major development, in that the buds of alveoli proliferate to form lobules (Lo) composed of numerous alveoli (Al). The interlobular **connective tissue** (CT) becomes reduced to thin sheets in regions, while elsewhere it maintains its previous character to support the increased weight of the breast. Observe that the connective tissue in the immediate vicinity of the ducts and lobules (arrows) retains its loose consistency. Compare this photomicrograph with Figure 1.

FIGURE 3 ■ *Mammary gland. Lactating. Human. Paraffin section.* × 132.

The active mammary gland presents numerous **lobules** (Lo) of **alveoli** (Al) that are tightly packed so that the **connective tissue** (CT) elements are greatly compressed. This photomicrograph clearly illustrates the crowded nature of this tissue. Although this tissue bears a superficial resemblance to the histology of the thyroid gland, the presence of ducts and branching alveoli (arrows), as well as the lack of colloid material, should assist in distinguishing this tissue as the active mammary gland.

Inset. **Mammary gland. Active. Human. Paraffin section.** × 270.

Observe the branching (arrows) of this alveolus, some of whose simple cuboidal **epithelial cells** (Ep) appear vacuolated (arrowheads). Note also that the lumen (L) contains fatty secretory product.

FIGURE 4 ■ *Mammary gland. Nipple. Human. Paraffin section.* × 14.

The large, conical nipple of the breast is covered by a thin **epidermis** (Ed), composed of stratified squamous keratinized epithelium. Although the nipple possesses neither hair nor sweat glands, it is richly endowed with **sebaceous glands** (SG). The dense irregular collagenous **connective tissue** (CT) core displays numerous longitudinally positioned lactiferous ducts that pierce the tip of the nipple to convey milk to the outside. The lactiferous ducts are surrounded by an extensive network of **smooth muscle** fibers (SM) that are responsible for the erection of the nipple, elevating it to facilitate the suckling process. The region immediately surrounding the nipple is know as the **areola** (Ar).

▨ KEY

Al	alveolus	D	duct	L	lumen
Ar	areola	dCT	dense connective tissue	Lo	lobule
BA	buds of alveoli	Ed	epidermis	SM	smooth muscle
CT	connective tissue	Ep	epithelium	SG	sebaceous gland

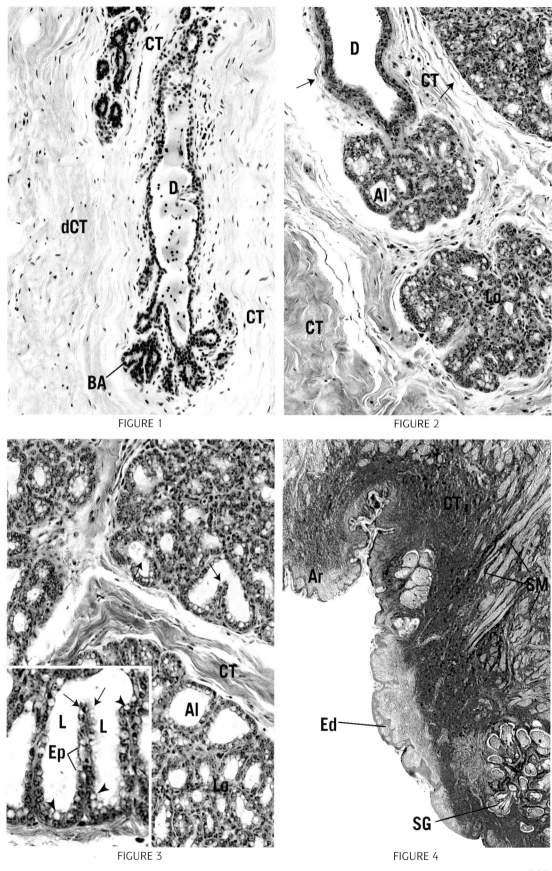

FIGURE 1

FIGURE 2

FIGURE 3

FIGURE 4

Female Reproductive System ■ **367**

Male Reproductive System

The male reproductive system (see Graphic 18-1) consists of the two testes (the male gonads), a system of genital ducts, accessory glands, and the penis. The male reproductive system functions in the formation of spermatozoa, the elaboration of male sex hormones, and the delivery of male gametes into the female reproductive tract.

TESTES

Each **testis** is an oval structure housed in its separate compartment within the scrotum. Its fibromuscular connective tissue capsule, the **tunica albuginea**, is thickened at the **mediastinum testis**, from which septa are derived to subdivide the testis into approximately 250 small, incomplete compartments, the **lobuli testis**. Each lobule houses one to four highly tortuous **seminiferous tubules** that function in the production of **spermatozoa**. The lumen of each seminiferous tubule is lined by a **seminiferous epithelium** several cell layers thick. The **basal cells** of this epithelium are composed of **Sertoli cells** and **spermatogonia**. The latter cells divide by mitotic activity to replicate themselves and to produce primary **spermatocytes**. These diploid primary spermatocytes enter the **first meiotic division**, forming **secondary spermatocytes** that, by completing **second meiotic division**, give rise to haploid **spermatids**. Subsequent to shedding much of their cytoplasm, reorganizing their organelle population, and acquiring certain specialized organelles, spermatids become **spermatozoa**, the **male gamete**. The differentiating cells are supported by Sertoli cells both physically and nutritionally. Moreover, occluding junctions between adjacent Sertoli cells establish a **blood-testis barrier** that protects the developing germ cells from autoimmune phenomena. The seminiferous epithelium sits on a basal membrane that is surrounded by a fibromuscular tunica propria.

The connective tissue surrounding the seminiferous tubules houses, in addition to neural and vascular elements, small clumps of **androgen-producing endocrine cells**, the **interstitial cells of Leydig**. These cells produce the male sex hormone **testosterone**. Prior to puberty, testosterone is not produced, but at the onset of puberty the pituitary gland releases **luteinizing hormone** (**LH**) and **follicle-stimulating hormone** (**FSH**). The former activates the interstitial cells of Leydig that release testosterone, whereas FSH induces the Sertoli cells to produce **adenylate cyclase**, which, via a cAMP intermediary, stimulates the production of **androgen-binding protein** (**ABP**). Testosterone binds to ABP, and the complex is released into the lumen of the seminiferous tubule, where the elevated testosterone concentration enhances **spermatogenesis**.

GENITAL DUCTS

A system of **genital ducts** conveys the spermatozoa and the fluid component of the semen to the outside. The **seminiferous tubules** are connected by short straight tubules, the **tubuli recti**, to the **rete testis**, which is composed of labyrinthine spaces located in the **mediastinum testis**. From here, spermatozoa enter the first part of the epididymis, the 15–20 **ductuli efferentes** that lead into the **ductus epididymis**. During their sojourn in the epididymis, spermatozoa mature. The head of the epididymis is composed of the ductuli efferentes, while the body and tail consist of the ductus epididymis, whose continuation is the **ductus deferens** (**vas deferens**) (Graphic 18-1). This thick, muscular structure passes through the inguinal canal, as a part of the spermatic cord, to gain access to the abdominal cavity. Just prior to reaching the prostate gland, the **seminal vesicle** empties its secretions into the ductus deferens, which terminates at this point. The continuation of the duct, known as the **ejaculatory duct**, enters the **prostate gland**. This gland delivers its secretory product into this duct. The right and left **ejaculatory ducts** empty into the **urethra**, which conveys both urine and **semen** to the outside. The urethra, which passes through the length of the penis, has three regions: prostatic, membranous, and cavernous (spongy) portions.

ACCESSORY GLANDS

The three **accessory glands** of the male reproductive system, which supply the fluid component of semen, are the two **seminal vesicles** and the **prostate gland**. Additionally, a pair of small **bulbourethral glands** deliver their viscous secretions into the cavernous (spongy) urethra. Each seminal vesicle is a long, narrow gland that is highly folded on itself. Each seminal vesicle produces a rich, nutritive substance with a characteristic yellow color. The prostate gland is composed of numerous individual glands that surround, and whose ducts pierce, the wall of the urethra. These glands are distributed in three regions of the prostate and are, therefore, categorized as mucosal, submucosal, and external (main) prostatic glands. The secretion of the prostate gland is a whitish, thin fluid containing proteolytic enzymes and acid phosphatase. **Prostatic concretions** are frequently found in the lumina of the prostate gland.

PENIS

The **penis**, the male organ of copulation, is normally in the flaccid state. During erotic stimulation, however, its three cylindrical bodies of erectile tissues, the two **corpora cavernosa** and the **corpus spongiosum**, become distended with blood. The fluid turgid pressure within the vascular spaces of the erectile tissues greatly enlarges the penis, causing it to become erect and hard. Subsequent to ejaculation or the termination of erotic stimulation, detumescence follows and the penis returns to its flaccid state.

Histophysiology

I. SERTOLI CELL FUNCTIONS

Sertoli cells sit on the basal lamina of the seminiferous tubule and form **zonulae occludentes** with one another, thus separating the lumen of the seminiferous tubule into an outer **basal compartment** and an inner **adluminal compartment**. By doing so, they isolate the adluminal compartment from connective tissue elements and thus protect the developing sperm cells from the immune system.

Prompted by follicle-stimulating hormone (**FSH**) secreted by the anterior pituitary gland, Sertoli cells secrete **androgen-binding protein** (**ABP**), which binds **testosterone** and releases it into the lumen of the seminiferous tubules, where it is maintained at a sufficiently high threshold level to permit spermatogenesis to occur. These cells also secrete the hormone **inhibin**, which blocks the release of FSH via a biofeedback mechanism.

Spermatocytes, spermatids, and spermatozoa are physically and metabolically **supported** by Sertoli cells. Moreover, cytoplasm discarded during **spermiogenesis** is **phagocytosed** by Sertoli cells. Sertoli cells also secrete a fructose-rich fluid that supports spermatozoa and provides a fluid medium for their transport through the seminiferous tubules and the genital ducts.

During embryonic development, Sertoli cells produce **antimüllerian hormone**, which prevents the development of the müllerian duct, thus ensuring the development of a male rather than a female embryo.

II. SPERMATOGENESIS

Spermatogenesis, the process of producing haploid male gametes, is dependent on several hormones, including **luteinizing hormone** (**LH**) and **FSH** from the adenohypophysis (see Graphic 18-2). LH induces interstitial cells of Leydig to secrete **testosterone**, and FSH causes Sertoli cells to release ABP. ABP maintains a high enough concentration of testosterone in the seminiferous epithelium for spermatogenesis to occur. Testosterone acts as a **negative feedback** for LH release, and **inhibin**, produced by Sertoli cells, inhibits the release of FSH. For spermatogenesis to proceed normally, the testes must be maintained at 35° C, a temperature that is slightly below normal body temperature.

Spermatogenesis occurs in a cyclic but asynchronous fashion along the length of the seminiferous tubule. These **cycles of the seminiferous epithelium** consist of repeated aggregates of cells in varying stages of development. Each aggregate is composed of groups of cells that are connected to one another by **intercellular bridges**, forming a synchronized syncytium that migrates toward the lumen of the seminiferous tubule as a unit. The three phases of spermatogenesis are spermatocytogenesis, meiosis, and spermiogenesis.

Spermatocytogenesis is a process involving mitosis, where **pale type A spermatogonia** divide to form more pale type A and **type B** spermatogonia, both of which are diploid. **Dark type A spermatogonia** represent a reserve population of cells that normally do not undergo cell division, but when they do, they form pale type A spermatogonia.

Type B spermatogonia divide via mitosis to form diploid **primary spermatocytes**. All spermatogonia are located in the **basal compartment**, whereas primary spermatocytes migrate into the **adluminal compartment**.

Meiosis phase starts when primary spermatocytes (4CDNA content) undergo the first meiotic division, forming two short-lived **secondary spermatocytes** (2CDNA content). Secondary spermatocytes do not replicate their DNA but immediately start the second meiotic division, and each forms two **haploid** (**N**) spermatids.

Spermiogenesis (Graphic 18-2) is the process of cytodifferentiation of the spermatids into spermatozoa and involves no cell division. Instead, the spermatid loses much of its cytoplasm (phagocytosed by Sertoli cells), forming an **acrosomal granule**, a long **cilium**, and associated **outer dense fibers** and a **coarse fibrous sheath**. The **spermatozoon** that is formed and released into the lumen of the seminiferous tubule is **nonmotile** and is incapable of fertilizing an ovum. The spermatozoa remain immotile until they leave the epididymis. They become capable of fertilizing once they have been **capacitated** in the female reproductive system.

III. ERECTION AND EJACULATION

The **penis** during **copulation** delivers spermatozoa-containing **semen** to the female reproductive tract. It is also the excretory organ for urine. The penis is covered by skin and is composed of three **erectile** bodies, the two **corpora cavernosa** and the ventrally positioned **corpus spongiosum (urethrae)**.

Each erectile body, housing large endothelially lined **cavernous spaces,** is surrounded by a thick connective tissue capsule, the **tunica albuginea.** The erectile bodies are supplied by **helicine arteries** that are usually bypassed via arteriovenous shunts, maintaining the penis in a flaccid state. **Parasympathetic impulses** to these shunts cause vasoconstriction, directing blood into the helicine arteries and thus into the cavernous spaces. The erectile bodies (especially the corpora cavernosa) become engorged with blood, and the penis becomes **erect.**

Subsequent to ejaculation or in the absence of continued stimulation, parasympathetic stimulation ceases; blood flow to the helicine arteries is diminished; blood slowly leaves the cavernous spaces; and the penis returns to its flaccid condition.

Ejaculation is the forceful expulsion of **semen** from the male reproductive tract. The force required for ejaculation is derived from rhythmic contraction of the thick smooth muscle layers of the **ductus (vas) deferens** and the rapid contraction of the **bulbospongiosus muscle.**

Each ejaculate contains spermatozoa suspended in **seminal fluid.** The accessory glands of the male reproductive system, the **prostate** and **bulbourethral glands,** as well as the **seminal vesicles** (and even the glands of Littré) contribute to the formation of the fluid portion of semen. Secretions of the bulbourethral glands lubricate the urethra, whereas secretions of the prostate assist the spermatozoa in achieving motility by neutralizing the acidic secretions of the ductus deferens and of the female reproductive tract. Energy for the spermatozoa is provided by fructose-rich secretions of the seminal vesicles.

Clinical Considerations ▪ ▪ ▪

Cryptorchidism
Cryptorchidism is a developmental defect where one or both testes fail to descend into the scrotum. When neither descends, it results in sterility because normal body temperature inhibits spermatogenesis. Usually, the condition can be surgically corrected; however, the patient's sperm may be abnormal.

Vasectomy
Vasectomy is a method of sterilization that is performed by making a small slit in the wall of the scrotum through which the ductus deferens is severed.
A normal **ejaculate** averages about 3 mL of semen that contains 60 to 100 million spermatozoa per mL. It is interesting to note that about 20% of the ejaculated spermatozoa are abnormal and 25% immotile. An individual producing less than 20 million spermatozoa per mL of ejaculate is considered **sterile**.

Benign Prostatic Hypertrophy
The prostate gland undergoes hypertrophy with age resulting in benign prostatic hypertrophy, a condition that may constrict the urethral lumen resulting in difficulty in urination. At age 50 about 40% of the male population is affected and at age 80 about 95% of the male population is affected by this condition.

Adenocarcinoma of the Prostate
Adenocarcinoma of the prostate affects about 30% of the male population over 75 years of age. Although this carcinoma is slow growing it may metastasize to bone. Analysis of elevated levels of **prostate specific antigen (PSA)** in the bloodstream is utilized as an early diagnostic test for prostatic cancer. Surgical removal of the gland with or without chemo- or radiation therapy is the usual treatment; however, complications may result in impotence and incontinence.

Testicular Cancer
Testicular cancer affects mostly men younger than 40 years of age. It is discovered upon palpation as a lump in the scrotum. If the lump is not associated with the testis it is usually benign, whereas if it is associated with the testis it is usually malignant; therefore, a lump noticed on the testis, whether or not it is painful, should be examined by a physician. Frequently, individuals with testicular cancer present with elevated blood **alpha-fetoprotein** and **human chorionic gonadotropin** levels. The common treatment for testicular cancer is surgical removal of the affected testis. If metastasis has occurred than the surgery is supplemented by radiation and chemotherapy.

Summary of Histological Organization

I. TESTES

A. Capsule

The fibromuscular connective tissue **capsule** of the testes is known as the **tunica albuginea**, whose inner vascular layer is the **tunica vasculosa**. The capsule is thickened at the **mediastinum testis** from which **septa** emanate, subdividing the testis into approximately 250 incomplete **lobuli testis**, with each containing one to four **seminiferous tubules** embedded in a connective tissue **stroma**.

B. Seminiferous Tubules

Each highly convoluted **seminiferous tubule** is composed of a fibromuscular **tunica propria**, which is separated from the **seminiferous epithelium** by a basal membrane.

1. Seminiferous Epithelium

The **seminiferous epithelium** is composed of sustentacular **Sertoli cells** and a stratified layer of developing **male gametes**. Sertoli cells establish a blood-testis barrier by forming occluding junctions with each other, thus subdividing the seminiferous tubule into **adluminal** and **basal compartments**. The basal compartment houses **spermatogonia A** (both **light** and **dark**), **spermatogonia B**, and the basal aspects of Sertoli cells. The adluminal compartment contains the apical portions of Sertoli cells, **primary spermatocytes, secondary spermatocytes, spermatids,** and **spermatozoa**.

2. Tunica Propria

The **tunica propria** consists of loose collagenous connective tissue, **fibroblasts**, and **myoid cells**.

C. Stroma

The loose vascular connective tissue **stroma** surrounding seminiferous tubules houses small clusters of large, vacuolated-appearing endocrine cells, the **interstitial cells** (of Leydig).

II. GENITAL DUCTS

A. Tubuli Recti

Short straight tubes, the **tubuli recti**, lined by Sertoli-like cells initially and **simple cuboidal epithelium** later, connect the seminiferous tubules to the rete testis.

B. Rete Testis

The **rete testis** is composed of cuboidal cell-lined labyrinthine spaces within the **mediastinum testis**.

C. Epididymis

1. Ductuli Efferentes

The **ductuli efferentes** compose the **head of the epididymis**, whose lumina are lined by **simple columnar** (tall ciliated and low nonciliated) **epithelium**. The walls of the ductules consist of fibroelastic connective tissue and **smooth muscle cells**.

2. Ductus Epididymis

The **ductus epididymis** comprises the **body** and **tail** of the **epididymis**. Its lumen is lined by a **pseudostratified** type of **epithelium** composed of short **basal** and tall **principal cells** bearing **stereocilia** (long microvilli). The epithelium is separated by a **basal membrane** from the connective tissue wall that houses **smooth muscle cells**.

D. Ductus (Vas) Deferens

The enlarged continuation of the ductus epididymis, the **ductus deferens**, is a highly muscular structure. The **mucosal lining** of its small **lumen** is composed of **pseudostratified stereociliated epithelium** lying on a thin fibroelastic **lamina propria**. Its thick muscular coat is composed of three layers of **smooth muscle**, an **inner** and **outer longitudinal** and a **middle circular** layer. A loose fibroelastic **adventitia** surrounds the outer longitudinal muscle layer.

III. ACCESSORY GLANDS

A. Seminal Vesicles

As the **seminal vesicles**, two highly convoluted tubular structures, join the ductus deferens, they form the paired **ejaculatory ducts**. The highly folded **mucous membrane** of the seminal vesicle is composed of a **pseudostratified epithelium**, whose columnar cells are interspersed with short **basal cells**, sitting on a fibroelastic **lamina propria**. The muscular coat is composed of **inner circular** and **outer longitudinal** layers of **smooth muscle** and is invested by a fibrous **adventitia**.

B. Prostate Gland

The ejaculatory ducts join the urethra as these three structures traverse the substance of the **prostate gland**, whose **capsule** is composed of fibroelastic connective tissue and **smooth muscle cells**. The dense **stroma** of the gland is continuous with the capsule. The **parenchyma** of the prostate is composed of numerous individual glands disposed in three layers: **mucosal**, **submucosal**, and **external** (**main**). The **lumina** of these three groups drain into three systems of **ducts** that lead into the expanded **urethral sinus**. The folded mucosa of the glands is composed of **simple cuboidal** to **columnar** (with regions of pseudostratified columnar) **epithelia** supported by fibroelastic vascular **stroma** displaying **smooth muscle cells**. Frequently, the lumina of the glands of older men possess round-to-ovoid **prostatic concretions** that are often lamellated and may become calcified.

C. Bulbourethral Glands

Each small **bulbourethral** (**Cowper's**) **gland** possesses a thin connective tissue **capsule** whose septa subdivide the gland into **lobules**. The **cuboidal-to-columnar cells** lining the lumen of the gland possess flattened, basally located **nuclei**. The main **duct** of each gland delivers its mucous secretory product into the **cavernous** (**spongy**) **urethra**.

IV. PENIS

The **penis**, ensheathed in **skin**, possesses a thick collagenous capsule, the **tunica albuginea**, that encloses the three cylindrical bodies of **erectile tissue**. The two dorsally positioned **corpora cavernosa** are incompletely separated from each other by **septa** derived from the tunica albuginea. The **corpus cavernosum urethrae** (**corpus spongiosum**) contains the spongy portion of the **urethra**. The vascular spaces of the erectile tissues are lined by **endothelium**.

V. URETHRA

The male **urethra** is subdivided into three regions: **prostatic**, **membranous**, and **spongy** (**penile**) urethra.

A. Epithelium

The **prostatic portion** is lined by **transitional epithelium**, whereas the **membranous** and **spongy portions** are lined by **pseudostratified-to-stratified columnar epithelium**. The **spongy urethra** frequently displays regions of **stratified squamous epithelium**. **Goblet cells** and **intraepithelial glands** are also present.

B. Lamina Propria

The **lamina propria** is composed of a type of **loose connective tissue** housing **elastic fibers** and **glands of Littré**. **Smooth muscle**, oriented longitudinally and circularly, is also evident.

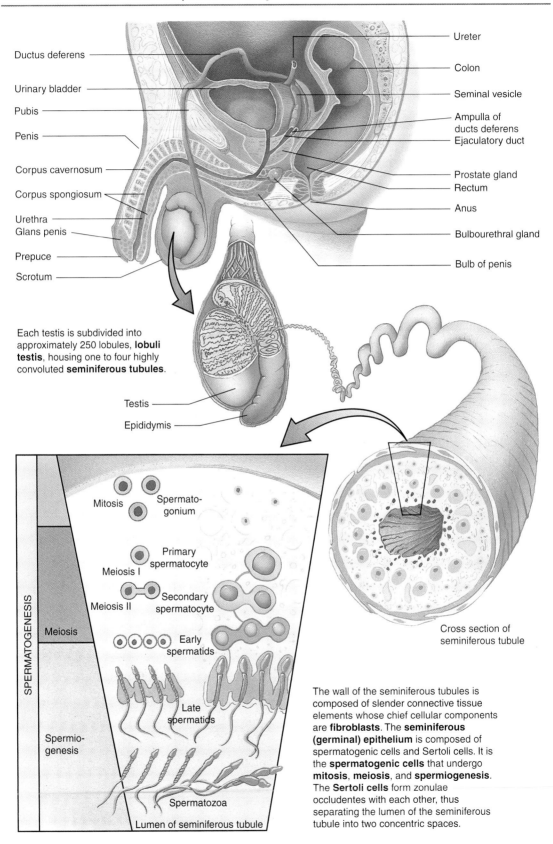

Ductus deferens

Urinary bladder

Pubis

Penis

Corpus cavernosum

Corpus spongiosum

Urethra

Glans penis

Prepuce

Scrotum

Ureter

Colon

Seminal vesicle

Ampulla of ducts deferens

Ejaculatory duct

Prostate gland

Rectum

Anus

Bulbourethral gland

Bulb of penis

Each testis is subdivided into approximately 250 lobules, **lobuli testis**, housing one to four highly convoluted **seminiferous tubules**.

Testis

Epididymis

Cross section of seminiferous tubule

SPERMATOGENESIS

Mitosis

Spermato-gonium

Primary spermatocyte

Meiosis I

Secondary spermatocyte

Meiosis II

Meiosis

Early spermatids

Late spermatids

Spermio-genesis

Spermatozoa

Lumen of seminiferous tubule

The wall of the seminiferous tubules is composed of slender connective tissue elements whose chief cellular components are **fibroblasts**. The **seminiferous (germinal) epithelium** is composed of spermatogenic cells and Sertoli cells. It is the **spermatogenic cells** that undergo **mitosis**, **meiosis**, and **spermiogenesis**. The **Sertoli cells** form zonulae occludentes with each other, thus separating the lumen of the seminiferous tubule into two concentric spaces.

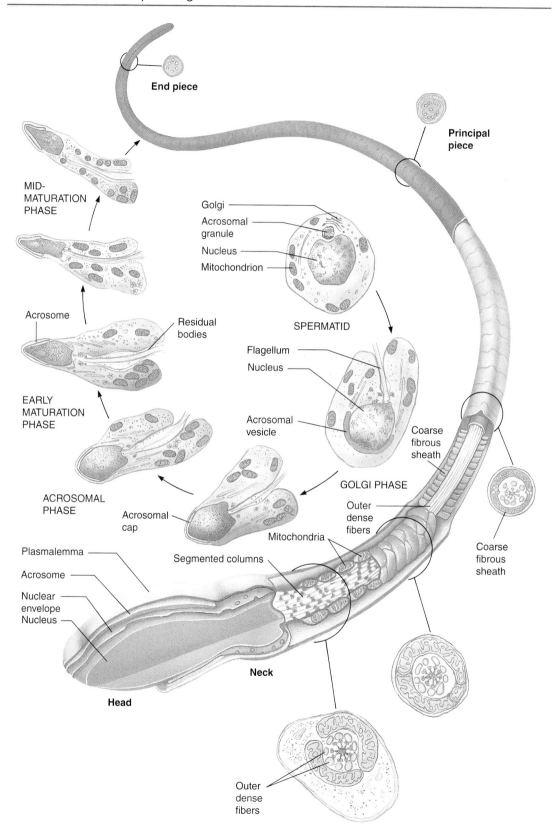

End piece

Principal piece

MID-MATURATION PHASE

Golgi

Acrosomal granule

Nucleus

Mitochondrion

SPERMATID

Acrosome

Residual bodies

Flagellum

Nucleus

Acrosomal vesicle

Coarse fibrous sheath

EARLY MATURATION PHASE

ACROSOMAL PHASE

Acrosomal cap

GOLGI PHASE

Mitochondria

Outer dense fibers

Coarse fibrous sheath

Plasmalemma

Acrosome

Nuclear envelope

Nucleus

Segmented columns

Neck

Head

Outer dense fibers

PLATE 18-1 ■ *Testis*

FIGURE 1 ■ *Testis. Monkey. Plastic section.* × 14.

This low magnification photomicrograph of the testis displays its thick **tunica albuginea** (TA), as well as the slender **septa** (Se) that attach to it. Observe that sections of **seminiferous tubules** (ST) present various geometric profiles, attesting to their highly convoluted form. Note that each **lobule** (Lo) is densely packed with seminiferous tubules, and the connective tissue stroma (arrows) occupies the remaining space. A region similar to the boxed area is presented at a higher magnification in Figure 2.

FIGURE 2 ■ *Testis. Seminiferous tubules. Monkey. Plastic section.* × 132.

This photomicrograph is a higher magnification of a region similar to the boxed area of Figure 1. Observe that the **tunica vasculosa** (TV) of the **tunica albuginea** (TA) is a highly vascular region (arrows) and that **blood vessels** (BV) penetrate the lobuli testis in connective tissue **septa** (Se). The walls of the **seminiferous tubules** (ST) are closely apposed to each other (arrowheads) although in certain regions the cellular **stroma** (St) is evident. Observe that the **lumen** (L) of the seminiferous tubule is lined by a stratified **seminiferous epithelium** (SE).

FIGURE 3 ■ *Testis. Seminiferous tubule. Monkey. Plastic section.* × 540.

The adjacent walls of two **seminiferous tubules** (ST), in close proximity to each other, are composed of **myoid cells** (MC), **fibroblasts** (F), and fibromuscular **connective tissue** (CT). The stratified **seminiferous epithelium** (SE) is separated from the tubular wall by a basal membrane (arrowheads). **Spermatogonia** (Sg) and **Sertoli cells** (SC) lie on the basal membrane, and are in the **basal compartment** (BC), while **primary spermatocytes** (PS), secondary spermatocytes, **spermatids** (Sp), and **spermatozoa** (Sz) are in the **adluminal compartment** (AC). Observe that the **lumen** (L) of the seminiferous tubule contains spermatozoa, as well as cellular debris discarded during the transformation of spermatids into spermatozoa. Compare the cells of the seminiferous epithelium with those of Figure 4.

FIGURE 4 ■ *Testis. Seminiferous tubule. Monkey. Plastic section.* × 540.

Observe that the fibromuscular walls of the two tubular cross-sections are very close to each other (arrows); however, in regions, **arterioles** (A) and **venules** (V) are evident. The **Sertoli cells** (SC) may be recognized by their pale nuclei and dense **nucleoli** (n). In comparing the **seminiferous epithelia** (SE) of the tubules in the right and left halves of this photomicrograph, as well as those of Figure 3, it should be noted that their cellular compositions are different, indicative of the cyclic stages of the seminiferous epithelium. Note also that three types of spermatogonia are recognizable by their nuclear characteristics: **dark spermatogonia A** (Ad) possessing dark, flattened nuclei; **pale spermatogonia A** (Ap) with flattened pale nuclei; and **spermatogonia B** (B) with round nuclei.

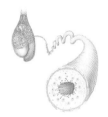

Testis, epididymis, and seminiferous tubule

KEY

A	arterioles	L	lumen	Sg	spermatogonia
AC	adluminal compartment	Lo	lobule	Sp	spermatid
Ad	dark spermatogonia A	MC	myoid cell	ST	seminiferous tubules
Ap	pale spermatogonia A	n	nucleoli	St	stroma
B	spermatogonia B	PS	primary spermatocyte	Sz	spermatozoa
BC	basal compartment	SC	Sertoli cell	TA	tunica albuginea
BV	blood vessel	SE	seminiferous epithelium	TV	tunica vasculosa
CT	connective tissue	Se	septum	V	venule
F	fibroblast				

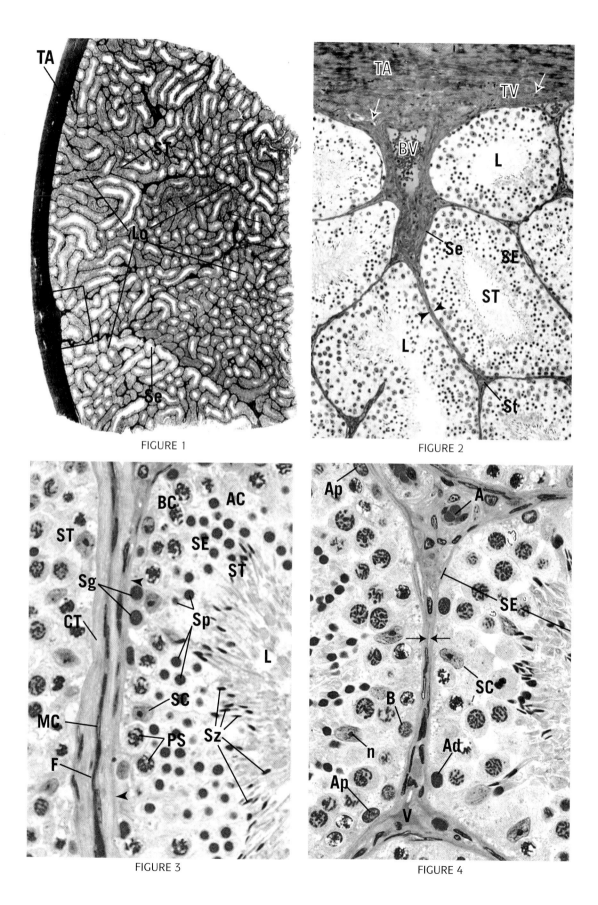

FIGURE 1

FIGURE 2

FIGURE 3

FIGURE 4

PLATE 18-2 ■ *Testis and Epididymis*

FIGURE 1 ▧ *Interstitial cells. Testis. Monkey. Plastic section.* × 270.

The **stroma** (St) surrounding **seminiferous tubules** (ST) possesses a rich **vascular supply** (BV), as well as extensive **lymphatic drainage** (LV). Much of the vascular elements are associated with the endocrine cells of the testis, the **interstitial cells of Leydig** (IC), which produce testosterone.

Inset. Interstitial cells. Testis. Monkey. Plastic section. × 540.

The **interstitial cells** (IC), located in small clumps, are recognizable by their round-to-oval **nuclei** (N) and the presence of lipid (arrow) within their cytoplasm.

FIGURE 2 ▧ *Rete testis. Human. Paraffin section.* × 132.

The **rete testis** (RT), located in the **mediastinum testis** (MT), is composed of labyrinthine, anastomosing spaces, lined by a simple cuboidal **epithelium** (Ep). The dense collagenous **connective tissue** (CT) of the mediastinum testis is clearly evident, as are the profiles of **seminiferous tubules** (ST). Spermatozoa gain access to the rete testis via the short, straight **tubuli recti** (TR).

FIGURE 3 ▧ *Ductuli efferentes. Human. Paraffin section.* × 132.

The first part of the epididymis, the **ductuli efferentes** (De), receives **spermatozoa** (Sz) from the rete testis. The lumina of the ductuli are lined by a simple columnar **epithelium** (Ep), composed of tall and short cells, which are responsible for the characteristic fluted (uneven) appearance of these tubules. The thick fibroelastic **connective tissue** (CT) wall of the ductuli houses numerous smooth muscle cells (SM).

FIGURE 4 ▧ *Ductus epididymis. Monkey. Plastic section.* × 132.

The **ductus epididymis** (DE) may be distinguished from the ductuli efferentes with relative ease. Note that the **nuclei** (N) of the pseudostratified **epithelial lining** (Ep) are of two types, oval and round, whereas those of the ductuli are round. Observe that the lumen contains numerous **spermatozoa** (Sz) and that the epithelium sits on a basal lamina. The connective tissue wall of the ductus epididymis may be differentiated easily from its circularly arranged **smooth muscle coat** (SM).

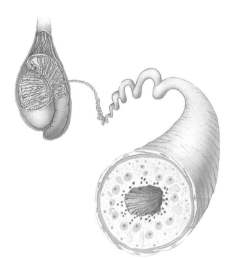

Testis, epididymis, and seminiferous tubule

KEY

BV	blood vessel	IC	interstitial cells of Leydig	SM	smooth muscle
CT	connective tissue	LV	lymphatic vessels	ST	seminiferous tubules
DE	ductus epididymis	MT	mediastinum testis	St	stroma
De	ductuli efferentes	N	nuclei	Sz	spermatozoa
Ep	epithelium	RT	rete testis	TR	tubuli recti

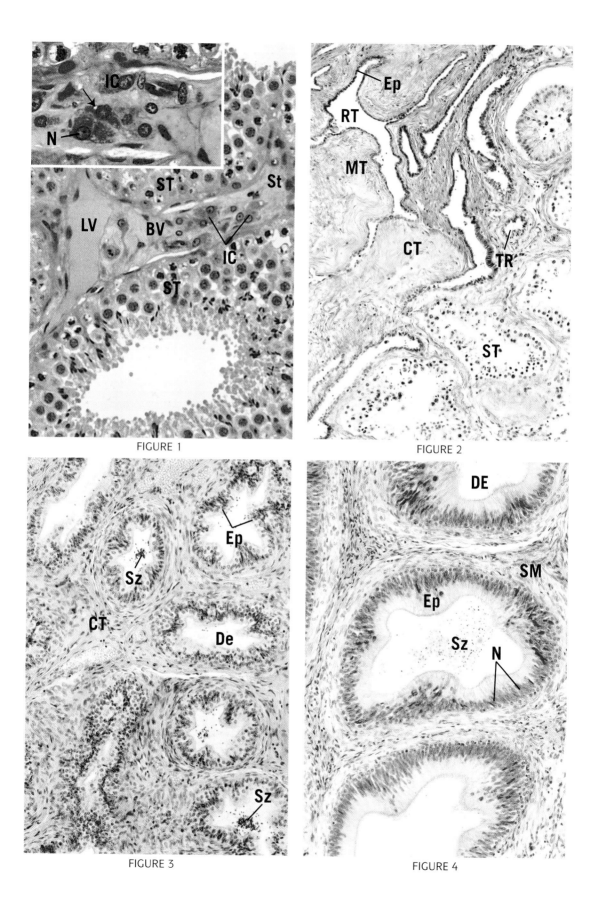

FIGURE 1

FIGURE 2

FIGURE 3

FIGURE 4

PLATE 18-3 ■ *Epididymis, Ductus Deferens, and Seminal Vesicle*

FIGURE 1 ■ *Ductus epididymis. Monkey. Plastic section.* × 270.

The pseudostratified stereociliated columnar **epithelium** (Ep) lining the lumen of the ductus epididymis is composed of two types of cells: short **basal cells** (BC), recognizable by their round nuclei, and tall columnar **principal cells** (PC), whose oval nuclei display one or more **nucleoli** (n). The **smooth muscle** (SM) cells, composing the wall of the epididymis, are circularly oriented and are surrounded by **connective tissue** (CT) elements.

Inset. Ductus epididymis. Monkey. Plastic section. × 540.

Observe the round nuclei of the **basal cells** (BC) and oval nuclei of the **principal cells** (PC). Clumped stereocilia (arrows) extend into the **spermatozoa** (Sz)-filled lumen.

FIGURE 2 ■ *Ductus deferens. Monkey. Plastic section.* × 132.

The ductus deferens is a thick-walled muscular tube that conveys spermatozoa from the ductus epididymis to the ejaculatory duct. The thick muscular coat is composed of three layers of smooth muscle: **outer longitudinal** (OL), **middle circular** (MC), and **inner longitudinal** (IL). The fibroelastic **lamina propria** (LP) receives its **vascular supply** (BV) from vessels (arrow) that penetrate the three muscle layers. A pseudostratified columnar **epithelium** (Ep) lines the spermatozoa-filled **lumen** (L).

Inset. Ductus deferens. Monkey. Plastic section. × 270.

A higher magnification of the pseudostratified columnar **epithelium** (Ep) displays the presence of **stereocilia** (Sc).

FIGURE 3 ■ *Seminal vesicle. Human. Paraffin section.* × 132.

The paired seminal vesicles are elongated tubular glands whose ducts join the ductus deferens just prior to the beginning of the ejaculatory ducts. The highly folded **mucous membrane** (MM) of the seminal vesicle is composed of pseudostratified **epithelium** (Ep) with a thin **connective tissue core** (CT). The folded membrane anastomoses with itself, partitioning off small spaces (asterisks) that, although continuous with the central lumen, appear to be discrete regions. A region similar to the boxed area is presented at a higher magnification in Figure 4.

FIGURE 4 ■ *Seminal vesicle. Monkey. Plastic section.* × 540.

This photomicrograph is a higher magnification of a region similar to the boxed area of the previous figure. Note that the tall **columnar cells** (CC) possess basally located round **nuclei** (N) and that their cytoplasm displays secretory granules (arrows). Short **basal cells** (BC) are occasionally present, which may function as regenerative cells for the epithelium. The secretory product is released into the **lumen** (L) as a thick fluid that coagulates in histological sections. Observe the presence of numerous **capillaries** (C) in the connective tissue core deep to the epithelium. Although **spermatozoa** (Sz) are frequently noted in the lumen of the seminal vesicles, they are not stored in this structure.

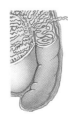

Testis and epididymis

■ **KEY**

BC	basal cell	L	lumen	OL	outer longitudinal muscle layer
BV	blood vessel	LP	lamina propria	PC	principal cell
C	capillaries	MC	middle circular muscle layer	Sc	stereocilia
CC	columnar cell			SM	smooth muscle
CT	connective tissue	MM	mucous membrane	Sz	spermatozoa
Ep	epithelium	N	nucleus		
IL	inner longitudinal muscle layer	n	nucleoli		

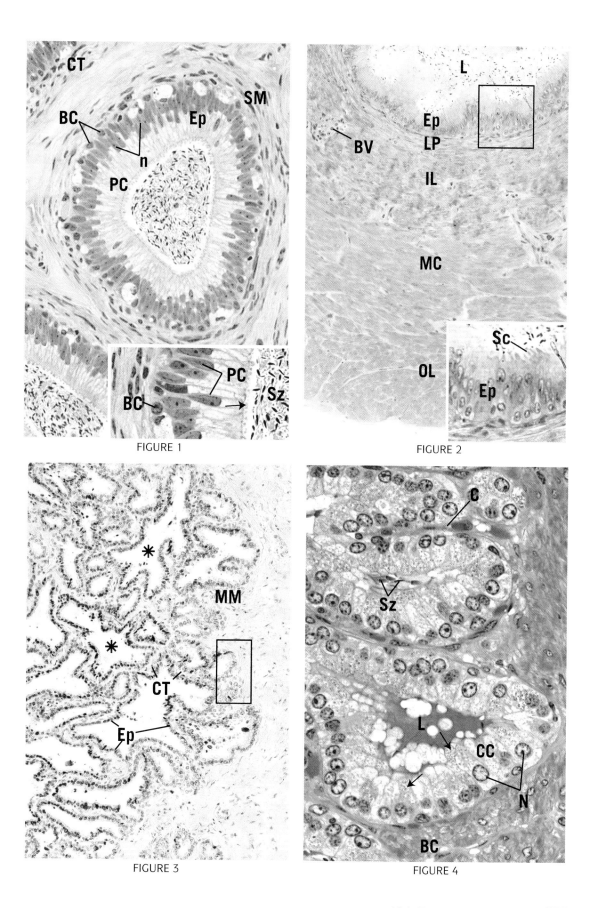

CT

BC

Ep

SM

n

PC

PC

BC

Sz

FIGURE 1

L

Ep

BV

LP

IL

MC

OL

Sc

Ep

FIGURE 2

MM

*

*

CT

Ep

FIGURE 3

C

Sz

L

CC

N

BC

FIGURE 4

PLATE 18-4 ■ *Prostate, Penis, and Urethra*

FIGURE 1 ■ *Prostate gland. Monkey. Plastic section.* × 132.

The prostate gland, the largest of the male reproductive accessory glands, possesses a thick fibroelastic connective tissue capsule with which the connective tissue **stroma** (St) is continuous. Note that the stroma houses **smooth muscle** (SM) and blood vessels. The secretory portion of the prostate gland is composed of individual glands of varied shapes, but consisting of a simple cuboidal-to-low columnar type of **epithelium** (Ep), although regions of pseudostratified columnar epithelia are readily apparent. A region similar to the boxed area is presented at a higher magnification in Figure 2.

FIGURE 2 ■ *Prostate gland. Monkey. Plastic section.* × 540.

This photomicrograph is a higher magnification of a region similar to the boxed area of the previous figure. Observe that the fibroelastic connective tissue **stroma** (St) presents numerous **blood vessels** (BV) and **smooth muscle cells** (SM). The parenchyma of the gland is composed of **columnar cells** (CC), as well as short **basal cells** (BC). Note that the dome-shaped apices (arrows) of some of the columnar cells appear to protrude into the lumen, which contain a **prostatic concretion** (Pc). The number of these concretions, which may calcify, increases with age.

FIGURE 3 ■ *Penis. Human. x.s. Paraffin section.* × 14.

The penis is composed of three erectile bodies: the two corpora cavernosa and the corpus spongiosum. The cross-section of the **corpus spongiosum** (CS) displays the **urethra** (U) that is surrounded by **erectile tissue** (ET) whose irregular, endothelially lined **cavernous spaces** (Cs) contain blood. The spongy tissue is surrounded by the thick, fibrous **tunica albuginea** (TA). The three cavernous bodies are surrounded by a looser connective tissue sheath to which the skin (removed here) is attached. The boxed area is presented at a higher magnification in Figure 4.

Inset. **Penis. Human. x.s. Paraffin section.** × 14.

The **cavernous spaces** (Cs) of the corpus cavernosum are larger than those of the corpus spongiosum. Moreover, the **fibrous trabeculae** (FT) are thinner, resulting in the corpora cavernosa becoming more turgid during erection than the corpus spongiosum.

FIGURE 4 ■ *Urethra. Human. Paraffin section.* × 132.

This photomicrograph is a higher magnification of the boxed area of the previous figure. Note that the spongy **urethra** (U) is lined by a pseudostratified columnar **epithelium** (Ep) surrounded by a loose **connective tissue sheath** (CT) housing a rich **vascular supply** (BV). The entire urethra is enveloped by the **erectile tissue** (ET) of the corpus spongiosum. Additionally, the mucous **glands of Littré** (GL) deliver their secretory product into the lumen of the urethra, lubricating its epithelial lining.

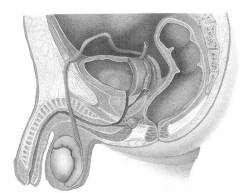

Male reproductive system

■ KEY

BC	basal cell	CT	connective tissue	Pc	prostatic concretion
BV	blood vessel	Ep	epithelium	SM	smooth muscle
CC	columnar cell	ET	erectile tissue	St	stroma
CS	corpus spongiosum	FT	fibrous trabeculae	TA	tunica albuginea
Cs	cavernous space	GL	glands of Littré	U	urethra

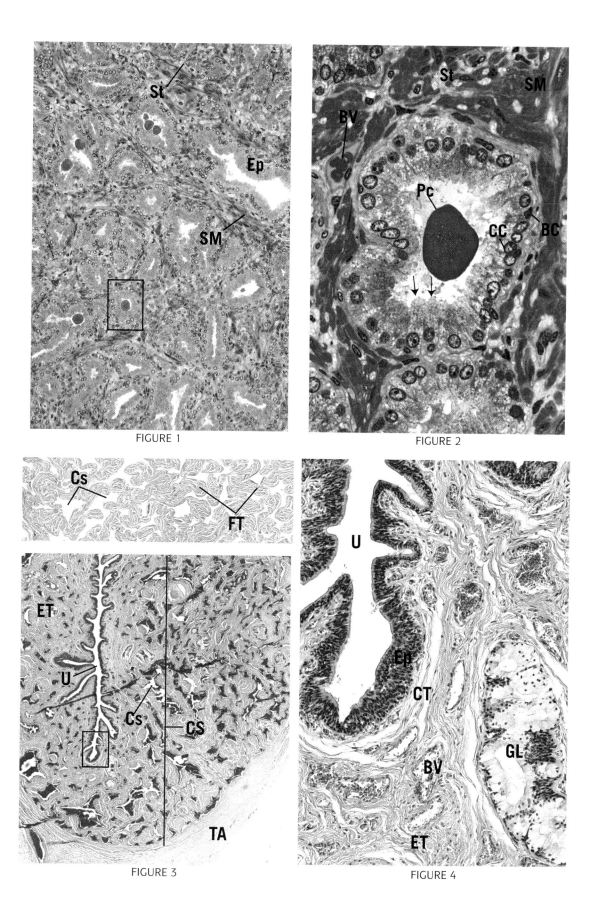

FIGURE 1

FIGURE 2

FIGURE 3

FIGURE 4

PLATE 18-5 ■ *Epididymis, Electron Microscopy*

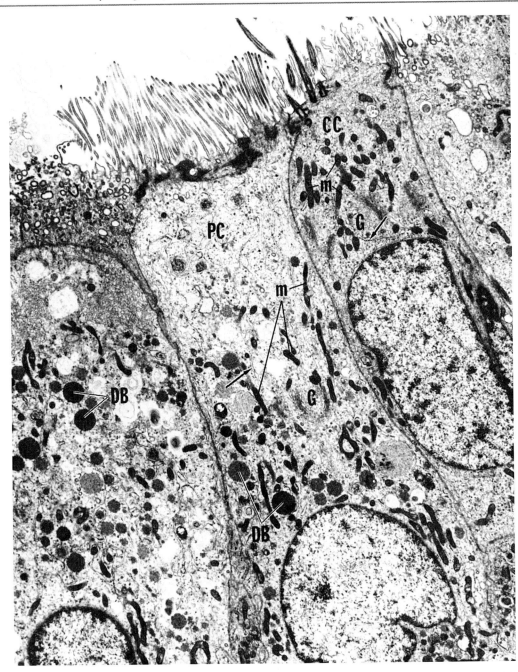

FIGURE 1 ■ *Epididymis. Rabbit. Electron microscopy.* × 7200.

The epithelial lining of the rabbit ductuli efferentes is composed of two types of tall columnar cells: **principal cells** (PC) and **ciliated cells** (CC). Note that both cell types possess numerous organelles, such as **Golgi** (G), **mitochondria** (m), and rough endoplasmic reticulum (arrows). Additionally, principal cells contain **dense bodies** (DB), probably a secretory material. (Courtesy of Dr. R. Jones.)

■ **KEY**

CC	ciliated cell	G	Golgi apparatus	PC	principal cell
DB	dense bodies	m	mitochondrion		

Special Senses

The organs of special senses include the gustatory, olfactory, visual, auditory, and vestibular apparatus. The gustatory apparatus, consisting of taste buds, is discussed in Chapter 13, and the olfactory epithelium is treated in Chapter 12. The present chapter details the microscopic morphology of the eye and the ear.

EYE

The **eye** is a sensory organ whose **lens** focuses rays of light reflected from the external environment on photosensitive cells of the **retina** (see Graphic 19-1). The intensity, location, and wavelengths of the transmitted light are interpreted by the visual cortex of the brain as three-dimensional color images of the external milieu. Each orb, protected by the eyelids, is movable by means of a group of extrinsic skeletal muscles that insert into the fibrous tunic of the orb, thus assisting in suspending it in its bony orbit. The anterior surface of the eye is bathed in **tears,** a fluid medium secreted by the **lacrimal gland.** Three coats constitute the wall of the orb: the outer fibrous tunic, the middle vascular tunic (uvea), and the inner retinal tunic.

The **fibrous tunic** (**corneoscleral layer**) is composed of the opaque, white **sclera** that covers the posterior aspect of the orb, and the transparent **cornea** that covers the anterior 1/6th of the orb. The junction between the sclera and the cornea is known as the **limbus.**

The **vascular tunic** is composed of several regions: the anteriorly positioned **iris** and **ciliary body** and the posteriorly located, highly vascular and pigmented **choroid.** Intrinsic muscles located in the iris function to adjust the aperture of the iris, whereas intrinsic muscles located within the ciliary body function to release tension on the lens, thus permitting near focus (accommodation) by altering its diameter.

The innermost **retinal tunic** is composed of 10 layers responsible for photoreception and impulse generation. The two photoreceptors are the **rhodopsin-synthesizing rods** and **iodopsin-forming cones,** with the former sensitive to dim and the latter sensitive to bright light. Axons of connecting neurons, located within the retina, leave the eye via the **optic nerve** to synapse in the brain.

The additional components of the orb are the **aqueous humor,** a fluid; the **vitreous body,** a gel; and the **lens,** all of which serve as parts of the refractive media.

EAR

The **ear** functions in the reception of sound, as well as in the perception of the orientation of the head and, therefore, the body in relation to the directional forces of gravity (see Graphic 19-2). To perform both functions of hearing and equilibrium (balance), the ear is subdivided into the external, middle, and inner ears.

The **external ear** is composed of a cartilaginous, skin-covered **auricle** (pinna) and the **external auditory meatus** with its cartilaginous outer and bony inner aspects, whose internal end is separated from the middle ear by the thin **tympanic membrane.**

The **tympanic cavity** of the **middle ear** houses the three **auditory ossicles:** outermost **malleus** (hammer), middle **incus** (stirrup), and innermost **stapes** (anvil). This cavity is connected to the **nasopharynx** via the cartilaginous **auditory (eustachian) tube,** which permits equalization of atmospheric pressures on either side of the tympanic membrane. Sound waves are funneled by the auricle to the tympanic membrane, whose vibrations are amplified and transmitted to the **oval window** of the inner ear's **cochlea** by actions of the ossicles.

The **inner ear,** concerned with both hearing and balance, is housed within a **labyrinth** in the petrous portion of the temporal bone. The region closest to the middle ear, the **bony cochlea,** houses the apparatus responsible for hearing, while its deeper aspect contains the structures responsible for vestibular function (balance).

The bony cochlea contains the **endolymph-filled cochlear duct**, which is surrounded by **perilymph**, housed in the superiorly located **scala vestibuli** and the inferiorly positioned **scala tympani**. The two scalae communicate with each other via the **helicotrema**, a small slit-like opening.

Within the **cochlear duct** is the **spiral organ of Corti** whose **inner** and **outer hair cells** are in close association with the **tectorial membrane**. Vibrations of the **basilar membrane**, induced by disturbances in the perilymph, result in stimulation of the **cochlear nerves** by the hair cells. Dendrites of the cochlear nerves lead to the spiral ganglion located in the modiolus. Oscillations set in motion at the **oval window** are dissipated at the secondary tympanic membrane covering the **round window** of the cochlea.

The bony labyrinth also contains the endolymph-filled **utricle**, **saccule**, and the three **semicircular canals**, membranous structures responsible for balance and orientation in three-dimensional space.

The principal functional components of the utricle and saccule, oriented perpendicularly to each other, are known as **maculae**. These structures house **neuroepithelial hair cells** whose **microvilli** and **kinocilia** (nonmotile cilia) project into the **otolith-containing proteinaceous otolithic membrane**. The utricle and saccule respond to linear acceleration.

A similar collection of hair cells is located on the **crista ampullaris** of the ampulla of each semicircular canal. The microvilli and kinocilia of these neuroepithelial cells also project into a proteinaceous material, the **cupula**, which contains no otoliths. Since each semicircular canal is oriented perpendicularly to the other two, angular acceleration along any of the three axes is registered and interpreted as a vector in three dimensions.

Histophysiology

I. EYE

A. Orb

The **eye** functions as the photosensitive organ responsible for vision. It receives light through the **cornea**, which is subsequently focused on the **retina** via the **lens**. It is here that specialized cells (**rods** and **cones**) recognize various patterns of the image for transmission to the brain via the **optic nerve**. **Extrinsic muscles** attached to the orb direct the pupil to the most advantageous position for perceiving the image viewed. Because the eyes are set apart, their visual fields overlap, thus enhancing three-dimensional imaging. **Intrinsic muscles** represented by the **sphincter pupillae** and **dilator pupillae muscles** adjust the aperture of the **iris**, and **ciliary muscles** manipulate the focal length of the lens for **accommodation** for close vision.

Melanocytes located in the epithelium and stroma of the iris block light from passing through the iris, except at the pupil. Additionally, eye color is related to the abundance of these melanocytes: large numbers of melanocytes impart dark eyes, whereas fewer melanocytes render the eyes light in color.

Aqueous humor, a plasma filtrate produced by the cells covering the ciliary processes passes from the posterior chamber of the eye into the anterior chamber via the opening between the lens and the pupil.

The wall of the orb is composed of three tunics: the **tunica fibrosa**, **tunica vasculosa**, and **tunica retina**. The tunica retina is responsible for **photoreception**. Although the retina displays 10 distinctive layers, most of its cells support and/or relay impulses to the optic nerve for transmittal to the brain. The two deepest layers, the retinal pigment epithelium and the layer of rods and cones, bear the major responsibility for photoreception.

Retinal pigment epithelium functions in **esterifying vitamin A** and transporting it to the rods and cones, **phagocytosing** the shed tips of rods and cones, and **synthesizing melanin**, which absorbs light after rods and cones have been stimulated.

Rods are sensitive to low light intensity and possess many flattened discs containing **rhodopsin** (an integral membrane protein **opsin** bound to **retinal**, the aldehyde form of **vitamin A**) in their outer segment. When light is absorbed by rhodopsin, it dissociates into **retinal** and **opsin** (bleaching), permitting diffusion of bound Ca^{2+} into the outer segment. Excess of Ca^{2+} hyperpolarizes the cell by closing Na^+ channels, thus preventing the entry of

Na^+ into the cell. The electrical potential thus generated is relayed to other rods via gap junctions and then along the pathway to the optic nerve. Dissociated retinal and opsin reassemble, and the Ca^{2+} ions are recaptured, establishing a normal resting potential.

Cones, sensitive to light of high intensity, producing **greater visual acuity**, are much more numerous than rods and produce **iodopsin**, the photopigment sensitive to red, green, or blue light. The mechanism of transducing photoenergy into electrical energy for transmission to the brain via the optic nerve is similar to that described in the rods.

The **optic disc**, the region where fibers of the optic nerve exit the orb, contains neither cones nor rods; consequently, it is called the **blind spot**. Just lateral to the blind spot is the **fovea centralis**, a depression in the wall of the orb. The fovea contains mostly cones that are packed so tightly that not all layers of the retina are present. This is the region of the retina where visual acuity is the greatest.

B. Accessory Structures

Accessory structures of the eye include the conjunctiva, eyelids, and lacrimal gland. The **conjunctiva** is a transparent mucous membrane that lines the eyelids and reflects on the orb. The **eyelids** contain modified sebaceous glands, **meibomian glands**, responsible for altering the surface tension of the watery tears, thus slowing evaporation. The **lacrimal glands** secrete tears that keep the conjunctiva and cornea moist. **Tears** also contain **lysozyme**, an antibacterial enzyme.

II. EAR

The **ear** is composed of three parts: the **external ear** (pinna and external acoustic meatus), which receives the sound waves; the **middle ear** (containing the bony ossicles), which transmits the sound waves; and the **inner ear** (containing the cochlea), where sound waves are transduced into nerve impulses and the sensation of equilibrium is achieved by the vestibular apparatus.

The **tympanic membrane**, located at the deepest aspect of the external acoustic meatus, transmits sound vibrations to the bony ossicles of the middle ear. The tympanic cavity of the middle ear contains the **malleus, incus,** and **stapes** (bony ossicles) connected in series to each other and between the tympanic membrane and the **oval window** of the bony wall. They greatly amplify and translate movements of the tympanic membrane to the oval window.

The **bony labyrinth** of the inner ear, subdivided into the **semicircular canals**, **vestibule**, and **cochlea**, is filled with perilymph. Loosely contained within it and all of its subdivisions is the **membranous labyrinth** containing endolymph. Movements of the fluid environment within this system are perceived by certain sensory cells contained within the membranous labyrinth and ultimately transduced to electrical impulses for transmission to the brain.

The **saccule** and **utricle**, specializations of the membranous labyrinth in the vestibule, contain **type I** and **type II hair cells** (**neuroepithelial cells** containing many **stereocilia** and a single **kinocilium**) whose free ends are embedded in the **otolithic membrane** containing **otoliths** (**otoconia**). **Static equilibrium** and **linear acceleration** are determined by movements in these hair cells, which synapse with nerve cells of the vestibular portion of the acoustic nerve.

Semicircular ducts, specializations of the membranous labyrinth in the semicircular canals, contain **neuroepithelial hair cells** located in the **cristae ampullares** (sensory regions) of the **ampullae**. Free ends of these hair cells are embedded in a glycoprotein, the **cupula**. Movements of the endolymph and the cupula are translated to the hair cells, which synapse with nerve cells of the vestibular portion of the acoustic nerve. This process is sensitive to **rotational acceleration** in any of the three directions of orientation of the semicircular canals.

The **endolymphatic sac** (terminal end of the **endolymphatic duct**) contains phagocytic cells in its lumen and may function in **resorption of endolymph**.

The **cochlear duct** contains the **spiral organ of Corti**, which is bordered by the **scala vestibuli** and the **scala tympani** (both scalae contain perilymph and communicate at the **helicotrema**). The **vestibular membrane** located between the scala vestibuli and the cochlear duct functions to maintain the **high ion gradient** between the perilymph and endolymph.

The **spiral organ of Corti**, sitting on the **basilar membrane**, contains, among other supporting cells, neuroepithelial **inner** and **outer hair cells** whose free ends are embedded in the gel-like **tectorial membrane**. Sound waves translated to the oval window set the perilymph of the scala tympani in motion, which displaces the basilar membrane, thus moving the hair cells but not the tectorial membrane. Bending of the hair cells causes them to release neurotransmitter substance, exciting the **bipolar cells** of the spiral ganglion, resulting in transmission of the impulse to higher centers of the brain. Although the basilar membrane vibrates at many frequencies, certain regions vibrate optimally at specific frequencies. For example, low frequency

sound waves are detected farther away from the oval window. It should be noted that loud sounds, such as those at rock concerts, create a great deal of energy within the hearing mechanism, such that it may take two or three days for the energy to be completely dissipated and the buzzing to stop.

Clinical Considerations ▪ ▪ ▪

Glaucoma
Glaucoma is a condition of high intraocular pressure caused by an obstruction that prevents aqueous humor from exiting the anterior chamber of the eye. If left untreated, blindness may result.

Cataract
Cataract, a common condition of aging, is caused by excessive UV radiation and by pigments and other substances accumulating in the lens, making it opaque and thus impairing vision. This condition may be corrected by excising the lens and replacing it with a plastic lens.

Detached Retina
Detached retina may result from a trauma where the neural and pigmented layers of the retina become separated. This condition may cause partial blindness, but it may be corrected by surgical intervention.

Conductive Hearing Loss
Conductive hearing loss may arise from a middle ear infection (otitis media), an obstruction, or osteosclerosis of the middle ear.

Nerve Deafness
Nerve deafness results from a lesion in the cochlear portion of the vestibulocochlear nerve (cranial nerve VIII). This condition may be the result of disease, prolonged exposure to loud sounds, and/or drugs.

Ménière's Disease
Ménière's disease is an inner ear disorder characterized by symptoms such as hearing loss due to excess fluid accumulation in the endolymphatic duct, vertigo, tinnitus, nausea, and vomiting. Many of the symptoms may be relieved by drugs that are prescribed for vertigo and nausea or in more severe cases vestibular neurectomy (cutting the vestibular nerve) may be performed. In very severe cases labyrinthectomy is the treatment of choice, where the semicircular canals and the cochlea are surgically removed.

Summary of Histological Organization

I. EYE

A. FIBROUS TUNIC

1. Cornea

The **cornea** is composed of five layers. From superficial to deep, they are

a. Stratified Squamous Nonkeratinized Epithelium

b. Bowman's Membrane

The outer, homogeneous layer of the stroma.

c. Stroma

A transparent, dense regular collagenous connective tissue housing **fibroblasts** and occasional **lymphoid cells**, comprising the bulk of the cornea.

d. Descemet's Membrane

A thick basal lamina.

e. Corneal Endothelium

Not a true endothelium, a simple **squamous-to-cuboidal epithelium**.

2. Sclera

The **sclera**, the white of the eye, is composed of three layers: the outer **episcleral tissue** housing blood vessels; the middle **stroma**, composed of dense regular collagenous connective tissue; and the **suprachoroid lamina**, a loose connective tissue housing **fibroblasts** and **melanocytes**.

B. Vascular Tunic

The **vascular tunic** (**uvea**) is a pigmented, vascular layer housing smooth muscles. It is composed of the **choroid membrane**, the **ciliary body**, and the **iris**.

1. Choroid Membrane

The **choroid membrane** is composed of four layers. The **suprachoroid layer** is shared with the sclera and houses **fibroblasts** and **melanocytes**. The **vascular** and **choriocapillary layers** house larger vessels and capillaries, respectively. The **glassy membrane** (of Bruch), interposed between the choroid and the retina, is composed of basal lamina, collagen, and elastic fibers.

2. Ciliary Body

The **ciliary body** is the region of the vascular tunic located between the ora serrata and the iris. The ciliary body is composed of the numerous, radially arranged, **aqueous humor-forming ciliary processes** that together compose the **ciliary crown** from which **suspensory ligaments** extend to the lens. Three layers of **smooth muscle**, oriented more or less meridianally, radially, and circularly, function in accommodation. The **vascular layer** and **glassy membrane** of the choroid continue into the ciliary body. The inner aspect of the ciliary body is covered by the inner nonpigmented and outer pigmented layers of the **ciliary epithelium**.

3. Iris

The **iris**, separating the **anterior** from the **posterior chamber**, is attached to the ciliary body along its outer circumference. The center of the iris is incomplete, forming the **pupil** of the eye. The iris is composed of three layers: the outer (frequently incomplete) **simple squamous epithelial layer**, a continuation of the corneal epithelium; the middle **fibrous layer**, composed of the nonvascular **anterior stromal** and vascular **general stromal layers** that house numerous **melanocytes** and **fibroblasts**; and the posterior **pigmented epithelium**. The **sphincter** and **dilator muscles** of the pupil are composed of myoepithelial cells derived from the pigmented epithelium.

C. Retinal Tunic

The **retinal tunic**, the deepest of the three layers, consists of the **pars iridica**, **pars ciliaris**, and **pars optica**. The last of these is the only region of the retina that is sensitive to light, extending as far anteriorly as the **ora serrata**, where it is continuous with the pars ciliaris.

1. Pars Optica

The **pars optica** is composed of ten layers.

a. Pigment Epithelium

The **pigment epithelium** is attached to the choroid membrane.

b. Lamina of Rods and Cones

The **outer** and **inner segments** of the photoreceptor cells form the first layer, while the remainder of these cells constitutes the next three layers.

c. External Limiting Membrane

The **external limiting membrane** is not a true membrane. It is merely a junctional specialization between the photoreceptor cells and processes of Müller's (supportive) **cells**.

d. Outer Nuclear Layer

The **outer nuclear layer** houses the cell bodies (and nuclei) of the photoreceptor cells. At the **fovea centralis**, only cones are present.

e. Outer Plexiform Layer

The **outer plexiform layer** is the region of synapse formation between the **axons** of photoreceptor cells and the processes of **bipolar** and **horizontal cells.**

f. Inner Nuclear Layer

The **inner nuclear layer** houses the **cell bodies of Müller, amacrine** (associative), **bipolar,** and **horizontal cells.**

g. Inner Plexiform Layer

The **inner plexiform layer** is the region of synapses between **dendrites** of **ganglia cells** and **axons** of **bipolar cells.** Moreover, processes of **Müller** and **amacrine cells** are also present in this layer.

h. Ganglion Cell Layer

The **ganglion cell layer** houses the **cell bodies** of **multipolar neurons,** which are the final link in the neuronal chain of the retina, and their **axons** form the optic nerve. Additionally, **neuroglia** are also located in this layer.

i. Optic Nerve Fiber Layer

The **optic nerve fiber layer** is composed of the **unmyelinated axons** of the **ganglion cells,** which will be collected as the optic nerve.

j. Inner Limiting Membrane

The **inner limiting membrane** is composed of the expanded terminal processes of **Müller cells.**

2. Pars Ciliaris and Pars Iridica Retinae

At the **pars ciliaris** and **pars iridica retinae** the retinal layer has been reduced to a thin epithelial layer consisting of a columnar and a pigmented layer lining the ciliary body and iris.

D. Lens

The **lens** is a biconvex, flexible, transparent disc that focuses the incident rays of light on the retina. It is composed of three layers, an elastic **capsule** (basement membrane), an anteriorly placed **simple cuboidal epithelium,** and **lens fibers,** modified epithelial cells derived from the **equator** of the lens.

E. Lacrimal Gland

The **lacrimal gland** is external to the eye, located in the superolateral aspect of the orbit. It is a **compound tubuloalveolar gland** producing a lysozyme-rich serous fluid with an alkaline pH.

F. Eyelid

The **eyelid** is covered by **thin skin** on its external aspect and by **conjunctiva,** a mucous membrane, on its inner aspect. A thick dense fibrous connective tissue **tarsal plate** maintains and reinforces the eyelid. Associated with the tarsal plate are the **tarsal**

glands secreting an oily sebum that is delivered to the margin of the eyelid. Muscles controlling the eyelid are located within its substance. Associated with the eyelashes are **sebaceous glands,** while ciliary glands are located between eyelashes.

II. EAR

A. External Ear

1. Auricle

The **auricle** is covered by thin skin and is supported by an **elastic cartilage plate.**

2. External Auditory Meatus

The **external auditory meatus** is a **cartilaginous tube** lined by skin, containing **ceruminous glands** and some fine **hair.** In the medial aspect of the meatus the cartilage is replaced by **bone.**

3. Tympanic Membrane

The **tympanic membrane** is a thin, taut membrane separating the external from the middle ear. It is lined by **stratified squamous keratinized epithelium** externally and low **cuboidal epithelium** internally and possesses a core of **collagen fibers** disposed in two layers.

B. Middle Ear

The **middle ear** is composed of the **simple cuboidal epithelium**-lined **tympanic cavity** containing the three **ossicles** (**malleus, incus,** and **stapes**). The tympanic cavity communicates with the nasopharynx via the cartilaginous and bony **auditory tube.** The medial wall of the middle ear communicates with the inner ear via the **oval (vestibular)** and **round (cochlear) windows.**

C. Inner Ear

1. Cochlea

The bony **cochlea** houses the endolymph-filled **cochlear duct** that subdivides the perilymph-filled cochlea into the superiorly positioned **scala vestibuli** and the inferiorly located **scala tympani.**

a. Cochlear Duct

The **cochlear duct** houses the **spiral organ of Corti** that lies on the **basilar membrane.** The spiral organ of Corti is composed of **cells of Claudius, cells of Boettcher,** and **cells of Hensen,** all of which assist in the formation of the **outer tunnel** along with the **outer hair cells** and **outer phalangeal cells.** The **tectorial membrane** lies over the outer hair cells, as well as the **inner hair cells,** thus forming the **internal spiral tunnel.** The region between the inner and outer hair cells is occupied by **pillar cells,** which assist in the formation of the **inner tunnel (of Corti).** The **stria** vascularis constitutes the outer wall of the cochlear duct. Nerve fibers lead to the **spiral ganglion** (housing pseudounipolar cells) in the **modiolus**.

b. Membranous Labyrinth

The **membranous labyrinth** is composed of the **utricle**, the **saccule**, and the three **semicircular canals**.

1. Utricle and Saccule

The **utricle** and **saccule** are both filled with **endolymph** and house **maculae**. Each **macula** is composed of simple **columnar epithelium** composed of two cell types, neuroepithelial **hair cells** and **supporting cells**. The free surface of the macula displays the **otolithic membrane** housing small particles called **otoliths**.

2. Semicircular Canals

The three **semicircular canals** are oriented perpendicular to each other. The **ampulla** of each canal houses a **crista**, a structure similar to a macula, composed of neuroepithelial **hair cells** and **supporting cells**. A gelatinous **cupula** is located at the free surface of the crista, but it contains no otoliths.

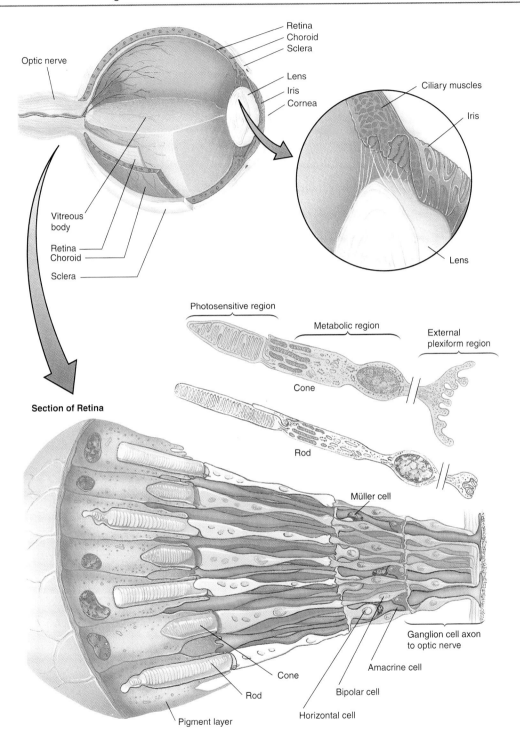

Optic nerve

Retina
Choroid
Sclera

Lens
Iris
Cornea

Ciliary muscles

Iris

Lens

Vitreous body

Retina
Choroid

Sclera

Section of Retina

Photosensitive region

Metabolic region

External plexiform region

Cone

Rod

Müller cell

Ganglion cell axon to optic nerve

Amacrine cell

Cone

Bipolar cell

Rod

Horizontal cell

Pigment layer

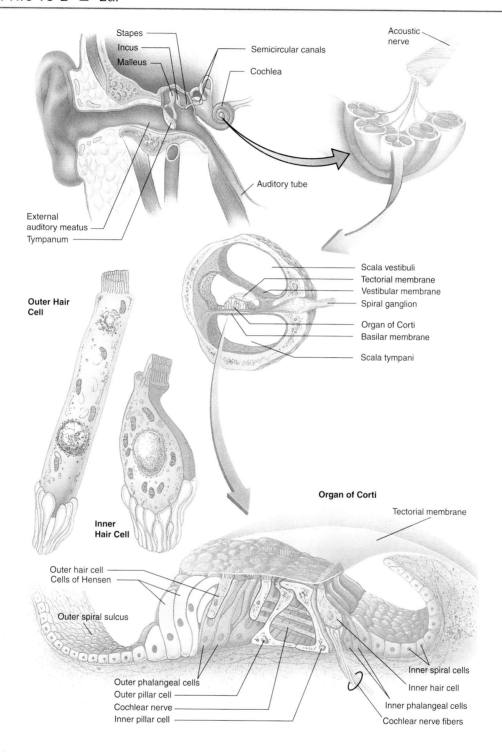

Stapes
Incus
Malleus
Semicircular canals
Cochlea
Acoustic nerve
Auditory tube
External auditory meatus
Tympanum

Outer Hair Cell

Scala vestibuli
Tectorial membrane
Vestibular membrane
Spiral ganglion
Organ of Corti
Basilar membrane
Scala tympani

Inner Hair Cell

Organ of Corti

Tectorial membrane

Outer hair cell
Cells of Hensen

Outer spiral sulcus

Inner spiral cells

Inner hair cell

Outer phalangeal cells
Outer pillar cell
Cochlear nerve
Inner pillar cell

Inner phalangeal cells
Cochlear nerve fibers

PLATE 19-1 ■ *Eye, Cornea, Sclera, Iris, and Ciliary Body*

FIGURE 1 ■ *Cornea. Monkey. Paraffin section.* × 132.

The cornea is a multilayered, transparent structure. Its anterior surface is covered by a stratified squamous nonkeratinized **epithelium** (Ep), deep to which is a thin, acellular Bowman's membrane. The bulk of the cornea, the **stroma** (St) is composed of regularly arranged **collagen fibers** (CF) and intervening fibroblasts, whose **nuclei** (N) are readily evident. The posterior surface of the cornea is lined by a simple squamous-to-cuboidal **epithelium** (Ep). A thin acellular Descement's membrane lies between the simple epithelium and the stroma.

Inset. **Cornea. Monkey. Paraffin section.** × 270.

A higher magnification of the anterior surface displays the stratified squamous **epithelium** (Ep), as well as the acellular **Bowman's membrane** (BM). Note the regularly arranged bundles of **collagen fibers** (CF) and intervening **fibroblasts** (F).

FIGURE 2 ■ *Sclera. Monkey. Paraffin section.* × 132.

The sclera is similar to and continuous with the cornea, but it is not transparent. Note that the **epithelium** (Ep) of the conjunctiva covers the anterior surface of the sclera. Deep to the epithelium is the loose **episcleral tissue** (ET), whose **blood vessels** (BV) are clearly evident. The **stroma** (St) is composed of thick **collagen fiber** (CF) bundles housing numerous **fibroblasts** (F). The deepest layer of the sclera is the **suprachoroid lamina** (SL) whose **melanocytes** (M) house melanin pigment.

FIGURE 3 ■ *Iris. Monkey. Paraffin section.* × 132.

The **iris** (I) separates the **anterior chamber** (AC) from the **posterior chamber** (PC). The medial border of this structure defines the **pupil** (P) of the eye. "The iris is composed of three layers: an outer discontinuous layer of melanocytes and fibroblasts; the middle **fibrous layer** (FL), housing **pigment cells** (Pc); and the posterior double layered **pigmented epithelium** (PEp)." The **sphincter** (sM) and dilatator muscles are composed of myoepithelial cells. The pupillary region of the iris contacts the **capsule** (Ca) of the **lens** (L) in living individuals.

FIGURE 4 ■ *Ciliary body. Monkey. Paraffin section.* × 132.

The ciliary body is composed of **ciliary processes** (CP), projecting into the **posterior chamber** (PC) from which suspensory ligaments extend to the lens. The bulk of the ciliary body is composed of **smooth muscle** (SM) disposed more or less in three layers, not evident in this photomicrograph. Numerous **pigment cells** (Pc) are present in this region. Note that the epithelium of the ciliary body is composed of two layers: an **outer pigmented** (OP) and an **inner nonpigmented** (IN) epithelium. The narrow **vascular layer** (VL) is evident between the epithelium and ciliary muscles.

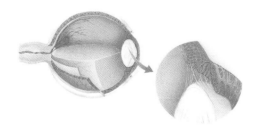

Eye, ciliary muscles, iris, and lens

■ **KEY**

AC	anterior chamber	FL	fibrous layer	Pc	pigment cells
BM	Bowman's membrane	I	iris	PEp	pigmented epithelium
BV	blood vessel	IN	inner nonpigmented layer	SEp	squamous epithelium
Ca	capsule	L	lens	SL	suprachoroid lamina
CF	collagen fibers	M	melanocytes	SM	smooth muscle
CP	ciliary process	N	nucleus	sM	sphincter muscle
Ep	epithelium	OP	outer pigmented layer	St	stroma
ET	episcleral tissue	P	pupil	VL	vascular layer
F	fibroblasts	PC	posterior chamber		

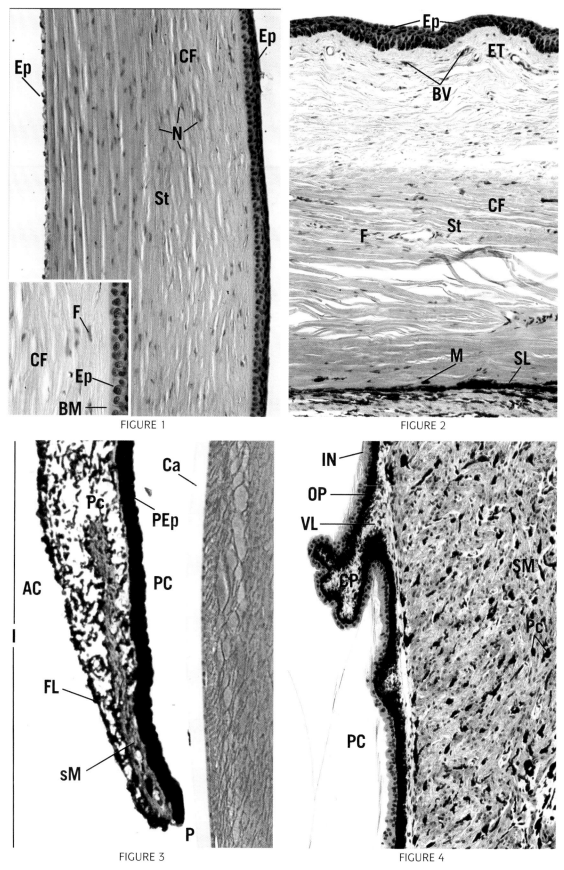

FIGURE 1

FIGURE 2

FIGURE 3

FIGURE 4

PLATE 19-2 ■ *Retina, Light and Scanning Electron Microscopy*

FIGURE 1 ■ *Tunics of the eye. Monkey. Paraffin section.* × 14.

This survey photomicrograph is of an anterolateral section of the orb, as evidenced by the presence of the **lacrimal gland** (LG). Note that the three layers of the orb are extremely thin in relation to its diameter. The **sclera** (S) is the outermost layer. The pigment **choroid** (Ch) and multilayered **retina** (Re) are easily distinguishable even at this magnification. The **posterior compartment** (PCo) houses the vitreous body. A region similar to the boxed area is presented at a higher magnification in Figure 2.

FIGURE 2 ■ *Retina. Pars optica. Monkey. Paraffin section.* × 270.

The pars optica of the retina is composed of 10 distinct layers. The **pigment epithelium** (1), the outermost layer, is closely apposed to the vascular and pigmented **choroid** (Ch). Various regions of the **rods** (R) and **cones** (C) form the next four layers. These are the **lamina of rods and cones** (2), **external limiting membrane** (3), **outer nuclear layer** (4), and **outer plexiform layer** (5). The **inner nuclear layer** (6) houses the cell bodies of various associative glial (Müller) and functional cells. The **inner plexiform layer** (7) is a region of synapse formation, while the **ganglion cell layer** (8) houses the cell bodies of multipolar neurons and neuroglia. Fibers of these ganglion cells form the **optic nerve fiber layer** (9), while the **inner limiting membrane** (10) is composed of the expanded processes of Müller cells. A region similar to the boxed area is presented in Figure 3, a scanning electron micrograph of the rods and cones.

FIGURE 3 ■ *Rods and cones. Monkey. Scanning electron microscopy.* × 6300.

This scanning electron micrograph of the monkey retina displays regions of several **cones** (C) and of a few **rods** (R). The inner segments of the **lamina of rods and cones** (2), **external limiting membrane** (3), and **outer nuclear layer** (4) are clearly recognizable.

The **microvilli** (Mv) noted in the vicinity of the external limiting membrane belong to the Müller cells, which were removed during specimen preparation. Observe the longitudinal ridges (arrows) along the surface of the inner segments. (From Borwein B, Borwein D, Medeiros J, McGowan J: *Am J Anat* 159:125–146, 1980.)

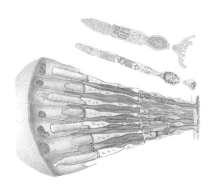

Section of retina

■ **KEY**

1	pigment epithelium	7	inner plexiform layer	LG	lacrimal gland
2	lamina of rods and cones	8	ganglion cell layer	Mv	microvilli
3	external limiting membrane	9	optic nerve fiber layer	PCo	posterior compartment
4	outer nuclear layer	10	inner limiting membrane	R	rods
5	outer plexiform layer	C	cones	Re	retina
6	inner nuclear layer	Ch	choroid	S	sclera

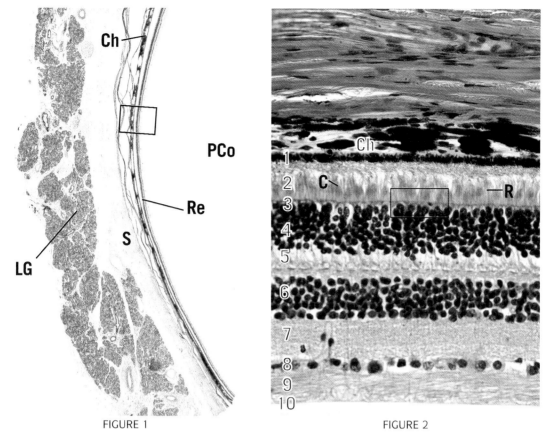

FIGURE 1

FIGURE 2

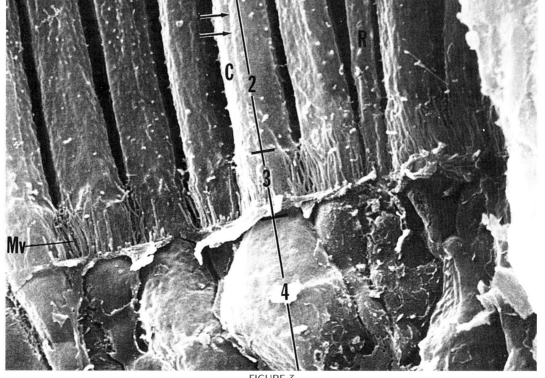

FIGURE 3

PLATE 19-3 ■ *Fovea, Lens, Eyelid, and Lacrimal Glands*

FIGURE 1 ■ *Fovea centralis. Monkey. Paraffin section.* × 132.

The retina is greatly reduced in thickness at the **fovea centralis** (FC) of the macula lutea. This is the region of greatest visual acuity, and **cones** (C) are the only photoreceptor cells in this area. Note that the retinal layers present are the **pigmented epithelium** (1), **lamina of cones** (2), **external limiting membrane** (3), **outer nuclear layer** (4), **outer plexiform layer** (5), **ganglion cell layers** (8), and **inner limiting membrane** (10). Observe the presence of the vascular **choroid** (Ch) whose pigment cells impart a dark coloration to this layer.

FIGURE 2A ■ *Lens. Monkey. Paraffin section.* × 132.

The lens is a biconvex, flexible, transparent disc covered by a homogenous **capsule** (Ca) deep to which lies the simple cuboidal lens **epithelium** (Ep). The fibers (arrows), constituting the bulk of the lens, are composed of closely packed, hexagon-shaped cells whose longitudinal axes are oriented parallel to the surface.

Inset. Lens. Monkey. Paraffin section. × 270.

Note the presence of the homogeneous **capsule** (Ca) overlying the simple cuboidal lens **epithelium** (Ep).

FIGURE 2B ■ *Lens. Monkey. Paraffin section.* × 132.

The equator of the lens displays the presence of younger cells that still possess their **nuclei** (N). Note the **suspensory ligaments** (SL), **capsule** (Ca), and the lens **epithelium** (Ep).

FIGURE 3 ■ *Eyelid. Paraffin section.* × 14.

The external aspect of the eyelid is covered by thin **skin** (Sk) and lined by a stratified columnar epithelium, the **palpebral conjunctiva** (pC). The substance of the eyelid is formed by the thick connective tissue **tarsal plate** (TP), whose **tarsal glands** (TG) are clearly evident. Two skeletal muscles are associated with the upper eyelid, the circularly disposed **orbicularis oculi** (OO) and the longitudinally oriented levator palpebrae superioris. Although the latter muscle is not present in this photomicrograph, its connective tissue aponeurosis is evident (arrow). Eyelashes and the sebaceous **ciliary glands** (CG) are present at the inferior tip of the lid.

FIGURE 4 ■ *Lacrimal gland. Monkey. Paraffin section.* × 132.

Lacrimal glands are compound tubuloalveolar glands, separated into lobes and **lobules** (Lo) by **connective tissue** (CT) elements. Since these glands produce a lysozyme-rich, watery secretion, they are composed of numerous **serous acini** (SA), as evidenced by the round, basally located **nuclei** (N) of the secretory cells.

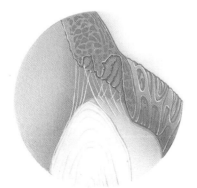

Ciliary muscles, iris, and lens

■ KEY

1	pigmented epithelium	Ca	capsule	OO	orbicularis oculi
2	lamina of cones	Ch	choroid	pC	palpebral conjunctiva
3	external limiting membrane	CG	ciliary gland	SA	serous acini
4	outer nuclear layer	CT	connective tissue	Sk	skin
5	outer plexiform layer	Ep	epithelium	SL	suspensory ligaments
8	ganglion cell layer	FC	fovea centralis	TG	tarsal glands
10	inner limiting membrane	Lo	lobule	TP	tarsal plate
C	cones	N	nucleus		

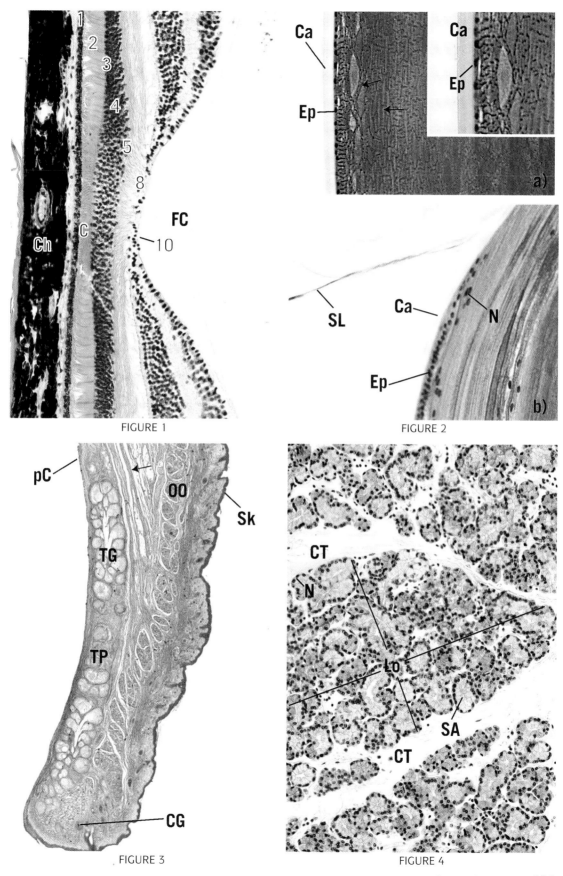

FIGURE 1

FIGURE 2

FIGURE 3

FIGURE 4

PLATE 19-4 ■ *Inner Ear*

FIGURE 1 ■ *Inner ear. Paraffin section.* × 21.

This photomicrograph is a survey section of the petrous portion of the temporal bone displaying the various components of the inner ear. At the extreme right, note the spirally disposed **bony cochlea** (BC) housing the endolymph-filled **cochlear duct** (CD) and the perilymph-filled **scala tympani** (ST) and **scala vestibuli** (SV). The apex of the cochlea displays the **helicotrema** (H), the space through which perilymph may be exchanged between the scala tympani and the scala vestibuli. Innervation to the **spiral organ of Corti** (OC), located within the cochlear duct, is derived from the **spiral ganglion** (SG), housed in the **modiolus** (M). Two cranial nerves, **vestibulocochlear** (VN) and **facial** (FN), are evident in this photomicrograph. The **vestibule** (V), as well as sections of the **ampullae** (A) of the semicircular canals containing the **crista ampullaris** (CA), are clearly recognizable. Finally, note one of the **auditory ossicles** (AO) of the middle ear.

Inset. **Crista ampullaris. Paraffin section.** × 132.

The **crista ampullaris** (CA) is housed within the expanded **ampulla** (A) of each semicircular canal. **Nerve fibers** (NF) enter the connective tissue core of the crista and reach the neuroepithelial **hair cells** (HC) that are supported by **sustentacular cells** (SC). Kinocilia and microvilli of the hair cells extend into the gelatinous **cupula** (Cu) associated with the crista.

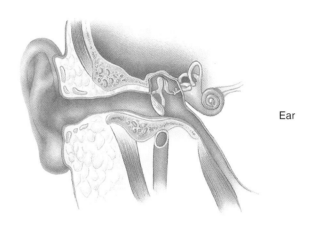

Ear

KEY

A	ampulla	FN	facial nerve	SC	sustentacular cells
AO	auditory ossicle	H	helicotrema	SG	spiral ganglion
BC	bony cochlea	HC	hair cells	ST	scala tympani
CA	crista ampullaris	M	modiolus	SV	scala vestibuli
CD	cochlear duct	NF	nerve fibers	V	vestibule
Cu	cupula	OC	spiral organ of Corti	VN	vestibulocochlear nerve

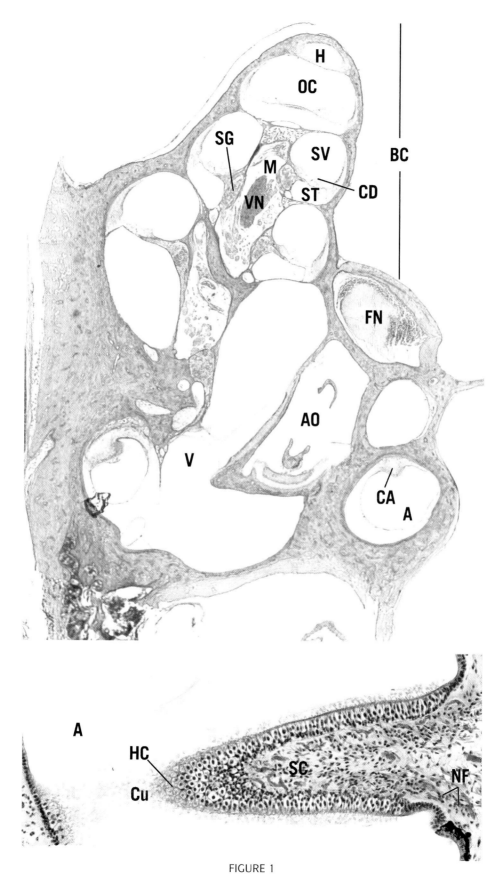

FIGURE 1

PLATE 19-5 ■ *Cochlea*

FIGURE 1 ■ *Cochlea. Paraffin section.* × 211.

This photomicrograph is a higher magnification of one of the turns of the cochlea. Observe that the **scala vestibuli** (SV) and **scala tympani** (ST), enclosed in the **bony cochlea** (BC), are **epithelially** (Ep) lined spaces, filled with perilymph. The **cochlear duct** (CD), filled with endolymph, is separated from the scala vestibuli by the thin **vestibular membrane** (VM) and from the scala tympani by the **basilar membrane** (BM). Within the bony casing is the **spiral ganglion** (SG), whose cell bodies are clearly evident (arrows). **Cochlear nerve fibers** (CNF) from the spiral ganglion traverse bony tunnels of the **osseous spiral lamina** (OL) to reach the hair cells of the **spiral organ of Corti** (OC). This structure, responsible for the sense of hearing, is an extremely complex entity. It rests on the basilar membrane, a taut collagenous sheet extending from the *spiral ligament* (SL) to the **limbus spiralis** (LS). Attached to the limbus spiralis is the **tectorial membrane** (TM) (whose elevation in this photomicrograph is an artifact of fixation) that overlies the spiral organ of Corti. Observe the presence of the **stria vascularis** (Sv), which extends from the vestibular membrane to the **spiral prominence** (SP). The stria vascularis possesses a pseudostratified **epithelium** (Ep) composed of basal, dark, and light cells, which are intimately associated with a rich capillary network. It is believed that endolymph is elaborated by some or all of these cells. The morphology of the spiral organ of Corti is presented at a higher magnification in Plate 19-6.

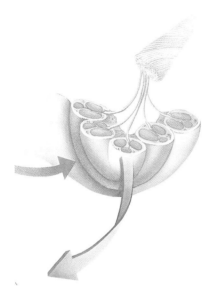

Cochlea and acoustic nerve

■ KEY

BC	bony cochlea	OC	spiral organ of Corti	ST	scala tympani
BM	basilar membrane	OL	osseous spiral lamina	SV	scala vestibuli
CD	cochlear duct	SG	spiral ganglion	Sv	stria vascularis
CNF	cochlear nerve fibers	SL	spiral ligament	TM	tectorial membrane
Ep	epithelium	SP	spiral prominence	VM	vestibular membrane
LS	limbus spiralis				

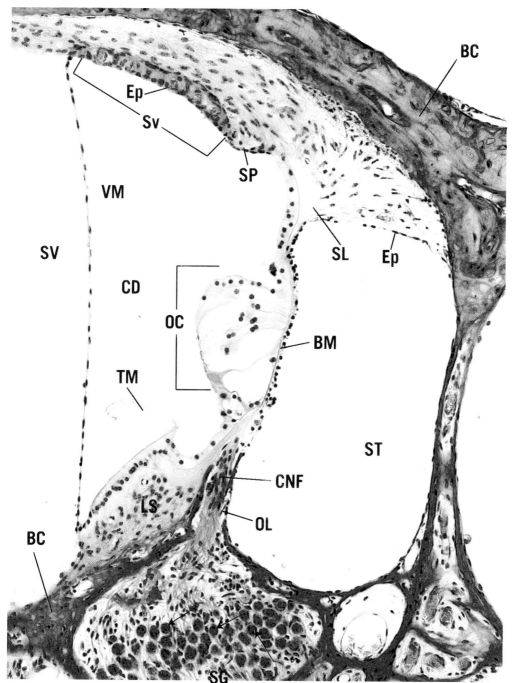

FIGURE 1

PLATE 19-6 ■ *Spiral Organ of Corti*

FIGURE 1 ■ *Spiral organ of Corti (Montage).*
Paraffin section. × 540.

The spiral organ of Corti lies upon the **basilar membrane** (BM), whose two regions, the **zona pectinata** (ZP) and **zona arcuata** (ZA), are delineated by the base of the **outer pillar cells** (OPC). The basilar membrane extends from the **spiral ligament** (SL) to the **tympanic lip** (TL) of the limbus spiralis, to whose **vestibular lip** (VL) the **tectorial membrane** (TM) is anchored. The tectorial membrane acts as a roof of the **internal spiral sulcus** (IS). Observe the **cochlear nerve fibers** (CNF) traversing the tunnels of the **osseous spiral lamina** (OL). The lateral wall of the internal spiral sulcus is formed by the single row of **inner hair cells** (IH), flanked by the **inner phalangeal cells** (IPh) and **border cells** (Bc). The floor of the internal spiral sulcus is formed by **inner sulcus cells** (IC).

Proceeding laterally, the **inner pillar cell** (IPC) and **outer pillar cell** (OPC) form the **inner tunnel of Corti** (ITC). The **spaces of Nuel** (SN) separate the three rows of **outer hair cells** (OH) from each other and from the outer pillar cells. Fine **nerve fibers** (NF) and **phalangeal processes** (PP) traverse these spaces. The outer hair cells are supported by **outer phalangeal cells** (OPh). The space between the **cells of Hensen** (CH) and the outermost row of outer phalangeal cells is the **outer tunnel** (OT). Lateral to the cells of Hensen are the darker staining, deeper positioned **cells of Boettcher** (CB) and the lighter staining, larger **cells of Claudius** (CC), which enclose the **outer spiral sulcus** (OSS). Note that the space above the spiral organ of Corti is the **cochlear duct** (CD), whereas the space below the basilar membrane is the scala tympani.

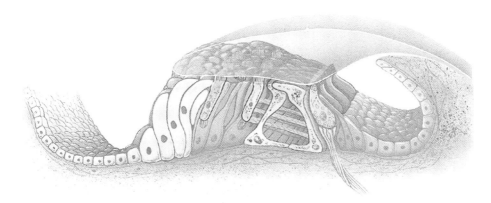

Organ of corti

■ **KEY**

Bc	border cells	IPh	inner phalangeal cells	OT	outer tunnel
BM	basilar membrane	IS	internal spiral sulcus	PP	phalangeal processes
CB	cells of Boettcher	ITC	inner tunnel of Corti	SL	spiral ligament
CC	cells of Claudius	NF	nerve fibers	SN	spaces of Nuel
CD	cochlear duct	OH	outer hair cells	TL	tympanic lip
CH	cells of Hensen	OL	osseous spiral lamina	TM	tectorial membrane
CNF	cochlear nerve fibers	OPC	outer pillar cells	VL	vestibular lip
IC	inner sulcus cells	OPh	outer phalangeal cells	ZA	zona arcuata
IH	inner hair cells	OSS	outer spiral sulcus	ZP	zona pectinata
IPC	inner pillar cells				

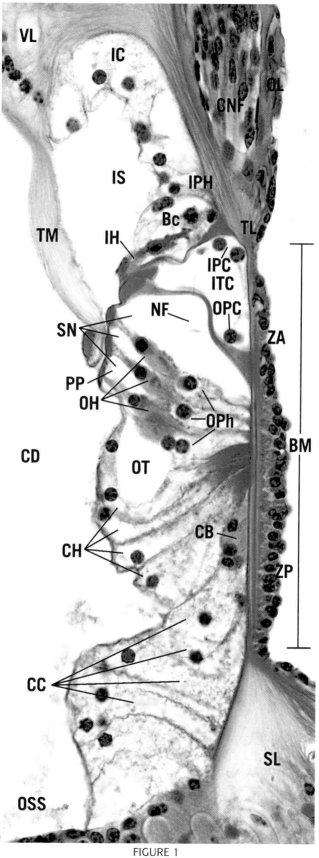

FIGURE 1

Index

In this index, page numbers in *italic* designate figures; page numbers followed by the letter "t" designate tables; (*see also*) cross-references designate related topics or more detailed subtopic lists.

Capillaries, 148, 150, 153, *155, 160–161*
  cerebral, *138–139*
  continuous, 148, 150, *155*
  discontinuous, 148
  ductus (vas) deferens, *382–383*
  fenestrated, 148, 150, *155*
  lung, *252–253*
  lymphatic, 148
  metabolic functions of, 150
  peripheral nerve, *142–143*
  sinusoidal, 150, *155*
  skeletal muscle, *110–111*
  smooth muscle, *118–119, 120–121*
  suprarenal gland, *212–213*
  terminal arterial, 168
  vaginal, *364–365*
Capillary beds, 147, *155*
Capillary loops, 221, *226–227, 228–229*
Capillary network
  peritubular, 323, *331*
  renal, *332–333*
Capillary permeability, 150
Capsular vessel, *332–333*
Capsule
  Bowman's, 323, 328, *331, 337*
  connective tissue, *40–41*
  ganglionic, *140–141*
  Glisson's, 306, *314–315*
  inner, *117*
  lens, *400–401*
  lymph node, 167, 173, *175, 182–183, 186–187*
  ocular, *396–397*
  outer, *117*
  pacinian corpuscle, *232–233*
  pancreatic, 306
  parathyroid gland, 199
  prostate gland, 374
  renal, 323, *332–333*
  splenic, 174
  suprarenal gland, *210–211*
  testicular, 373
  thymic, 174, *188–189*
  thyroid, 199, *208–209*
  tonsillar, 173, *184–185*
Carbaminohemoglobin, 237
Carbohydrates, digestion and absorption, 280
Carbonic anhydrase, 237
Carcinoma
  basal cell, 220
  squamous cell, 220
Cardia, 278, *285, 288–289*
Cardiac gland, 277, 279
Cardiac muscle, 104, 107, *109, 122–124, 162–165*
Cardiac muscle fibers, *122–123, 124*
Cartilage, 65–88
  clinical considerations, 69
  of ear, 388, *395*
  elastic, 65, 66t, 68, 70, *76–77*
  embryonic, 70
  fibrocartilage, 65, 66t, 68, 70
  histological organization of, 70
  histophysiology of, 68

  hyaline, 65, 66t, 68, 70, 74–75, *86*, 235, 239, *246–247*
  laryngeal, *244–245*
  types, 65, 66t
Cartilage degeneration, 69
Cartilage matrix, 65, 68, 70
Catalase, 2
Cataract, 390
Catecholamines, 196
Caveola, *120–121*
Cavernous (spongy) urethra, 374
Cavity
  infraglottic, 235, 239, *244–245*
  marrow, *72*
  medullary, 84–85
  nasal, 239, *244–245*
  oral, 255–275, *260, 261*
  thoracic, 237
  tympanic, 388, *395*
CD (cluster of differentiation) molecules, 92, 170
Cecum, 278, *286*
Cell body
  multipolar (motor), 129
  neuron, 125–126
  postganglionic, *294–295*
Cell cycle, 3
Cell-mediated immune response, 167, 170
Cell nests, 68
Cells, 1–24
  acidophilic, 195
  adipose (fat), *40–41*, 49, *246–247, 298–299*
  amacrine, 392
  androgen-producing, 369
  antigen-presenting (APCs), 168, 170, *178, 179*
  B, 167–168 (*see also* B lymphoctes)
  basal (*see* Basal cells)
  basket (myoepithelial), 29, *136–137*
  blood (*see* Blood cells *and specific types*)
  B memory, 171, *177*
  of Boettcher, *406–407*
  bone, 68, 70
  border, *406–407*
  cardiac muscle, 107
  cartilage, 70
  centroacinar, 304, *308, 312–313*
  chief (*see* Chief cells)
  chondrogenic, 65
  chromaffin, 195, *212–213*
  ciliated, *14–15*
    columnar tracheal, *248–249*
    epididymal, *386*
    oviductal, *358–359*
  Clara, 236, 239, *250–251, 252–253*
  of Claudius, 392, *406–407*
  clear, 225, 234
  clinical considerations, 5
  columnar, *294–295, 300, 384–385*
    uterine, *362–363*
  connective tissue, 46, 49–50, *53, 110–111*
  contractile, 46
  cytoplasm, 1–3, *6, 10–11, 20–21, 22*
  dark, 225, 234, *272–273*
  decidual, *364–365*

D

Follicle maturation, 345
Follicles
    atretic, 347
    Graafian, 343, 347, *350, 352–353, 354–355*
    hair, *63, 221, 225, 228–229, 230–231*
    ovarian, 343, 347, *350, 352–353, 354–355*
    thyroid gland, *208–209*
Follicle-stimulating hormone (FSH), 194, 343, 345,
        369, 371
Follicular atrophy, 347
Follicular cells, 192, *202, 352–353*
    parathyroid, *208–209*
    thyroid, *208–209*
Follicular fluid, *352–353*
Follicular (proliferative) phase, of endometrium, 344, 348
Folliculostatin, 345
Folliculostellate cells, *215*
Foramen, apical, *260*
Fovea centralis, 389, 391, *400–401*
Foveolae (gastric pits), 278, *285, 290–291, 292–293*
Fragmentins, 170, *178*
FSH (follicle-stimulating hormone), 194, 343, 345, 371
Fundic gland, 279, *290–291, 292–293*
Fundus
    gastric, 278, *285*
    uterine, 344
Fungiform papillae, 258, *261*

G

GABA (gamma-aminobutyric acid), 128
G actin, 105
GAGs (glycosaminoglycans), 45, 47
Galactorrhea, 198
Gallbladder, 303, 304, 306–307, *316–317*
Gallstones (biliary calculi), 305
GALT (gut-associated lymphoid tissue), *175*, 280
Gamete, male, 369
Ganglion (ganglia), 126
    dorsal root, 130
    sensory, 140–141
    spiral, *402–403, 404–405*
    sympathetic, 140–141
Ganglion cell layer, retinal, 392, *398–399*
Gap junctions, 25, *30*, 68, 104, *109*
    myometrial, 345
Gaseous exchange, *243*
    mechanism of, 237
Gastric glands, 279, *290–291*
    cells of, 282
Gastric inhibitory peptide, 278, 280t
Gastric mucosa, 282
Gastric pits (foveolae), 278, *285, 290–291, 292–293*
Gastrin, 278, 280t, 305
Gastrin intrinsic factor, 279
Gastrinoma, 305
Gated/ungated ion channels, 4
G cells, 305
G-CSF (granulocyte colony-stimulating factor), 91–92
Gene rearrangement, 172
Genital ducts, 369–370
    female, 343–344, 347–348
    male, 369–370, 373

Germinal centers, 167, *180–181, 182–183, 184–185, 190–191*
Germinal epithelium, 343, 347, *352–353, 376*
Gingiva (gum), 257, *260, 266–267*
Gingival margin, *266–267*
Gingival sulcus, *266–267*
Gingivitis, necrotizing ulcerative, 256
Glands, 25–26 (*see also* Endocrine system *and individual glands*)
    accessory male reproductive, 373–374
    apocrine, 348
    Bowman's, *244–245*
    branched alveolar holocrine, 221
    bulbourethral (Cowper's), 370, 372, 374, *376*
    cardiac, 277, 279
    ciliary, *400–401*
    circumanal, 285
    compound tubuloacinar (alveolar)
        mixed, *42–43*
        serous, *42–43*
    of digestive system, 303–321
    duodenal (Brunner's), 278, 280, 285, *294–295*
    endocrine, 25–26, 29 (*see also* Endocrine system *and
        individual components*)
    esophageal, 278, *288–289*
    exocrine, 25–26, 29
        compound, 29
        multicellular, 29
        pancreas, *42–43*
        simple, 29
        unicellular, 29
    fundic, 279, *290–291, 292–293*
    gastric, 279, 282, *290–291*
    histological organization, 29
    intraepithelial, *274–275*
    respiratory, *244–245*
    lacrimal, *384*, 387, 389, 392, *398–399, 400–401*
    of Littré, 324, *384–385*
    liver, 303, *309*
    male reproductive accessory, 372
    mammary, 344, 346, 348, *366–367*
    meibomian, 389
    mucous of palate, *272–273*
    pancreas, 303, *308*
    parathyroid, 198
    pineal body, 197
    pituitary (hypophysis) (*see* Pituitary gland)
    prostate, 369, 370, 372, 374, *376, 384–385*
    pyloric, 279, *292–293*
    salivary, *31*, 255, 257, 303, 304, 306, *310–311, 318–319*
    sebaceous, *40–41*, 218, 221, 222, *225, 228–229, 230–231,
        262–263*, 348, *366–367*, 392
    seromucous, 173, 235, 239, *246–247*
    serous of von Ebner, 258, *270–271, 272–273*
    sublingual, *42–43*
    submandibular, *42–43*
    suprarenal, 197, 198
    sweat, *56–57*, 218, 221, 222, *224, 225, 228–229, 230–231,
        232–233, 234*, 348, *366–367*
        eccrine, *40–41*
    tarsal, 392, *400–401*
    thyroid, 198
    tubuloacinar (alveolar) mucous, *42–43*
    urethral intraepithelial, 324
    uterine, *360–361, 362–363*

Hemopoietic growth factors, 91
Henle, loop of, 323, 324, 325, 328, *330, 332–333, 338–339*
Henle's layer, 221, *225*
Hensen, cells of, 392, *406–407*
Heparan sulfate, 45, 325
Hepatic artery, *314–315*
Hepatocytes, 303, 304, *309, 314–315, 316–317*
Hering, canals of, 306
Hernia, hiatal, 281
Herpetic stomatitis, 256
Herring bodies, 194, *206–207*
Hexosamine, 47
Hexuronic acid, 47
Hiatal hernia, 281
Hilum, renal, 323
His, bundle of, 149
Histamine, 148, 150
Histiocytes (macrophages), 46
Histological organization
    alimentary canal, 282–284
    blood, 93
    blood circulation, 153–154
    cartilage, 70
    connective tissue, 49–50
    ear, 392–393
    endocrine system, 199–200
    epithelium, 29
    eye, 391–392
    heart, 153
    hemopoiesis, 93–94
    integument, 221
    lymphoid tissue, 173–173
    oral region, 257–258
    respiratory tract, 239–240
    urinary system, 328–329
Histophysiology
    alimentary canal, 279–281
    blood, 91–92, 149–150
    cartilage, 68
    connective tissue, 47–48
    digestive glands, 304
    ear, 389
    endocrine system, 196–198
    epithelium, 27–28
    extracellular fluid, 48
    extracellular matrix, 47–48
    eye, 389
    female reproductive system, 345–346
    integument, 219–220
    lymphoid tissue, 170–172 (*see also* Immune response)
    male reproductive system, 371–372
    muscle, 105–106
    nerve tissue, 127–129
    oral region, 256
    respiratory system, 237
    urinary system, 325
HLA molecules, 170
Hodgkin's disease, 172
Hopewell-Smith, hyaline layer of, *274–275*
Horizontal cells, 129
Hormonal influences, on bone, 69
Hormones, 193
    antidiuretic (ADH, vasopressin), 326

antimüllerian, 371
of DNES cells, 278
of elementary canal, 280t
follicle-stimulating (FSH), 343, 345, 369, 371
gonadotropin-releasing, 345
luteinizing (LH), 194, 369
mechanism of action, 196
nonsteroid-based, 196
paracrine, 279
parathyroid (PTH), 195, 196
pituitary, 194, *201*
steroid-based, 196
thyroid, 196–197
Hormone-sensitive lipase, 48
Horns
    dorsal, 129, *134–135*
    ventral, 129, *134–135*
Howship's lacunae, 66, 70, *88*
Human chorionic gonadotropin (hCG), 345, 346, 372
Human chorionic mammotropin, 345
Human leukocyte antigen (HLA) molecules, 170
Humorally-mediated immune response, 92, 170, 171
Huntington's chorea, 128
Huxley's layer, 221, *225*
Hyaline cartilage, 65, 66t, 68, 70, 74–75, *86*, 235, 239, *246–247*
    embryonic, 74–75
Hyaline cartilage plates, 239
Hyaline layer of Hopewell-Smith, *274–275*
Hyaline membrane disease, 237
Hyaluronic acid, 45, 47, 68
Hydrolytic enzymes, 2
Hydroxyindole, 219
Hydroxylation, 47
Hydroxylysine, 47
Hydroxyproline, 47
Hyperparathyroidism, 198, 327
Hyperthyroidism, 198
Hypertonicity, 326
Hypertrophy, benign prostatic (BPH), 372
Hypodermis, 219, *224, 228–229*
Hyponychium, 218, 222, *225*
Hypophyseal portal system, 193
Hypophysis (*see* Pituitary gland)
Hypothalamo-hypophyseal tract, 194
Hypothalamus, *204–205*
Hypotonicity, 326
H zone, 103, *110–111, 112–113*

◆ **I**

I bands, 103, 105, 107, *108, 110–111, 112–113, 114–116*
Icterus (jaundice), 305
Ileum, 278, *285, 296–297*
Immature cells, *292–293*
Immune response, 92
    cell-mediated, 167, 170 (*see also* Lymphocytes)
    humorally-mediated, 170, 171
Immune tissue
    cells, 170–171, *178*
    lymph nodes, 171, *178*
    spleen, 171–172
Immunoglobulin A (IgA), 279, 304, 346
Immunoglobulins, surface (SIGs), 92, 171

Kidneys, 323–324, 328, *330, 332–333*
   general morphology, *332–333*
Kidney stones (nephrolithiasis), 327
Killer cells
   cytotoxic T, 167, 170, *178*
   natural (NK), 92, 170
Kinase, myosin light-chain, 106
Kinesin, 3
Kinocilium, 390
Knot
   enamel, 256
   syncytial, *364–365*
Krause's end bulbs, 221
Kupffer cells, *58–59*, 304, 306, *309, 316–317*

L

Labyrinth
   auditory, 388, *395*
   bony, 390
   membranous, 390, 393
   renal cortical, 328, *332–333, 334–335*
Lacrimal glands, *384, 387*, 389, 392, *398–399, 400–401*
Lactating mammary gland, 348, *366–367*
Lacteals, *180–181*, 278, 281, *294–295, 296–297*
Lactiferous ducts, 348
Lactiferous sinuses, 348
Lactoferrin, 304
Lacunae
   bone, 66, 68
   cartilage, 65, 68, 70
   Howship's, 66, 70, *88*
Lamella (lamellae)
   of bone, 66
   circumferential, 66
     inner, *72*
     outer, *72*
   interstitial, 66
Lamellar bodies, *243*
Lamellar systems, of bone, 71
Lamina (laminae) (*see also* specific types)
   basal, 25, 27 (*see also* Basal lamina)
   dental, 258, 260, *268–269*
   elastic, *58–59*
     external, *156, 158–159*
     internal, *158–159*
   external, *120–121*
   osseous spiral, *404–405, 406–407*
   of retinal rods and cones, *398–399, 400–401*
   succedaneous, *268–269*
   suprachoroid, *396–397*
Lamina densa, 27, 46, 325
Lamina lucida, 27, 46
Lamina propria, *244–245*
   bladder, 329, *340–341*
   bronchiolar, *250–251*
   ductus (vas) deferens, *382–383*
   duodenal, *294–295*
   esophageal, 282, *288–289*
   gallbladder, 307
   intestinal, 283
   oviduct, *358–359*
   palatal, *272–273*

seminal vesicles, *373–374*
   stomach, 282, *290–291, 292–293*
   tracheal, *246–247*
   urethral, 374
   vaginal, *364–365*
Lamina rara, 325
Lamina reticularis, 27
Laminin, 46
Langerhans cells, 218, 221, *224*
Langerhans, islets of, 303, 304, 306, *308, 312–313, 321*
Large intestine, 278, 284–285, *286, 298–299*
Large ribosomal subunit, 9
Laryngeal cartilage, *244–245*
Laryngeal ventricle, 235, *244–245*
Laryngeal vestibule, 235, 239, *244–245*
Larynx, 235, 239, *244–245*
Late endosomes, 2, 4, *8*
Layers (*see also* Laminae)
   basal uterine, *360–361*
   cartilage, 65
   corneal, *396–397*
   corneoscleral (fibrous tunic), *384*, 387
   fibrous ocular, *396–397*
   functional uterine, *362–363*
   granular
     external, *138–139*
     internal, *138–139*
   Henle's, 221, *225*
   Huxley's, 221, *225*
   hyaline of Hopewell-Smith, *274–275*
   molecular, *136–137, 138–139*
   odontoblastic, *264–265*
   optic nerve fiber, 392
   papillary, *226–227, 228–229*
   parietal, kidney, *334–335*
   Purkinje cell, *136–137*
   pyramidal, *138–139*
   reticular, 221, *226–227, 228–229*
   retinal
     ganglion cell, 392, *398–399*
     nuclear, 391
     pigmented, *396–397*
     plexiform, 392, *398–399, 400–401*
Leaflets, valve, *162–165*
Lens, *384*, 387, 389, 392, *396–397, 400–401*
Leukocytes, *12–13*, 46, 89, 90t (*see also* Lymphocytes)
Leukotrienes, 46
Leydig cells, 373, *380–381*
LH (luteinizing hormone), 194, 369
Lieberkühn, crypts of, 278, 279, 283, *285, 286, 294–295,*
     296–297, 298–299, 300, 301
Ligaments
   broad, *350, 356–357*
   ovarian, *350*
   periodontal, 257, 260, *266–267, 274–275*
   spiral, *404–405, 406–407*
   suspensory ocular, 391, *400–401*
Ligands, 4
Light cells, *272–273*
Light chains, myosin, 105, 106
Light meromyosin, 105, 106
Limbus, ocular, *384, 387*

◆ M

Pancreatic lipase, 281, 303
Paneth cells, 278, 279, *285, 294–295, 296–297*
Papanicolaou (Pap) smear, 346
Papillae, *228–229, 230–231*
    circumvallate, 258, *270–271, 272–273*
    dermal (dermal ridges), 217, 221, *268–269*
    filiform, 257, *261, 270–271*
    foliate, 258
    fungiform, 258, *261*
    renal, 328, *338–339*
    vallate, *261*
Papillary layer, *226–227, 228–229*
Paracortex, lymph node, 168, 171, 173, *182–183*
Paracrine hormones, 279
Parafollicular cells, *208–209*
Parakeratotic epithelium, 257
Parasympathetic nervous system, 125
Parathormone, 68
Parathyroid gland, 194–195, 199, *202, 208–209*
    clinical considerations, 198
Parathyroid hormone (PTH), 195, 196
Paraventricular hypothalamic nuclei, 194
Parenchyma, 25–26
    prostate gland, 374
Parenchymal cells
    pineal body, 200
    thyroid, 199
Parietal cells, 279, *290–291, 292–293*
Parietal layer, kidney, *334–335*
Parietal pleura, 237
Parkinson's disease, 128
Parotid glands, 304, 306, *310–311*
Pars ciliaris, 391, 392
Pars iridica, 391, 392
Pars optica, 391, *398–399*
Pars recta, 324, 325, *332–333*
Particles
    elementary, 1, *7*
    signal recognition, *9*
Passive transport, 4
Patches, Peyer's, *180–181*, 278, 280, *285, 296–297*
Pedicels, 323, *330, 331, 337*
Peg cells, *14–15, 358–359*
Pegs, interpapillary, *226–227, 228–229*
Pelvic inflammatory disease (PID), 346
Pelvis
    renal, 328
Pemphigoid, bullous, 28
Pemphigus vulgaris, 28
Penicillar arteries, 168
Penile bulb, *376*
Penis, 370, 374, *376, 384–385*
    glans, *376*
Pepsin, 278, 280
Peptidase, signal, 5
Peptide
    gastric inhibitory, 278, 280t
    vasoactive intestinal (VIP), 280t
Peptide bonds, 4, *9*
Perforins, 170, *178*
Periarterial lymphatic sheath (PALS), 168, 171–172, *190–191*
Periaxial space, *117*

Perichondrium, 65, 70, 71, *246–247*
Pericytes, 46, 148
Perikaryon, 125–126
Perilymph, 388, *395*
Perimysium, 103, 107, *109, 110–111*
Perineurium, 126, 130, *131*
    peripheral nerve, *142–143*
Periodontal ligament, 257, *260, 266–267, 274–275*
Periosteal bud, 67, *73*
Periosteum, 70, *72, 82–83, 84–85*
Peripheral nerves, 126, 130, *131, 142–143, 144–145*
Peripheral nervous system, 125
Peritendineum, *56–57*
Peritubular capillary network, 323, *331*
Perlacan, 46
Permeability
    capillary, 150
    selective, 150
Peyer's patches, *180–181*, 278, 280, *285, 296–297*
Phagocytosis, 1, 46, 89, 167
    ocular, 389
    Sertoli-cell, 371
Phagolysosomes, 2
Phalangeal cells, 392
    inner, *406–407*
    outer, *406–407*
Phalangeal processes, *406–407*
Phalanx (phalanges), distal, *232–233*
Pharyngeal tonsils, 168, 173, *184–185*
Pharynx, 255–256
Pheomelanin, 219
Phosphorylation, *9*
Photoreception, 389
Photoreceptors (rods and cones), *384, 387*
Pia mater, 125, 129, *134–135, 136–137, 138–139*
PID (pelvic inflammatory disease), 346
Pigment cells, *396–397*
Pigmented corneal epithelium, *396–397, 400–401*
Pigmented corneal layers, *396–397*
Pigment epithelium, 391
Pillar cells, 392
    inner, *406–407*
    outer, *406–407*
Pineal body (epiphysis), 195, 197, 200, *202, 212–213*
Pinealocytes, 195, 200
Pinocytic vesicles, *144–145*
Pinocytosis, 1
Pits, gastric (foveolae), 278, *285, 290–291, 292–293*
Pituicytes, 194, *206–207*
Pituitary gland (hypophysis), 193–194, 198, 199, *201, 204–207, 215*
    clinical considerations, 198
    pars anterior, 193–194, 199, *204–205, 214*
    pars intermedia, 194, 199, *204–205, 206–207*
    pars nervosa, *204–205, 206–207*
    pars nervosa and infundibular stalk, 194, 199
    pars tuberalis, 194, 199, *204–205*
Pituitary hormones, *201*
Placenta, 344, 348, *351, 364–365*
Plaque regions, of bladder, 324
Plasmablasts, *180–181*

Pyloric gland, 279, *292–293*
Pyloric sphincter, 282
Pylorus, 278, *285*
Pyramidal cells, 129, *138–139*
Pyramidal layer
    external, *138–139*
    internal, *138–139*
Pyramids, renal, 323

R

Ranvier, node of, 130, *131, 142–143*
Rappaport, acinus of (liver acinus), 306
Raynaud's disease, 152
Rays, renal medullary, 328, *332–333*
RBCs (red blood cells) (*see* Erythrocytes)
Receptor-mediated endocytosis, 1, 4, *8*
Receptor-mediated transport, 128
Receptors, 4, *8*
    acetylcholine, 127
    aldosterone, 325
    dihydropyridine-sensitive (DHSRs), 105
    hormone, 196
    ryanodine (calcium channels), 105
    T cell, 170
    transferrin, 128
Rectae spuriae, 323, *331*
Recycling endosomes, 2, *8*
Red blood cells (RBCs) (*see* Erythrocytes)
Red bone marrow, 90
Red pulp, 168, 172, 174, *190–191*
Refractory period, 127
Regenerative cells, 278, 279, *286*
Regulated secretion, 1
Relaxation, muscle, 105
Relaxed transitional epithelium, *31*
Relaxin, 345
Renal calculi (nephrolithiasis), 327
Renal calyx (calyces), 324, 328
Renal capsule, 323
Renal columns of Bertin, 323
Renal corpuscle, 323, *331*
Renal cortex, *332–333, 334–335*
Renal cortical labyrinth, *332–333, 334–335*
Renal failure, acute, 327
Renal filtration barrier, 325
Renal medulla, *332–333, 338–339*
Renal papillae, 328, *338–339*
Renal papillary ducts, *338–339*
Renal pelvis, 328
Renal pyramids, 323
Renin, 278, 325–326
Reproductive system
    female, 343–367, *360* (*see also* Female reproductive system *and individual structures*)
    male, 369–386, *376* (*see also* Male reproductive system *and individual structures*)
RER (*see* Rough endoplasmic reticulum)
Residual bodies, 2, 4, *8*
Respiration, mechanism of, 237
Respiratory bronchioles, 236, 239, *242, 243, 250–251, 252–253*
Respiratory system, 235–254
    clinical considerations, 237–238
    conducting portion, 239, *242,* 245–246

histological organization, 239–240
    histophysiology, 237
    respiratory portion, 236, 239–240, *243*
    summary table, 241t
Resting potential, 127
Rete ridges, *262–263, 272–273*
Rete testis, 369–370, 373, *380–381*
Reticular cells, 49, *54–55,* 167–168, 168
    thymic, *188–189*
Reticular connective tissue, 46, *54–55*
Reticular fibers, 45, 47, 49, *54–55,* 107, 173, 174
    splenic, *190–191*
Reticular layer, *228–229*
Reticulocytes, 94, *97*
Reticulum
    endosplasmic (*see* Rough endoplasmic reticulum; Smooth endoplasmic reticulum)
    sarcoplasmic, 103, 105
    stellate, *268–269*
Retina, *384,* 387, 389, *398–399*
    detached, 390
Retinal, 389
Retinal tunic, *384,* 387, 391–392
Rhodopsin, 389
Rhodopsin-synthesizing rods, *384,* 387
Ribophorins, 1, 5
Ribosomal subunit
    large, *9*
    small, *9*
Ribosomes, 1, 3, 6, *20–21, 22*
Ridges
    dermal (dermal papillae), 217, 221, *228–229*
    epidermal, 221, *226–227*
    rete, *262–263, 272–273*
Ring, tonsillar, 168, 255
RNA synthesis, 3
Rods and cones, *384,* 387, 389, 391, *398–399, 400–401*
Rokitansky-Aschoff sinuses, 307
Root hair plexus, *224, 225*
Roots
    dorsal, *134–135*
    hair, 221, *230–231*
    ventral, *134–135*
Rotational acceleration sense, 390
Rough endoplasmic reticulum (RER), 1–2, 2–3, 4, 6, *7, 18–19, 20–21, 36–37, 60*
    adipocyte, *63*
    hyaline cartilage, *86*
    liver, *320*
    osteoblast, *86*
    peripheral nerve, *144–145*
    tracheal, *248–249*
Round window, 388, *395*
Ruffled border, 88
Ryanodine receptors (calcium channels), 105

S

Saccule, 388, 393, *395*
Sacs
    alveolar, 236, 240, *252–253*
    dental, *268–269*
    endolymphatic, 390
Saliva, 255, 304